The Handbook of Assistive Technology

Gregory Church, M
The Kennedy Institute

Sharon Glennen, PhD
The Kennedy Institute
The Johns Hopkins University
School of Medicine

———

———

SINGULAR PUBLISHING GROUP, INC.
SAN DIEGO, CALIFORNIA

To the many individuals and families who sought our assistive technology advice yet taught us more than we can ever return.

To my parents, Mary and William Church, and to Bill, Tim, and Kathy, for their patient understanding and support throughout this project.

To Matthew who took long afternoon naps and to Wayne who watched him when he was awake. Without both of you, my life and this book would be incomplete.

Published by Singular Publishing Group, Inc.
4284 41st Street
San Diego, California 92105

© 1992 by Singular Publishing Group, Inc.

Typeset in 10/12 Times by CFW Graphics
Printed in the United States of America by McNaughton & Gunn

Library of Congress Cataloging-in-Publication Data

Church, Gregory, 1960-
    The handbook of assistive technology / Gregory Church, Sharon Glennen.
        p.   cm.
    ISBN 1-879105-53-5
    1. Self-help devices for the disabled.   2. Rehabilitation.
I. Glennen, Sharon.   II. Title.
RM698 . C47   1991
617.1'03 — dc20   91-29485
                                                                        CIP

Contents

Acknowledgments

The material for this handbook has been developed over a period of years by the authors from their deep conviction that a functional handbook is critical to the application and implementation of technology with disabled users. Developing effective and practical technology solutions for individuals who are disabled is not an easy task, primarily because technology has the potential to affect many facets of the user's cognitive, physical, social, and emotional development. Therefore, it was necessary to seek the help of others. We wish to thank the professionals who helped us complete this work. Many individuals from The Kennedy Institute, The Johns Hopkins University, and The Johns Hopkins School of Medicine reviewed the manuscript and gave us advice. We thank them for their support on this project.

Preface

The application of assistive technology has the potential to give individuals who were previously destined to live isolated, dependent lives the ability to move into the mainstream and become full and productive citizens. Although assistive technology has great potential for improving the quality of life for individuals who are disabled, it frequently is not applied to solving functional client needs or is applied inappropriately. In this text, the reader will look at individuals whose disabilities have prevented them from participating fully in educational, community, vocational, or work activities. Through the use of appropriate technologies, these individuals are able to benefit fully from their use of practical, integrated approaches to assistive technology service delivery.

This book emphasizes an interdisciplinary perspective on the practical application of assistive technology for children and young adults with disabilities. This approach distinguishes it from other texts written on the subject. This collaboration, developed by the authors over many years of working together, offers the reader unique experiences and practical knowledge for implementing assistive technology service programs.

The Handbook of Assistive Technology presents professionals in rehabilitation technology, physical and occupational therapy, speech-language pathology, special education, and related services with an interdisciplinary perspective for planning, implementing, and managing assistive technology service delivery to persons who are disabled in home, school, and community settings. This approach provides professionals, advocates, and parents with relevant learning experiences developed from many professional disciplines. This collaborative professional partnership provides the reader with unique perspectives on how to effectively use technology to meet the needs of individuals who are disabled. The interdisciplinary approach of this text also gives service providers and clients an innovative service delivery viewpoint. By bringing together the knowledge and expertise of medicine, psychology, education, physical therapy, occupational therapy, speech-language pathology, and related services, professionals can better assist individuals with disabilities to reach their full potential.

Given the enormous challenge associated with assistive technology service delivery, the participant authors have synthesized their various experiences and practices to provide the reader with practical guidelines for reaching the full potential of today's and tomorrow's technology. This textbook focuses on several areas of assistive technology: computer access, augmentative communication, seating and power mobility, adaptive play and environmental control, and the integration of technology into the client's home, school, and community.

What makes this resource especially appealing to practitioners is its thoroughness in responding to questions that occur daily as they work to establish, maintain, or expand assistive technology services for individuals with developmental and acquired disabilities. The authors are active assistive technology service delivery providers who have specialized training in the treatment of children and young adults with developmental and acquired disabilities. They bring to this book unique experiences that emphasize the questions that must be addressed in planning, developing, and implementing assistive technology service delivery programs. Much of the book's content has been presented for critical review at national and international conferences to bring a practical and functional resource to its audience rather than new theories that have limited testing and application.

Chapter 1, written by Greg Church and Sharon Glennen, addresses issues associated with assistive technology service delivery. These issues include service delivery constraints, consumer awareness, technology availability, training, and funding. The authors identify and compare different models of service delivery, giving the reader insight into the complexities and dynamics of various service models.

Chapter 2, written by Greg Church, is a general introduction to microcomputer technology. Nontechnical discussions of computer system components provide a functional foundation on how computer systems work and how they affect assistive technology solutions.

Chapter 3, written by Susan Harryman and Lana Warren, gives a dual perspective on the challenges of providing appropriate client seating and power mobility. Seating and support systems are discussed in detail to provide practical guidelines for effecting optimal seating. Power mobility systems, control options, and transportation issues also are addressed.

Chapter 4, written by Sharon Glennen, discusses augmentative and alternative communication aids and evaluation methods. Consideration is given to the wide array of augmentative communication systems. Pragmatic guidelines and suggestions provide the reader with strategies for evaluating, training, and developing the client's skill in operating communication aids.

Chapter 5, written by Greg Church, identifies and discusses the complexities associated with interfacing assistive technology with microcomputers. A comprehensive nontechnical approach explains the operation and use of adaptive computer equipment. Vignettes illustrate the variety of programming issues associated with the application of assistive technology with children and adults with disabilities. This chapter also provides detailed listings of commercially available computer products for many types of microcomputer systems.

Chapter 6, coauthored by Sharon Glennen and Greg Church, extends the use of technology to adaptive play and environmental control applications. Types of adaptive play are discussed as well as technology systems that may be utilized with children who are disabled. Alternative environmental systems also are explored as a means of providing individuals who are disabled with increased independence in leisure, home, and work activities.

Chapter 7, written by Joan Carney and Cindy Dix, addresses the issues associated with the integration of assistive technology into home, school, and community settings. The authors discuss issues related to the integration team, community acceptance, staff preparation, peer preparation, physical environment, and development of student integration plans.

Chapter 8, written by Sharon Glennen, is a guide to the selection of assistive technology products for special education and rehabilitation. The chapter helps readers quickly identify specific products that have been mentioned throughout the text. The products are organized by their function. A description of each device is given, along with vendor information.

Chapter 9, written by Greg Church, expands the resource listings of the text. Professionals, consumers, and advocates will find this chapter helpful for locating technology vendors, private and nonprofit organizations, professional journals, magazines, newspapers, databases, and information networks dedicated to the application of assistive technology with persons who are disabled.

Chapter 10, written by Greg Church, is a glossary of assistive technology terminology commonly used to describe equipment and related concepts. It provides a quick reference for readers who require a brief review of some of the terminology used throughout the book.

The Handbook of Assistive Technology is a comprehensive resource that includes material suitable for the novice as well as the seasoned professional. The text's illustrations clarify the concepts presented in the chapters, which explore the many complex and confusing facets of assistive technology service delivery. It is a resource guide that uses a nontechnical approach and is intended for professionals, practitioners, and advocates who wish to design and implement assistive technology for children and young adults with cognitive and physical disabilities.

Contributors

Joan Carney, MA
Educational Consultant
Assistive Technology Center
The Kennedy Institute
Educational Specialist
Pediatric Neurorehabilitation
  Unit
The Kennedy Institute
Baltimore, Maryland

Gregory Church, MS, MAS
Computer Coordinator
Special Education Division
The Kennedy Institute
Computer Coordinator
Assistive Technology Center
The Kennedy Institute
Baltimore, Maryland

Cynthia Dix, MS, CCC-SLP
Speech–Language Pathologist
Augmentative Communication
  and Technology Team
Howard County Public Schools
County Diagnostic Center
Columbia, Maryland

Sharon Glennen, PhD, CCC-SLP
Assistant Director of
  Communicative Sciences
  and Disorders
The Kennedy Institute
Instructor in Otolaryngology
The Johns Hopkins University
  School of Medicine
Baltimore, Maryland

Susan Harryman, MS, RPT
Director of Physical Therapy
The Kennedy Institute
Instructor in Pediatrics
The Johns Hopkins University
  School of Medicine
Baltimore Maryland

Lana Warren, MS, OTR/L, FAOTA
Director of Occupational
  Therapy
The Kennedy Institute
Instructor in Rehabilitation
  Medicine
The Johns Hopkins University
  School of Medicine
Baltimore, Maryland

1

Assistive Technology Program Development

■ Gregory Church, MS, MAS ■
■ Sharon Glennen, PhD ■

The National Institute on Disability and Rehabilitation Research (NIDRR) estimates that over 32 million noninstitutionalized persons living in the United States have a chronic health disability that limits their ability to participate fully in life. In addition, a significant number of individuals with acquired severe neurogenic disorders and spinal cord injuries also require technology services and equipment. The number of potential consumers of assistive technology as the result of traumatic injury is growing rapidly as local, state, and regional acute medical trauma networks expand. These hospitals and acute care facilities provide comprehensive state-of-the-art medical care. The results have been impressive; today more individuals are surviving catastrophic traumatic injuries than ever. However, in many instances, the individuals who survive have severe functional losses with persistent disabilities, even after extensive medical rehabilitation services. The large number of individuals surviving catastrophic traumatic injuries necessitates the need for expanded related services and assistive technology on a short- and long-term basis.

1

Both the heightened awareness of the apparent need for assistive technology and the observable increase in the interaction among various technology-related organizations, health professionals, and advocates have created many different models of service delivery. Further, the variety, complexity, and often quality of these approaches raises concern over the focus of technology and the continuity of services needed to appropriately apply technology. The service provider must consider many program variables when designing and implementing new assistive technology services. Without first identifying potential issues involved with assistive technology service delivery, the planned benefits of technology can fall far short of the program's expected objectives. Service providers often see problems manifest themselves in administrative policy, client programming, professional training, service delivery approaches, referral process, resource availability, staff roles, interagency cooperation, or communications. Consequently, before embracing any new technology plans, administrators and service providers should carefully evaluate assistive technology issues as they relate to proposed service delivery innovations.

ASSISTIVE TECHNOLOGY PROGRAM DEVELOPMENT ISSUES

For service providers, administrators, and advocates interested in developing new technology programs, preliminary program planning requires examination of a variety of major environmental and program planning issues. Acknowledging the array of programming issues early in the planning process facilitates the assessment of their impact on service delivery and greatly reduces the risks involved with technology implementation. The following sections will discuss important assistive technology issues related to service delivery approaches, client population needs, training and staff development, integration of technology services, interagency communication and cooperation, information and program awareness, technology availability, and funding programs and equipment. Some of these issues are within the control of the assistive technology team whereas others are outside the program's control. To a large extent, these issues may have both positive and negative influences on the effectiveness of assistive technology initiatives. A newly developing assistive technology program should seek to recognize any constraining factors and to develop the best possible program within those limitations. Rather than trying to develop an all encompassing assistive technology program that tries to do all things for all persons, the team should limit services to those areas which can be performed well. Once service providers are confident that all relevant program issues have been identified, careful consideration should be given to the development of planning and policy making decision processes that provide for the management of both the positive and negative effects of these issues.

The Client Population

One of the first issues to be examined is the selection of the client population. The purpose of analyzing client populations is to formulate a clear understanding of the clients' service needs. An assistive technology program, given certain organizational constraints, cannot be expected to provide comprehensive technology services to all disabled individuals. Clearly, service providers must differentiate the client population in order to serve individual client needs more effectively.

To begin, service providers should make every effort to identify and collect database information about client demographics, population trends, and current level of services in the service delivery system. This analysis should clearly define the variety and incidence of disabilities found within the anticipated service area. In addition, an effective needs analysis of the client population will identify not only what services are available to the community, but also what new or related services are needed in the community. The information collected can then be used by service providers to determine what types of services are needed. This analysis should also include an estimate of the size, scope, and duration of the services needed by the client population.

Another emerging issue for service providers is the development of tracking systems for client populations. These systems emphasize reliable, valid, and cost-effective methods for identifying current and future service needs, define accurate incidence rates, and serve a variety of other purposes, including case management, client planning, justifying services, program evaluation, and determining professional training needs. The challenge for service providers is to develop client tracking systems that include effective identification, monitoring, and referral mechanisms, which are designed to ensure that individuals who are disabled and their families receive continuous and appropriate services.

Professional Training and Development

There is a lag between the development of promising technological innovations and their application in the rehabilitation environment. This lag can be partially accounted for by a scarcity of assistive technology professionals who are trained to understand, use, and teach others to use the new technology. The problem is further complicated by professional training that focuses on theoretical rather than applied instruction as it relates to practical uses of assistive technology.

Many university- and college-level programs continue to offer more traditional training, with little attention given to improving the understanding of applications in assistive technology. In addition, even with increasing professional interest, few university or college programs offer degree programs in the area of assistive technology.

Technology teams require highly trained professionals who specialize in the field (Cohen, 1986). Many professional positions requiring assistive technology expertise remain unfilled in a variety of service environments. For example, educational systems, particularly in more rural areas, must contract for services, as skilled technology professionals simply are not available. In classroom situations, the lack of appropriate professional training in the arrangement, application, and maintenance of assistive technology devices can result in under-utilization or even non-utilization by the client.

There is also a great need for cross-field training of service professionals. Many therapists and clinicians have highly specialized technology training in their respective fields. However, the prescription and application of assistive technology should have specific relevance to all aspects of the client's environment, including school, work, and community. Cross-field training provides professionals with broader insights into evaluation, treatment, and the implementation of technology interventions.

Quality technology teams consist of professionals who are capable of crossing discipline boundaries to provide thorough services (Yorkston & Karlan, 1986). Because assistive technology is a relatively new field, traditional disciplinary boundaries often are ignored. For example it is not unusual to find augmentative communication technology specialists who are speech-language pathologists, special educators, or occupational therapists. Powered mobility might be the specialty of a physical or occupational therapist. Table 1–1 lists assistive technology areas and the professionals who typically provide services in each area.

The multidisciplinary model of providing assistive technology services requires coordination across disciplines. A team leader is needed to coordinate services and to resolve team differences. The team leader needs to be familiar with technology issues across all team areas but does not need to be an expert in each discipline.

The Service Delivery Environment

In addition to issues involving the client population, service providers should also take a critical look at the service delivery environment. All organizations, large or small, private or nonprofit, must deal with the realities of their operating environment. The assistive technology ser-

Table 1–1. Assistive Technology Professional Areas

Technology Area	Responsible Professions
Academic and vocational skills	Special Education Vocational Rehabilitation Psychology
Augmentative communication	Speech-Language Pathology Special Education
Computer technology	Computer Technology Vocational Rehabilitation Special Education
Daily living skills	Occupational Therapy Special Education
Engineering	Computer Technology Rehabilitation Engineering
Mobility	Occupational Therapy Physical Therapy
Seating and positioning	Occupational Therapy Physical Therapy
Written communication	Speech-Language Pathology Special Education

vice environment, like any environmental setting, has a set of operating constraints. The service provider must understand that there are implied operating conditions that exist for all organizations operating in the service delivery environment. These environmental constraints might include, for example, geographic location, social or economic influences, or unique client demographics.

The service environment is an issue that often cannot be controlled by the assistive technology team. However, through analysis of the service delivery system, service providers can identify the types, quantity, and scope of organizations currently providing services. The careful and accurate evaluation of the service environment can provide professionals with information on the condition of insufficient and/or overlapping services. More importantly, service professionals also may identify needs that extend beyond the current capabilities of the service delivery system. Technology providers then can then focus on developing new or related services for clients that "fall through the cracks" of the existing service delivery system. For example, technology programs have been established in traditional school settings, residential schools, outpatient clinics, hospitals, and as itinerant traveling teams. The service delivery environment often dictates the focus and scope of the program's services (Cohen, 1986). An assistive technology team operating at a residential school would have different program goals than a team operating at a rehabilitation hospital.

In addition to issues encompassing the service delivery environment, technology providers must familiarize themselves with issues related to the specific technology program. Assistive technology programs have unique constraints that further define the boundaries of their service delivery potential. For example, assistive technology programs can specialize in evaluating clients, treating clients, providing evaluation and treatment services, or disseminating product or service information. In addition, programs can specialize in one specific area of assistive technology, or can provide a broad range of services across many technology areas. Technology areas might include augmentative communication, powered mobility, seating and positioning, written communication, academic or vocational skills, and technology for individuals who are visually impaired or hearing impaired. For example, an assistive technology program in a school setting might provide evaluation and treatment services only for children using augmentative communication systems and computer systems for written language use. Children in the school who need technology assistance in areas such as power mobility would be referred to other programs.

The scope of the program and operating environment often control which professional disciplines are included on the assistive technology team. Typically the technology team consists of several professionals who form the core of the team, with other professionals called in as needed. The core team of professionals needed may vary from client to client. For example, some clients require powered mobility and also require augmentative communication systems. These clients would need to be seen by specialists in both areas. However, other clients who require powered mobility are capable of speaking normally and do not need an augmentative communication device. They would not need to be seen by the augmentative communication specialist even though this professional may be a core member of the assistive technology team.

ASSISTIVE TECHNOLOGY SERVICE DELIVERY MODELS

Assistive technology service delivery approaches can be classified by a wide range of differentiating factors. Some assistive technology models are differentiated by the nature of their functional services, for example, seating and positioning, augmentative communication, special education technology services, or adaptive equipment design and engineering. Other models may delineate service delivery by advocating and administering to specific disabilities. Examples of these programs include the United Cerebral Palsy Foundation, Muscular Dystrophy Association, or the Association for Children with Learning Disabilities. Here service delivery typically specializes in serving only specific types of acquired or developmental disabilities. The variety of service delineations for these types of programs are broad. Assistive technology service models may also categorize programs based on the organization's mission. Some agencies may provide clients with comprehensive evaluation and treatment services. These service programs may further delineate services by concentrating on either short- or long-term care approaches. The mission objective of other service programs might be to provide funding or information resources to other service delivery programs in a predefined geographic service area.

Whatever service delivery approach is taken, the service provider generally can identify two major categories of service delivery models: indirect and direct service delivery systems. Indirect service models focus on staff training, information dissemination, and public awareness, whereas direct models provide service delivery including assessment, software and assistive equipment prescriptions, and the implementation of technology with clients. A fundamental planning issue for the service provider is developing a service delivery system that is compatible with the organization's goals. Each type of service model has its own benefits and drawbacks in technology service delivery.

The following section outlines various models of service delivery. Each model varies in the proportion of services allocated to indirect and direct services and in the scope of direct services provided. Specific assistive technology programs may incorporate characteristics of more than one model of service delivery. The five models are: (1) Information and Demonstration Centers, (2) Short-Term Evaluation Centers, (3) Short-Term Evaluation and Training Centers, (4) Long-Term Evaluation and Training Centers, and (5) Long-Term Training Centers.

Information and Demonstration Center Model

Information and Demonstration Centers are usually grant-supported regional centers which serve as "libraries" for assistive technology equipment and information. Information and Demonstration Centers are often located in college and university settings, or are operated by state-wide technology resource agencies. These programs are staffed by professionals with strong clinical and technical skills. Professionals and clients can make appointments to go to the center to try out various pieces of equipment or software. Some centers allow professionals to borrow equipment for short periods of time to try with clients. These centers often provide valuable training to professionals in a variety of assistive technology fields. Most Information and Demonstration Centers do not provide direct evaluation or training services to clients. Instead, centers serve as referral resources by linking clients to appropriate assistive technology service providers in an area.

Strengths and Weaknesses

Information and Demonstration Centers are useful programs for assistive technology professionals. These centers provide professionals with a means of accessing up-to-date technology and serve an important training function. However, they are extremely costly to develop and maintain. These centers must have state-of-the-art equipment kept in good working condition at all times. In addition, if the center has an equipment loan program, it needs to have duplicate pieces of equipment and software available for use. These costly requirements make it necessary to fund Information and Demonstration Centers through grants. Any program that is grant funded will be affected by budget restrictions, resource limitations, and changing mandates as the granting sources change their priorities. Grant funding often is available for establishing new programs but is difficult to obtain for continuing programs. Because the funding is tied to specific time periods, Information and Demonstration Centers often have difficulty maintaining equipment and services after the initial grant monies have been spent.

Short-Term Evaluation Center Model

Short-Term Evaluation Centers typically evaluate clients for assistive technology needs in a one- or two-day period. These centers are often established at hospitals or at outpatient programs such as centers sponsored by the Easter Seal Society, Muscular Dystrophy Association, or United Cerebral Palsy Association. Some state programs have established short-term evaluation centers as part of a state-wide service delivery system. These programs often provide a wide range of technology services and are sometimes considered regional assistive technology evaluation centers (Shane & Yoder, 1981). Assistive technology services usually are offered as a component service within the organization's broad spectrum of comprehensive rehabilitation services. These programs provide comprehensive patient care based on an interdisciplinary approach in which many professionals work together.

The operational model for a Short-Term Evaluation Center consists of an interdisciplinary evaluation by the assistive technology team. These evaluations typically take place on site, or the team may travel to the client to provide services. Programs with large regional client populations have developed traveling itinerant assistive technology teams which operate using the short-term evaluation model (Cohen, 1986). Following the evaluation, the team confers to develop a technology prescription and recommendations for the client. Usually the team assists the client in seeking funding for equipment and in ordering equipment.

Once the ordered technology equipment arrives, the client typically is brought back to the short-term evaluation center to fit the equipment. This is usually done in one or two days. Parents and others who interact regularly with the client are shown how to operate the equipment, since they will be responsible for long-term training.

Because the assistive technology team is not actively involved in long-term training, it is important that assistance be provided to persons who interact regularly with the client. This can be done through periodic follow-up visits. The purpose of the follow-up visit is to provide ongoing assessment of technology needs, and to resolve any problems that may arise with the prescribed equipment. In addition the team may provide videotapes, phone consultations, and on-site visits for follow-up purposes. Videotapes that detail how to set up and operate equipment, along with training tips, have been found to be especially useful for follow-up training.

Strengths and Weaknesses

The primary strength of a Short-Term Evaluation Center is the use of an interdisciplinary evaluation approach. The evaluation, prescription, and fitting of equipment is viewed from a variety of clinical perspectives. This holistic approach to patient care is much more successful than programs that make recommendations in clinical isolation. Multidisciplinary approaches to evaluation are costly. However, because the client is evaluated in a relatively short period of time, personnel costs for each assessment are low. This translates into savings for the client, or for third-party payers who may be funding the assessment.

Another strength of this model is the timeliness of decision making by the technology team. Typically, a prescription for equipment is made by the team after all of the evaluations are completed. Because the assessment is completed in one or two days, the team can quickly develop a prescription for the client and begin seeking funding and ordering equipment. This speeds up the time that the client has to wait before actually receiving the prescribed technology.

The speed of decision making is also one of the weaknesses of the Short-Term Evaluation Center model. It is sometimes difficult to make an accurate prescription for severely involved clients in such a short time. Some clients need repeated practice with equipment before learning to use it well; others have changing needs which need to be evaluated over longer periods of time before a final technology prescription is made.

The final weakness of the Short-Term Evaluation Center model is its reliance on others for long-term training. The model works well when the client has community contacts who will be able to carry out training. However, some clients do not have families or others who are capable of assisting with this process. The authors have had numerous experiences with families who do not feel a need to use technology at home, school personnel who are not given sufficient time for client training, and group homes with frequent staff turnovers. While follow-up services can overcome some of these problems, it cannot solve them completely.

Short-Term Evaluation and Training Center Model

Short-Term Evaluation and Training Centers offer assistive technology assessments which can last up to one or two weeks. These programs usually are established in rehabilitation hospitals, or other hospital settings. These programs can be funded at a federal or state level, such as a hospital run by the state Department of Vocational Rehabilitation or a Veteran's Hospital. However, most regional rehabilitation hospitals provide care financed by third-party payers.

A client typically stays at a Short-Term Evaluation and Training Center throughout the entire evaluation process. Because the evaluation takes place over an extended period of time, the client receives ongoing training with assistive technology equipment as part of the evaluation process.

The assistive technology team at a Short-Term Evaluation and Training Center typically provides an initial evaluation during the first few days at the center. The team then meets to confer about technology recommendations. The client is given opportunities to use the recommended technology for one to two weeks while the team provides training and monitors progress. At the end of this period the team re-evaluates its recommendations and makes a final prescription for the client.

Similar to the Short-Term Evaluation Model, the team typically assists the client with funding and ordering equipment. Once the equipment arrives the client returns to the center to receive initial training with the equipment. This can occur in a single day, or may require another one- to two-week stay at the facility. Parents and other professionals who interact regularly with the client are responsible for long-term training. Once the client leaves the facility with the prescribed technology, periodic follow-up visits are scheduled to monitor progress.

Strengths and Weaknesses

Centers that operate their assistive technology teams using this model often make excellent technology prescriptions for their clients. The extended evaluation period gives the team a chance to try out several technology options to determine which will work best. It also gives the client a chance to show improvement over time with a particular software program or piece of equipment. Individual client problems with equipment can be studied and corrected before the final prescription is made.

The extended evaluation period is also a weakness of this model. The length of the evaluation makes the total personnel cost for the assessment process excessive. These costs are certainly justified for clients who have severe disabilities that make them difficult to evaluate. However clients with less severe disabilities often do not require a one- or two-week evaluation. These clients are best served by a program that provides evaluation services in a shorter time period.

Finally, similar to the Short-Term Evaluation Center model, this model does not provide long-term training. This is a major weakness of the model since the team has to rely on others in the client's environment to provide long-term training.

Long-Term Evaluation and Training Model

Programs that offer long-term evaluation and training initially evaluate the client during a one- to two-week assessment period, then provide ongoing client training for an indefinite time. Unlike the Short-Term Evaluation Centers, these programs serve a limited population of clients who attend the center for a long period of time. Long-Term Evaluation and Training Centers typically are established in rehabilitation centers and Veteran's Hospitals. The Education of the Handicapped Act (Public Law 94-142, Amended) has encouraged the growth of a number of assistive technology programs in special education settings. These school-based programs are evolving in response to the recognition that schools often have multiple, complex service needs that go far beyond the bounds of education. These programs recognize that availability, access, and coordination of specialized technology services are essential to serving and maintaining handicapped children in the least restrictive environment. These programs are most often organized at a school district level to provide services to individual schools within the district.

The assistive technology team at a Long-Term Evaluation and Training Center assesses the client over a one- to two-week period, and then makes an initial technology prescription. The client receives training with the equipment with periodic re-evaluations from the team. In some centers the assistive technology team provides client training services. However, other personnel employed by the center may also provide ongoing client training. For example, in a school setting a centralized assistive technology team completes the initial evaluation while a specific clinician or teacher at the child's school provides ongoing training for the child. After a lengthy trial training period, a final prescription is made by the team. The team then assists with funding and ordering equipment. Follow-up services occur naturally because the client is receiving long-term training services at the center.

Strengths and Weaknesses

The Long-Term Evaluation and Training Center model works well for clients who are difficult to assess in a short period of time. For example, many rehabilitation clients have changing technology needs as they progress from the initial to the final stages of recovery. Depending on the client, this progression may take several months or years. A facility that operates under this model can monitor the client's progress over time during the training process and make changes in the prescribed technology as needed. The ability to train clients to use technology is also a strength of this model because the assistive technology team actually provides the training or closely monitors others at the facility who provide training. This ensures that clients will benefit from any prescribed technology by learning to use it to the best of their abilities.

Similar to the Short-Term Evaluation and Training Center, a major weakness of this model is the cost of providing evaluation services. Many clients do not need a lengthy evaluation period before a technology prescription can be made. In addition, programs operating under this model have high equipment costs. Equipment is needed for evaluations and to loan to clients during the initial stages of training. The program needs to have duplicates of popular equipment and software available for client use at all times.

Long-Term Training Model

Assistive technology teams that operate using a Long-Term Training Model provide only training services. These teams usually are located at facilities such as public schools, residential schools, and vocational training programs. A facility that provides only long-term training must work in conjunction with a program that can provide assistive technology evaluations. For example, a client might be sent to a regional assistive technology center that operates using the Short-Term Evaluation Model. The Short-Term Evaluation Center evaluates the client, develops a technology prescription, seeks funding for equipment, and initially fits the client with the ordered equipment. Assistive technology team members from the Long-Term Training facility may or may not participate in this process.

Once the client is fitted with equipment, the Long-Term Training Center provides ongoing training and follow-up services. Assistive technology team members at the Long-Term Training Center usually are responsible for training the client as well as parents or other involved professionals on how to use the prescribed technology.

Strengths and Weaknesses

A strength of the Long-Term Training Model is the low cost of providing services. Personnel costs per client are low, because team members provide training services to many clients at once. Equipment costs are also relatively low. An assistive technology program that provides only training does not need to have a storeroom of available technology to use with clients. The program needs only a few backup systems for clients to use if their equipment needs repair. The involvement of the assistive technology team in on-site training ensures good carryover of learned skills to the client's home, classroom, or job. The team can closely monitor technology use on a day-to-day basis and provide ongoing training for others who interact with the client on a regular basis.

The major weakness of the Long-Term Training Center model is its reliance on other professionals for evaluation services. Using another program to evaluate clients can work well if there is a good flow of information between the evaluation center and the long-term training program. However, conflicts between the two programs sometimes occur. Team members at the Long-Term Training Center may make a referral to an evaluation center with recommendations about what technology should be prescribed. However, the evaluation center may disagree with those recommendations and prescribe other equipment. Other areas that can cause conflicts between the two programs include responsibility for client follow-up, training strategies, and responsibility for equipment maintenance.

Summary of Service Delivery Models

There are many different models for establishing assistive technology teams. Technology service providers can be found in university settings, outpatient clinics, acute care hospitals, rehabilitation hospitals, schools, and state resource centers. Programs can be funded through private grants, third-party insurance payers, or federal and state taxes. Each assistive technology team will need to determine which model best fits their facility and client population before developing an assistive technology program. In addition the team needs to consider how to integrate its services within the existing assistive technology framework. Factors that need to be considered are listed in Figure 1-1. This questionnaire is designed to help the assistive technology team consider some of the major factors that will have an effect on the eventual structure and focus of the program. No single assistive technology program can provide all services to all clients. The team should focus on developing quality programs in areas in which it can provide effective and needed services.

INTEGRATION OF TECHNOLOGY SERVICES

Some communities, states, and even regional areas are fortunate to have aggressive private sector service delivery systems, progressive public sector service delivery systems, as well as a number of private, nonprofit service organizations. However, these delivery systems frequently are few in number and often face numerous environmental constraints that limit the breadth of service delivery options. Other technology programs, to remain competitive in difficult market areas, may decide to offer overlapping services. Unfortunately, these operational constraints do result in service delivery obstacles for technology consumers. Repercussions of these operational constraints include variable and inconsistent assistive technology service delivery. Figure 1-2 shows a model of service delivery integration on a state level.

As Figure 1-2 indicates, the variety of assistive technology service delivery programs operating at the state and local levels can be diverse. In addition, the working relationships among various service providers is often intricate and varies significantly between agencies. Most technology service providers acknowledge the need for assistive technology service integration. This integration effort must be addressed on several different levels. Consideration must be given to the technology service environment, client programming, and the client transition process.

The assistive technology service environment consists of a variety of different service models and unique service providers. Service providers have resource limitations which put unique restrictions on service potential. Effective technology programs therefore must be judicious in resource allocation. It is important for technology service providers to understand and identify where fragmented technology services exist,

Client Population

1. What client population does your facility currently serve?
2. Does your facility want to expand services to other client populations?
3. What technology areas of expertise are needed to help this population?
4. How long can clients stay at your facility?
5. How will clients be referred to your program?
6. How many clients does your program expect to serve during the first year, the second year, the third year?
7. How much will it cost your program to provide evaluation and/or training services to a single client?
8. Who would fund the client's cost for evaluation and training services?

Professional Expertise

1. Are there currently professionals at your faciity who could serve on the assistive technology team?
2. What other professionals would be needed to serve your current population?
3. What other professionals would be needed to serve an expanded client population?
4. Is funding available to hire additional professionals?
5. Is funding available for ongoing professional training?

Equipment

1. What assistive technology equipment is currently available at your facility?
2. What equipment would be needed to serve your current population?
3. What equipment would be needed to serve an expanded population?
4. Is funding available to purchase new equipment?
5. Is funding available to maintain old equipment and purchase new equipment on a continuing basis?
6. Is there space to store the equipment at your facility?

Administrative

1. Is there administrative and financial support from the facility to establish and maintain an assistive technology program?
2. Who would be placed in charge of the program?
3. Would your program duplicate services already provided by another assistive technology program in the area?

Figure 1-1
Assistive Technology Program Development Questionnaire

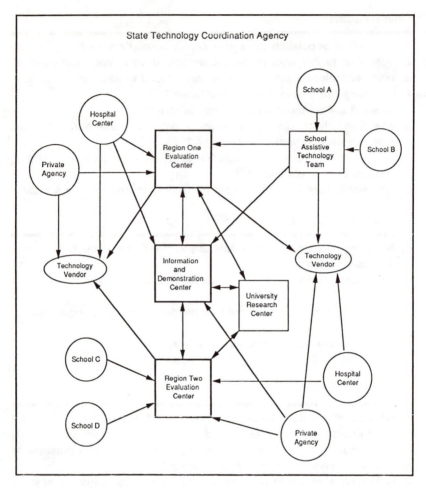

Figure 1–2

Model of Assistive Technology Service Delivery Integration on a State Level

and work toward integrating service segments to provide continuity and comprehensive service delivery. In instances where no services exist, programming efforts may involve the vertical integration of a new service program within the framework of an existing service delivery model. For example, a comprehensive clinical rehabilitation hospital might consider adding a seating and positioning clinic to the hospital's existing occupational or physical therapy department.

If segmented services are maintained across several service providers, the integration effort may involve developing new working relationships between service agencies. Often, this integration approach requires strong interagency cooperation, excellent community relations, and supportive working affiliations with other competitive organizations. Unfortunately, significant communication problems among state agencies and the private sector do exist, thus making the delivery of services to individuals with disabilities extremely variable and inconsistent. This fragmentation results in numerous service gaps, overlaps, and general breakdowns in the delivery of services. Unfortunately, interagency rivalry, dissimilar missions, poor program awareness, or different service timetables often impede service delivery integration.

The integration of services at the client programming level requires attention to daily organizational activities associated with providing assistive technology services. For example, client programming requirements include integrating referral procedures, preassessment activities, evaluation procedures, communicating assessment findings, implementing recommendations, and coordinating follow-up strategies. Administrative procedures and policy breakdowns also restrict the integration of client programming. For example, professionals may experience integration problems when attempting to provide the most appropriate and effective service program, especially to severely handicapped individuals with multiple needs. Further, problems can proliferate as service providers simultaneously operationalize complex procedural and regulatory requirements associated with assistive technology service delivery.

The client transition process also requires careful attention to the integration of technology services. Specifically, the client transition process involves integrating technology services across service delivery systems as disabled individuals leave one service system and enter another. As an example, this transition process might involve the provision of technology evaluation and treatment services to a client leaving a rehabilitation medical facility and entering the school special education system. Under these circumstances, an important service issue might be defining responsibility for training teachers and related support staff. Similarly, issues might arise with respect to accountability for prescribing client equipment when problems arise in the user's environment. From a fiscal perspective, funding for newly prescribed technology can become an issue as third-party payer justification changes from medical needs to educational needs. Finally, questions regarding the appropriateness of equipment recommendations also can become an issue between medical and educational service delivery systems.

In another example, the transition process may involve technology services for a developmentally disabled client leaving one secondary school-based service model and entering a postsecondary vocational education program. Related service issues might involve the adequacy of client placement, appropriateness of referrals, integration of vocational goals with technology service prescriptions, adequacy of client and support staff training, and responsibility for equipment customization, adaptations, and maintenance.

COOPERATION AND PROGRAM AWARENESS

There is generally an across-the-board communication and information gap among developers, providers, and users of assistive technology. At issue are the problems associated with lack of awareness of each service provider, the inability of technology providers to completely understand the needs of clients, and the clients' inability to understand the relevant applications of assistive technologies. This general lack of awareness leaves the potential for variable and inconsistent services which can result in the existence of service gaps, overlaps, and unidentified service needs. The repercussions on the assistive technology service environment can include a myriad of services and systems that are neither consumer friendly nor efficient in disseminating information. It can become extremely difficult for consumers, parents, and clinicians to access the system. Further, as the pace and breadth of technology transfer to disabled populations increases, the need for timely information will only escalate.

The impact of local and state cooperative agreements is important for the effectiveness of assistive technology service delivery efforts. First, these agreements allow for greater communication and awareness of the agencies involved. In addition, cooperative efforts can reduce the territorialism of participating agencies within the same service environment. Cooperative efforts also help develop liaisons that can facilitate service delivery in assessment, treatment, and transition services. The benefits of cooperative agreements can be seen in more effective long-range planning for new technology programs and the increase in joint funding for such cooperative efforts.

Service providers should also be concerned with barriers that currently limit cooperation between medical, special education, vocational education, vocational rehabilitation, and related service providers. These service organizations have distinct histories and operate under different legislative mandates. In addition, they have different goals and priorities, and their time frames for client contact and service provision are different. As a result, technology service providers must be aware of a variety of issues concerning interagency cooperation. For example, definitional problems associated with handicapping conditions can hinder the eligibility or continuation of services to the client. Interagency cooperation and coordination in the delivery of services to disabled individuals not only provides a continuum of treatment and support, but also can decrease service duplication in the assistive technology service environment.

The need for promoting consumer awareness is another important task in planning and implementing effective assistive technology programs. Consumer awareness efforts should include disseminating information on the organization's mission, goals, and objectives. The distribution effort should also ensure that consumers understand the range of services available to meet their needs. For example, this could include information on professional qualifications, comprehensiveness of facilities, classification and duration of technology services available, and descriptions on how technology assessments, prescriptions, and treatment interventions are conducted. Similarly, information on the referral process, treatment waiting periods, and service fees should also be included.

Information and promotion activities often require different approaches for dissimilar audiences. As an example, in organizations that provide awareness programs to other service agencies in the hope of obtaining new referrals, service providers usually develop very different information packages. These awareness programs might include information on rehabilitation licensing, state certifications, definitions of target populations, technical descriptions of the clinical staff, policy and procedure statements for interagency access to services, or detailed descriptions of the comprehensive nature of the service delivery program.

In addition to service information, both clients and service providers are constantly in need of updated database information on new products that improve performance, increase reliability, and provide more general flexibility to the user. A number of regional and local demonstration centers are being established to address these information needs. These sites function much like libraries in that assistive devices can be loaned to consumers, their families, and service providers. These centers also can provide training and technical assistance to professionals, clients, and their families who may have questions regarding the use of assistive technology equipment.

ASSISTIVE TECHNOLOGY EQUIPMENT AVAILABILITY

The successful use of technology by disabled individuals can only be achieved through personal use of an assistive device on a full-time basis. In many instances, disabled children in school settings are exposed to assistive devices for just a few hours each day. The school equipment generally cannot leave the school premises. As a result, the child is without the benefits of technology when he or she attempts to function in the home and community environment. This is a profound loss to a child who depends on such a system for daily social interaction and personal communications. As a result of budget constraints, other technology programs may purchase a single communication system, and proceed to share it with multiple children during the school day. Equipment availability also becomes an issue when individuals who are handicapped exit from the secondary school program and enter the workforce. Interagency coordination for transitional technology planning and programming is vital if they are to work and live independently. Coordinated programming among special education, vocational rehabilitation, and postsecondary vocational training agencies is needed to provide the support services necessary to facilitate the transition of youth who are disabled from school to work and community.

Regional and local demonstration centers can play an important role in providing technical assistance to consumers and professionals. Lending library systems are now being utilized to establish short- and long-term loans of assistive technology equipment. This allows individuals who are disabled to use a particular device over an extended day-to-day period of time in their homes, schools, and communities. The system has two important strengths in terms of assistive device availability. First, it allows the client and service provider to evaluate alternative systems in real-life situations. Second, it also can provide access to loaner equipment while funding sources for the purchase of equipment for clients are explored.

ASSISTIVE TECHNOLOGY FUNDING ISSUES

One of the most pervasive programming issues facing assistive technology service providers is funding. Due to finite funding levels, service delivery capacity is often severely compromised. It is not uncommon for service agencies to have their funds exhausted in the first several months of the fiscal year. The realities of limited financial resources demand that organizations make rigorous fiscal decisions. These pragmatic funding decisions determine the allocation of funds to services and ultimately produce some degree of funding restriction. These restrictions have a wide variety of impacts on the provision of services. For example, funding restrictions can constrain agencies in the number of part- and full-time staff positions specifically dedicated to the assessment and prescription of technology. Similarly, few organizations have the funding support necessary to provide comprehensive long-term training to all staff on technology and related issues. In addition, the drastic state-to-state variations in funding policies can greatly influence the eligibility requirements for clients in highly mobile family units. These policy variations frustrate any national effort at service integration.

The funding equation has two major components that must be addressed by service providers. These include funding issues associated with the costs of delivering technology services and funding issues associated with locating, cultivating, and acquiring third-party payment sources. In addition, service providers should understand that both components of the funding equation are dynamic in nature. Therefore, service providers require sensitivity and flexibility in order to manage both successfully. Regulations, interpretations, and qualifications are constantly changing as new sources of funding continue to become available.

Funding Assistive Technology Programs

The costs associated with developing new technology programs start with the estimation of "start-up" costs. There are a wide range of cost estimates associated with new technology initiatives, from several thousand to several million dollars. Funding levels will depend on the scope of the service model being developed and the fiscal objectives being pursued. However, despite program complexity, all programs will transition through a time period of initial start-up to operational status. Service providers should plan and estimate start-up costs based on a planning time frame of several years. When developing financial estimates for program start-up costs, service providers should consider the constraints of the service and organizational environment. These constraints will necessitate the use of a variety of resources that require up-front, short-, and long-term funding approaches.

Direct start-up costs typically fall into two areas: equipment and personnel. Equipment costs will vary with the focus of the program. Programs that specialize in evaluation services require appropriate technology for client assessment. Over time, the program will need to purchase new equipment as it becomes available and maintain old equipment as it needs repair and replacement. Considering the rapid pace of changing technology, ongoing equipment costs for an evaluation center can be quite high. Programs that provide only treatment services have much lower equipment costs. Typically, each client has his or her own equipment, which is funded by grants, insurance, or other sources. Ideally, the program should have backup equipment for devices that are used by several clients.

Start-up costs for personnel vary with the focus of the assistive technology program. Teams that provide technology services in more than one area need more professionals on the team to provide services. Personnel costs also vary depending on the percentage of time team members devote to assistive technology team functions. For example, a physical therapist might work half-time on the assistive technology team, and half-time seeing other clients. Overall personnel costs per client will be related to the total number of clients served and the extensiveness of the team's services. Other program start-up costs that service providers might consider include expanded administrative support services, office materials, expanded facilities, personnel and fringe benefits, licensing or certification expenses, and indirect costs associated with organizational change.

In addition to program start-up costs, service providers must also analyze and estimate both indirect and direct operational service costs. This includes developing cost structures for evaluation and assessment services, prescription and implementation services, client and support staff training, related follow-up services, and information and awareness efforts.

Funding of Assistive Technology Services and Equipment

The payment side of the funding equation requires considerable reflection on the part of service providers. Although financial resources are often scarce, funding should not limit the assistive technology team's services or equipment recommendations for a given client. Resourceful professionals who are willing to seek out all possible funding sources can almost always find money. A brief overview of some of the major third-party funding sources will give the reader some insight into the array of funding sources that exist at the federal, state, and private levels.

Third-Party Funding Sources

EDUCATIONAL PROGRAMS. The Education of the Handicapped Act (Public Law 94-142, as Amended) ensures that all handicapped children receive the free appropriate public education to which they are entitled. Each state and local education agency is required to develop special education programs for children who are eligible for special education services. The definition of children who are eligible is very broad. It includes children aged 3 to 21 years old, unless state practices do not provide service to 3- to 5-year-old or 18- to 21-year-old age groups. In addition, eligibility is also extended to children presently receiving services from any federally funded program, whether they are younger or older than the state school age. The eligibility requirements cover any disability category required by state or court order. This comprehensive law

law applies to all children regardless of their residence, including, for example, children living with their natural parents, children in foster homes, institutionalized children, or children living in group homes. Some states have established state-wide service delivery systems through the state Department of Education which fund assistive technology for children through state grants (Haney, 1990). Other states have provided seed money to local or regional districts to develop assistive technology services in the schools.

VOCATIONAL REHABILITATION. The federal government assists states in providing vocational rehabilitation services to help individuals who are handicapped become employable by providing assessment, treatment, and training. A state's guidelines and its resource base determine the range of services offered to clients. In general, these rehabilitation services are usually very individualized and are allocated according to recommendations by vocational counselors. Some states require that the individual be evaluated by professionals at a state Vocational Rehabilitation Center before funding assistive technology equipment.

THE DEVELOPMENTALLY DISABLED PROGRAM (DD). This federally funded state grant program is designed to help states improve the quality of services through comprehensive service planning and coordination of state resources. This program provides services to children with severe chronic mental and physical impairments that are manifested before the age of 22. This program utilizes the existing service delivery system to provide diagnosis, evaluation, and treatment to individuals who are handicapped.

CHILDREN'S MEDICAL SERVICES (CMS). This is a jointly funded federal and state program offering medical and related services to children who are handicapped from birth to age 21 and who meet certain financial requirements. This program provides free medical diagnosis and evaluation for all children. However, the range and cost of additional services varies from state to state. Some state CMS programs actively fund assistive technology equipment for children who qualify for CMS services.

MEDICARE. This is a federally funded health insurance program designed to help individuals over age 65 and individuals who are severely disabled under age 65 pay the cost of their health care. Medicare has two parts: (1) mandatory hospital insurance (Part A); and (2) optional medical insurance (Part B). Part A is designed to help pay for *inpatient* hospital care and specific follow-up care after patients leave the hospital. Part B covers a broader range of medical benefits, including *outpatient* hospital services, diagnostic tests, physicians' services, extremity braces, artificial limbs, and the purchase of outpatient durable medical equipment (DME). Currently, Medicare will pay for some assistive technology equipment if it is prescribed by a physician.

MEDICAID. This is a jointly funded federal and state program designed to provide medical insurance for individuals and families with low incomes. This program is administered by participating states within federal guidelines. These federal laws require certain basic services such as hospital and laboratory services. In addition, states may provide additional services at their own discretion. As a result, there are wide variations in the scope of state services offered. Various state Medicaid programs have been known to cover assistive technology devices when a physician's authorization is obtained. The Early Prevention Screening Diagnosis and Testing (EPSDT) program for children from birth to age 21 specifically states that durable medical equipment is funded under program guidelines. Lastly, because many Medicaid members are aged and/or disabled they often qualify for coverage under Medicare.

CHAMPUS. The Civilian Health and Medical Program of the Uniformed Services (CHAMPUS) is another federally funded program that provides medical benefits to spouses and children of active duty, retired, and deceased active duty and retired uniformed service personnel. The *Program for the Handicapped,* a component service of this program, provides financial assistance to active duty personnel for the care, training, and rehabilitation of a spouse or child who is seriously physically handicapped or moderately to severely mentally retarded. Through this program, CHAMPUS provides funding for assistive technology that is deemed medically necessary. CHAMPUS operates its programs through various insurance companies that have been contracted to provide health coverage in a designated region. When seeking coverage for assistive technology equipment, the application request must be sent to the insurance center located in the equipment vendor's region, not the client's region.

PRIVATE INSURANCE. This potential source of funding includes health insurance, long-term disability insurance, worker's compensation, and similar types of insurance. Private insurance plans vary greatly in terms of insurance coverage and the levels of payments. However, in general, the level of service provided by private insurance carriers depends on the terms of the contract or policy and the interpretation of the policy by the insurance carrier. Most private insurance companies will fund only assistive technology that is medically necessary and prescribed by a physician.

PRIVATE FUNDING. Private funding sources include volunteer agencies, small and large corporations, large private foundations, or even national ad-

vocacy groups. These private funding sources can provide direct dona-
tions, support philanthropic events, supply lobbying services, or volunteer staff time. Service providers can find a wide variety of private
funding opportunities in the local community and regional service area.

Most third-party funding sources have specific guidelines and
forms which must be completed to obtain funding. It is often useful to
contact a representative of the funding agency by telephone before
sending any paperwork. The representative can provide information
on the probability of obtaining funding and the process for obtaining
funding. If possible, ask for the name of a specific person at the funding agency to direct the request to. Most agencies require sending specific agency forms plus copies of any evaluation reports.

Funding agencies that are health-oriented often require a physician's prescription which states that assistive technology equipment is
medically necessary. These funding sources typically will not fund
equipment for educational or social needs. Therefore, all supporting
documents should be oriented toward establishing a medical need for
the equipment. Because most assistive technology services and equipment are novel to third-party payers, including descriptive brochures
with a funding request is often useful.

Guidelines for Third-Party Funding

Most third-party funding sources are large organizations that process hundreds of claims each week. Because of the volume of paper, it
is not suprising that funding requests are sometimes lost in the system.
Before sending any paperwork to a third-party payer, copies should be
made of all forms. Once the paperwork is sent, the funding agency
should be given 1 month to respond. If no response is received after 1
month, begin calling the agency to determine the status of the funding request.

If a third-party funding source denies paying for assistive technology services or equipment, the denial should be challenged by asking
for an appeal. The appeal is often directed to a special review board in
the funding agency which then examines the request and makes a final
decision. An appeal board will often ask for additional documentation
or may contact the assistive technology team with additional questions
about the funding request.

SUMMARY

When considering the implementation of assistive technology, service
providers must recognize and manage a wide variety of program issues. This chapter highlighted some of the major issues regarding the
planning and use of technology with individuals who are disabled.

Some of these issues include service constraints, consumer awareness, technology availability, training, and funding. Without proper attention, these and other issues often develop into major barriers to successful assistive technology initiatives.

Professionals planning new technology programs have many service delivery models available to use as guides for service implementation. Each service model has distinct benefits and drawbacks. There is no one approach that will meet all planning and program objectives. The selection of service delivery models will depend on the needs of the organization, the complexity of the technology project, the dynamics of the service environment, and the formal and informal structures of the service facility.

REFERENCES

Cohen, C. (1986). Total habilitation and life-long management. In S. B. Blackstone & D. Ruskin (Eds.), *Augmentative communication: An introduction.* Rockville, MD: ASHA Press.

Haney, C. (1990, November). *100 local augmentative specialists respond to statewide survey.* Paper presented at the American Speech-Language-Hearing Association annual convention, Seattle, WA.

Shane, H., & Yoder, D. (1981). Delivery of augmentative communication services: The role of the speech-language pathologist. *Language Speech and Hearing Services in Schools, 12,* 211–215.

Yorkston, K., & Karlan, G. (1986). Assessment procedures. In S. Blackstone & D. Ruskin (Eds.), *Augmentative communication: An introduction.* Rockville, MD: ASHA Press.

Introduction to Microcomputers

■ Gregory Church, MS, MAS ■

Assistive technologists working with microcomputers require practical information regarding the function and operation of computer technology. Through nontechnical explanations on such subjects as microcomputer processing, input, output, and storage, technologists can better understand the capabilities of microcomputers. These explanations can eliminate much of the confusion over various equipment standards, technical jargon, and the application of assistive technology aids. In addition, gaining information on current technologies is helpful for making product evaluations regarding appropriate client equipment prescriptions.

The purpose of this chapter is to introduce the reader to some of the fundamental concepts and basic terminology associated with microcomputer technology that will be used in this book. Throughout, the reader will encounter the terms "hardware" and "software" in descriptions of various computer systems and assistive devices. The **hardware** component of a microcomputer system or related assistive device is defined as anything that can be seen and touched. Any external hardware component that is attached to a computer is referred to as a **peripheral device**. Examples include a disk drive, printer, or keyboard. The **software** component of a computer, in contrast, is intangible and consists of the set of instructions to the hardware that is used to operate or perform some process. For instance, software might control a speech synthesizer, a computer operating system, or a software application like a word processor.

Assistive technology professionals utilize many different types of microcomputers as part of their service delivery approach. For example, service providers may develop technology solutions based on the Apple II series, Commodore, IBM, or Tandy computers in school settings. In a vocational rehabilitation or business setting, a technology solution might involve an Apple Macintosh, IBM *PS/2,* PC compatible, or Tandy system. Personal computer vendors package computers using a variety of different approaches. The desktop microcomputer system is a very popular computer system for home, school, and business applications. Desktop systems are the most prevalent microcomputers in use (see Figure 2–1). Desktop designs put the major hardware components into one large "box" or case. Other designs may separate each component part, placing each in its own box. These systems average about 30 to 90 pounds. The design approach makes for large, expansive microcomputer systems that are generally dedicated to a large desk or work station space. The weight and bulk of desktop systems generally restricts their portability.

Popular desktop computers include the IBM *PS/2,* IBM *PC* and *AT,* Tandy, Compaq *Deskpro,* Leading Edge *Model D,* Apple *Macintosh,* Commodore *Amiga,* Atari *1040ST,* Epson *Equity,* Apple *IIe* and *IIgs,* and Zenith systems. These are just of few the many systems available to consumers for home, school, and business use. Individuals who are disabled often find these systems useful in situations where portability is not an issue. Desktop systems can be found in classrooms where the user may be developing reading, writing, and math skills. Similarly, individuals who are handicapped successfully use desktop computers in office settings for word processing, drafting, or other work-related tasks.

Vendors also package microcomputers in a variety of portable configurations. Transportable computers are small desktop microcomputers that are lightweight enough to move, but still need an external alternating current (AC) power supply to operate (see Figure 2–1). True portable systems, which are small and lightweight enough to be carried around easily, use either replaceable or rechargeable batteries. Some have the option of using either batteries or AC power. Although features vary from computer to computer, some portable systems have the same full range of features as a desktop computer.

Laptop and notebook computers are a further refinement of portable microcomputer systems. Utilizing this approach, vendors miniaturize hardware components into a microcomputer with a footprint

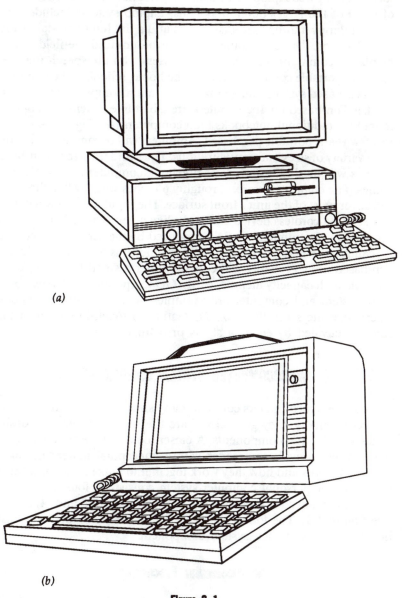

(a)

(b)

Figure 2-1

(a) Standard desktop microcomputer with separate system unit box, keyboard, and monitor.
(b) Portable microcomputer with integrated monitor, system unit, and keyboard.

the size of a sheet of paper, measuring only a few inches high, and weighing just several pounds (see Figure 2–2). Yet the capabilities and performance of these laptop and notebook personal computers rival those of some of the larger desktop systems. Laptop systems include small built-in floppy and/or hard-disk drives and a flat liquid crystal display (LCD) screen. These computers have revolutionized the field of augmentative communication by offering users who are speech impaired access to portable communication in the home, school, and community.

Pen-based systems are a new class of microcomputers entering the market. Pen-based microcomputers are tablet-like systems that operate more like traditional notebooks than computers (see Figure 2–2). Within a few years, portable pen-based computers will become available in a wide variety of sizes and configurations. The standard size of pen-based systems will be similar to today's notebook computers, about 8½ × 11 inches. The computer's screen, roughly 6 inches wide by 8 inches high, will cover most of the unit's front surface. The input method will consist of a stylus, a cordless device that looks like a pen. The stylus will interact with an electromagnetic field produced by the screen. The computer can sense where the stylus is and whether it is touching the screen. Pen-based units probably will contain either a small hard disk or removable high capacity memory cards. GO Corporation's *PenPoint* operating system and computer are examples of new pen-based systems. MicroSlate Inc.'s *Datellite 300L PC* features a touch-input screen that can be activated by either a stylus or a finger.

MICROCOMPUTER SYSTEM COMPONENTS

Although microcomputers come in many sizes and are made by many different vendors, they generally share the same fundamental design characteristics and components. A closer look at these computer components will provide the reader with a conceptual understanding of how each works and how they work together to make a microcomputer function. The personal computer system consists of four major hardware components: (1) processing, (2) input, (3) output, and (4) storage (see Figure 2–3). The following sections provide the reader with basic information about each system component.

Microcomputer Processing

The first major component of a microcomputer involves control and data processing. All microcomputers are built around a **system unit**, which controls all of the computer's functions and data-processing (Church & Bender, 1989). The typical system unit consists of three main

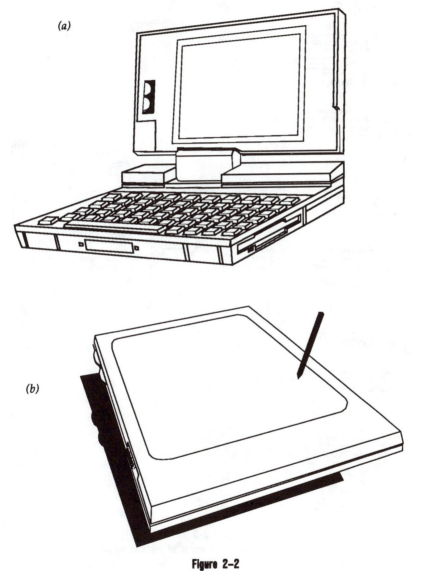

Figure 2–2
(a) Laptop microcomputer with built-in floppy disk drive and LCD screen. (b) Pen-based tablet microcomputer with stylus input.

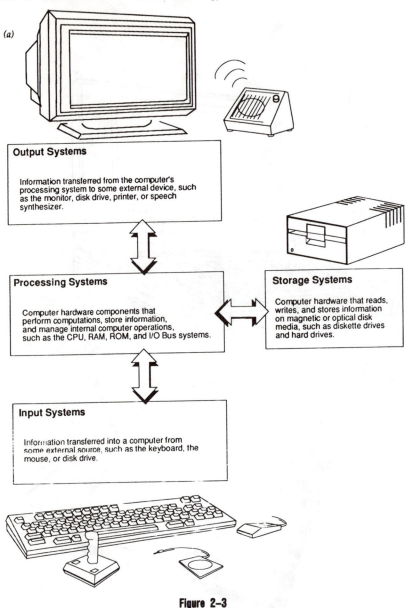

(a)

Output Systems

Information transferred from the computer's processing system to some external device, such as the monitor, disk drive, printer, or speech synthesizer.

Processing Systems

Computer hardware components that perform computations, store information, and manage internal computer operations, such as the CPU, RAM, ROM, and I/O Bus systems.

Storage Systems

Computer hardware that reads, writes, and stores information on magnetic or optical disk media, such as diskette drives and hard drives.

Input Systems

Information transferred into a computer from some external source, such as the keyboard, the mouse, or disk drive.

Figure 2–3
The four major system components of microcomputers.

parts: (1) microprocessor, (2) memory, and (3) input/output interface. The system unit is built on a printed circuit board located inside the microcomputer's case. This board is often called the **mother board** or **main system board**.

Microprocessor

The microprocessor or **central processing unit** (CPU) is the heart of the microcomputer. The CPU is responsible for the control of all the computer's major functions. These functions include controlling access to computer memory, interpreting instructions, directing and passing data to and from the computer, performing mathematical and logical operations, and establishing the timing of events (Church & Bender, 1989).

The computer's CPU performs all of its functions using just two digits: 0 and 1. Each binary digit is called a **bit** and is the smallest piece of data that can be recognized and used by a computer. A grouping of eight bits is a **byte**. The byte is used to measure the size of computer memory. It is commonly represented by the kilobyte (K) meaning 1,024 bytes, and megabyte (MB) meaning 1,048,576 bytes. For practical purposes however, users usually think of K as 1 thousand and MB as 1 million.

The computer's microprocessor uses two internal communication channels for transferring and communicating data. These communication channels are referred to as the address bus and the data bus. Each bus consists of a series of electrical circuits on the computer's mother board. The **address bus** is a communication channel internal to a computer by which the CPU can access particular input devices, output devices, or locations in memory. The **data bus** is a communication channel internal to a computer by which the CPU can exchange data and programs with peripherals.

Microprocessors are designed to handle internal data as a group of adjacent bits in a unit called a **word**. The word is manipulated within the computer's CPU. For example, some CPUs manipulate data in a 8-bit word, whereas newer systems handle word lengths of 16 and 32 bits. IBM and IBM-compatible computers use the Intel series of CPUs: 8088 (8-bit), 80286 (16-bit), 80386 (32-bit), and 80486 (32-bit) microprocessors. Apple II series computers use the 6502 (8-bit) series. Apple *Macintosh* and Commodore *Amiga* computers use the Motorola series of CPUs: 68000 (16-bit), 68020 (32-bit), 68030 (32-bit), and 68040 (32-bit) microprocessors.

The microcomputers just mentioned differ significantly in the speed and power at which they work. Speed generally is affected by three major factors. First, the larger the word length that a CPU can handle, the faster the system. For example, a 16-bit computer usually is faster than an 8-bit computer. Second, the computer system is built around a **system clock** that determines how fast CPU operations can be performed by the computer. System clocks are measured in millions of cycles per second, or megahertz (MHz). Microcomputers generally operate in a range from 1.2 MHz to over 40 MHz. Some systems offer the user several speed settings. A computer with a speed rating of 8 MHz can be expected to perform operations about twice as fast as a 4 MHz computer. Lastly, microcomputers incorporate **coprocessors** into the system unit. The coprocessor is designed to relieve the computer's CPU of some major functions, allowing it to perform other tasks. Math coprocessors, for example, take the burden off the CPU for performing mathematical and logical operations.

Computer speed considerations are important when assistive technology devices share the processing power of the computer's CPU. For example, speech recognition systems often require faster microcomputers to simultaneously process speech and run application software. Some computers do not have the capability to manage multiple operations effectively.

Memory

Microcomputers use two types of primary data storage: random access memory (RAM) and read only memory (ROM).

RAM is where data and program instructions are held, temporarily while being manipulated or executed. Because RAM is volatile, all data is lost when the computer's power is turned off. Thus, all data and program files must be transferred from RAM to a storage device such as a diskette. The amount of usable memory available to a computer can vary considerably. For example, an 8-bit system can address a maximum of 64K of RAM, a 16-bit system can access a maximum of 1 MB of RAM, and a 32-bit microprocessor a maximum of 16 MB of addressable storage.

ROM is used to hold permanent programs and information needed by the computer. This information can be read, but cannot be changed by the user. The contents of ROM may contain information on how to start the computer and even instructions for the entire operating system. For instance, IBM PC computers include the BASIC program language in ROM. In addition, many laptop computers include the disk operating system (MS-DOS, PC-DOS) in ROM to reduce the need for extra storage device requirements.

In assistive technology applications, RAM is a very important commodity. As an example, a physically disabled user may be using a headstick to operate a word processor while word prediction and abbreviation expansion software utilities, operating in the background, help the user generate text in the word processor. Many of these software aids are written as **Terminate-and-Stay-Resident** (TSR) programs. The technique allows software programs to remain a RAM-resident and active in the background while other software runs in the foreground. TSR programs also are referred to as memory-resident software. With the trend toward larger software programs, the need for additional RAM resources will increase (Church & Bender, 1989).

Because the computer's address bus and disk operating system impose memory limitations, a number of hardware and software schemes have evolved to overcome RAM limitations. Some older 8-bit computers get around their storage limitation by using **bank switching**. For example, although the Apple *IIe* can use 128K, it cannot address all 128K at any one time; instead, it uses two separate banks of 64K RAM. To use all 128K, the Apple switches between banks to give the user the illusion of using 128K.

IBM PCs and IBM-compatible computers face similar memory restrictions. For instance, the computer's disk operating system (DOS) can only recognize from 0 to 640K of RAM, despite the amount of memory installed in the computer. This lower 640K range of memory is called **conventional memory**. Any additional RAM between conventional memory (640K) and 1MB is called **high-DOS** memory. All hardware and software schemes designed to increase usable memory must work with or around DOS conventional memory. Ultimately, these schemes must make as much room as possible for software applications to run in DOS's 640K area, while loading as many TSR programs, expansion card software, and data blocks into RAM high-DOS memory.

For example, the Lotus, Intel, and Microsoft companies have developed a method that uses sections of high-DOS memory for running software programs under a scheme called "Lotus, Intel, Microsoft-Expanded Memory Specification" (LMS-EMS). To use this method, 80286-based computers must include memory expansion cards and software that complies with the LIM-EMS standard. Newer 80286, 80386, and 80486-based microcomputers include extra memory called **extended memory**, RAM located above 1 MB.

Input and Output Interface

The third major part of the system unit is the computer's input/output (I/O) interface. These facilities are designed to exchange information with the outside world. This information exchange involves both putting data into the computer (input) and receiving data from the computer (output) (Church & Bender, 1989). Assistive technology devices take advantage of these facilities by utilizing either serial or parallel I/O to communicate with microcomputers.

SERIAL I/O. The **serial** interface is used for transmitting data, sequentially, one bit at a time, one bit after the other, over a single data line. Serial data transmission is analogous to a single-lane road where each car must follow the other to travel from place to place. The speed at which bits travel on a serial data line is controlled by the CPU. The transmission speed is called the **baud rate** and is equivalent to the number of bits sent per second. Common speed ratings found in computers and assistive devices include 300, 1200, 2400, and 9600 baud. Serial I/O is the slowest of the two major types of computer I/O.

Typical microcomputer serial connectors use the Electronics Industries Association's written standards for defining serial functions. The two major written standards are called Recommended Standard number 232, version C, which is often referred to as the "RS-232C serial interface" (see Figure 2–4) and Recommended Standard number 422, known as "RS-422 serial interface." Assistive technology devices often use these inexpensive interfaces for accessing a microcomputer. The technologist or computer specialist will often come across various types of serial connectors (see Figure 2–4). The DB-(n) notation describes certain connectors, where (n) is the number of pins for male, or sockets for female, in the connector. For example, a DB-9 connector has a nine-pin configuration. The reader should be aware that peripheral manufacturers may or may not conform to the Electronic Industries Association's standards. As a result, it is suggested that technologists check with vendors and peripheral documentation for cable connector type and pin assignment to assure computer compatibility.

PARALLEL I/O. The **parallel** interface is used for transmitting data in sets of usually eight bits at a time, side by side, over multiple data lines. The parallel I/O concept is analogous to a short eight-lane highway supporting only one-way travel. The bits in each set must travel parallel with one another, and only one set of eight bits is allowed to use the parallel line at any one time. The parallel interface is often called a "Centronics" connector, after the company that developed it for its line of printers (see Figure 2–4). The parallel interface is designed for high-speed communications. Parallel printers and external disk drives often are connected to this interface.

Microcomputer Input

The most common input device for personal computers is the keyboard. Most keyboards consist of a matrix of letter, number, and symbol keys. In general, computer keyboards are not standardized in terms of numbers, layout, size, or shape of keys. Individuals whose impairments leave them unable to type on a regular keyboard often face difficulties controlling all the functions of the computer. There-

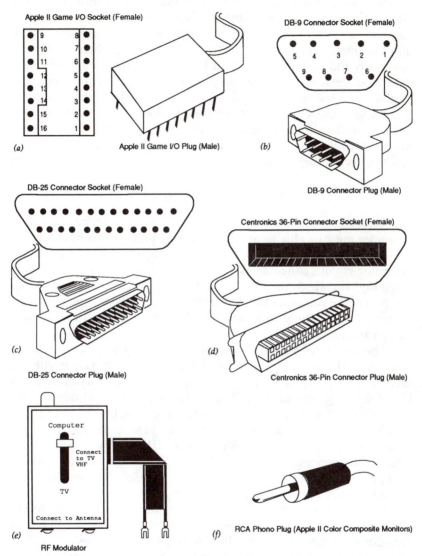

Figure 2-4

Microcomputer input/output interfaces. (a) Internal Apple II game I/O socket found on the main logic board. (b) Typical DB-9 serial interface port. (c) Typical DB-25 parallel interface port. (d) Centronics parallel interface port. (e) Radio Frequency (RF) modulator for connecting a microcomputer to a standard TV. (f) RCA phone plug used with color composite computer monitors.

fore, these potential users may not be able to access the same computer and software opportunities as the rest of the world. Fortunately, many alternate solutions are available to disabled users. These alternative assistive aids communicate with the microcomputer using a variety of input methods. Some systems replace the keyboard, others modify the computer, and still others work in tandem with the computer's standard input devices. The complexity of solutions varies from product to product, which demands different levels of expertise on the part of the technologist and client to set up, troubleshoot, and operate. Consequently, for the clinician, input hardware becomes critically important when evaluating the complexity, performance, and appropriateness of assistive technology solutions.

Buses and Expansion Slots

To receive and process information from an assistive device, the microcomputer must be able to move data to any piece of peripheral hardware connected to the system. The data travels across the computer on electronic circuits called a **bus**. One can think of a bus as a multi-lane "highway" on which data travel, exchanging electronic signals, from one part of the computer to another. Buses vary greatly from computer to computer, resulting in a number of different hardware standards and incompatibilities.

The classic IBM AT bus is known as Industry Standard Architecture (ISA). This early bus became an acknowledged standard with the early success of IBM's AT desktop computer. The ISA bus can send 16 bits of data over its data bus. Shortly after the AT was introduced and computers moved to higher data processing speeds, the shortcoming of the AT bus became apparent. It was too slow to keep up with the needs of microprocessors running faster than 8 MHz. This bus design continues to be very popular among IBM-compatible computer makers. Computers using this bus design include Compaq's *Deskpro,* HP's *Vectra 386,* NEC's *PowerMate,* and Olivetti's *M386* systems.

IBM's answer to the AT bus was the introduction of the Micro Channel Architecture (MCA) bus. The MCA bus can send 32 bits of data down its data bus at speeds near 14.5 MHz. As a result, this bus design greatly increases a microcomputer's speed and performance. Unfortunately, computer users who have a large financial investment in older ISA hardware cannot use these expansion boards in a MCA bus computer. The IBM *PS/2 Model 70, PS/2 Model 80,* and Advanced Logic Research's *ALR Power Cache 4* systems are examples of desktop MCA bus microcomputers.

The Enhanced Industry Standard Architecture (EISA) bus was developed by a consortium of leading IBM-compatible personal computer makers. EISA's features essentially duplicate the best elements of the MCA bus. In addition, EISA provides backward compatibility with older ISA hardware. As a result, the EISA bus will accommodate both ISA and EISA expansion boards, but it is a one-way compatibility. EISA hardware cannot be used in ISA bus computers. The Compaq *Systempro* and the Tandon *486 EISA* microcomputer are examples of microcomputers using the EISA bus.

Lastly, Apple Macintosh microcomputers offer two additional buses to the personal computer market. These buses are called the Processor-Direct slot (PDS) and the NuBus. The PDS bus operates at 20 Mhz and has direct access to the computer's microprocessor. As a result, the hardware used in this bus operates at very high speeds. Examples of computers using the PDS bus include the Apple *Macintosh SE* and *Macintosh LC*. The NuBus operates at 10 MHz, supports a 32-bit data bus, and provides the unique feature of "self-configuration" for NuBus specific expansion boards. Therefore, the user does not have to set special expansion board switches to set up and use peripherals. Microcomputer systems using the NuBus design include the Apple *Macintosh II, IICX, IIFX,* and *IISI* systems.

Buses vary greatly from computer to computer, but even ISA, MCA, EISA, PDS, and NuBus designs can be categorized in two basic types of systems: (1) open bus and (2) closed bus. The bus system is built on a printed circuit board located inside the microcomputer. This circuit board is often called the **main logic board** or the **mother board**.

The **open bus** system is designed for microcomputers that allow physical access to or direct expansion of the mother board. Open bus computers contain **expansion slots**, long, thin sockets on the mother board, that allow the user to install boards that expand the microcomputer's capabilities (see Figure 2–5). The Apple *IIe* and IBM AT desktop computers, for example, each have eight expansion slots. In addition, Compaq's *LTE 386/20,* Sharp's *PC-6220,* and Toshiba's *T-1600* laptop computers, to name a few, also have open bus designs. Depending on the bus, disabled users can use these slots to add peripherals such as a modem, a printer, a speech recognition unit, an alternative keyboard, or an environmental control unit to the microcomputer. When adapting computers, assistive technologists should identify the computer's bus design to assure expansion board compatibility. Alternative assistive technology vendors often make different versions of a product to accommodate various computer bus designs.

The **closed bus** system is designed for microcomputers that do not allow physical access to or direct expansion of the mother board. Instead, closed bus computers provide input capabilities through established ports that accept cables. A **port** is a socket on the back panel of the computer where you can plug in a cable to connect a peripheral

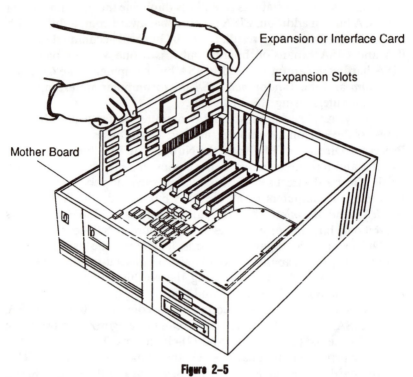

Figure 2-5

Open bus microcomputers contain expansion slots that accept interface cards. These cards expand the microcomputer's capabilities.

device (see Figure 2-4). The closed bus system usually defines the particular type of function or configuration each port may handle. For example, a video port is limited to video signals that are sent to the computer's external screen. In addition, other ports, such as serial or parallel ports, provide microcomputers with added functionality. IBM and IBM-compatible microcomputers usually label serial ports as COM1 and COM2 and parallel ports as LPT1 and LPT2. The Apple *Macintosh Plus* and Commodore *64* desktop computers are examples of closed bus systems. Many laptop and notebook computers also incorporate closed bus designs; the Zenith *MinisPort* and Toshiba *T1000* microcomputers are two examples.

In general, closed bus systems make it easier for the user to connect and configure peripherals than open bus systems with internal slots. Expanding closed bus computers is not a problem until all the ports are filled or until one wishes to add an assistive device or controller that cannot be accommodated by the computer's ports.

Microcomputer Output

The primary output device used with microcomputer systems is the monitor. The monitor gives the user a visual display of computer information. Recent developments in assistive computer technology have enhanced and expanded opportunities for users who are visually impaired or blind. Software and hardware solutions include large print systems which provide screen magnification for computer users with impaired vision. Speech synthesizers with screen review software now make computer monitor information accessible to users who are blind. In addition to video output, microcomputers can output information to a wide variety of peripherals, including printers, disk storage devices, speech synthesizers, and braille embossers, to name a few.

Video Output

Two kinds of video systems are used with computer displays: (1) cathode-ray tube (CRT) and (2) flat-panel displays. Monitor resolution, based on the number of picture elements or "pixels," contained on a screen, is used as a measure of display quality. The more pixels, the sharper the display image. Video display systems are either built into the computer's case or may be added as separate peripherals. The Apple *Macintosh Plus, Classic,* and *SE/30* models are a few examples of desktop systems with built-in CRT monitors. Similarly, Dolch's *P.A.C. 286* and *386DX* portable computer systems include built-in video display systems. Microcomputers with built-in CRT display screens can make users' systems more compact and easier to set up. Conversely, the attachable monitor requires connecting through either the computer's bus or its built-in video port. Some microcomputers provide users with both video expansion options.

Many laptop and notebook computers also provide built-in, flat-panel displays. However, these systems use lightweight displays called **liquid crystal displays** (LCDs). Many laptop systems use supertwist LCDs, which are generally easy to read in offices and classrooms with good lighting. **Supertwist** technology bends the screen's light to produce sharp, high contrast images. However, in poor lighting conditions, a standard supertwist LCD display can become difficult to read. As a result, assistive technology prescriptions that require a wide variety of lighting conditions should consider "backlit" LCDs. **Backlit** LCDs provide a lighting source behind the screen image to increase readability. These displays provide users with good readability in most lighting conditions. Backlighting, however, is a major source of power consumption in battery operated laptop systems.

Microcomputers can be adapted to use a wide range of video display systems. Home televisions, for example, can be used with a computer, but a **radio frequency (RF) modulator** is required to translate the video signals from the computer into a form the television can display (see Figure 2–4). In addition, many microcomputers provide support for a composite color monitor. The **composite video** signal is similar to a television signal, but the video signal can be transmitted directly through a single wire to either the computer or television monitor. RCA phono jacks can be used as composite video connectors between the computer and monitor (see Figure 2–4). Examples of computers using the composite signal include the Apple *II Plus,* Apple *IIe,* and Apple *IIGS* systems. The number of different video display standards available to IBM and IBM-compatible microcomputers is broad. Table 2–1 summarizes the major IBM and IBM-compatible video display standards.

Table 2–1. IBM and IBM-compatible Video Standards

Year	Display Type	Resolution	Display Modes	Colors	Compatibility Modes
1981	Monochrome Display Adaptor (MDA)	720 × 350	Text	1	None
1981	Color Graphics Adaptor (CGA)	640 × 200	Text	16	None
		320 × 200	Text	16	
		160 × 200	Graphics	16	
		320 × 200	Graphics	4	
		640 × 200	Graphics	2	
1982	Hercules Monochrome Graphics Adaptor (MGA)	720 × 350	Text	1	MDA
		120 × 348	Graphics	1	MDA
1984	Enhanced Graphics Adapter (EGA)	640 × 350	Text	16	CGA, MDA
		720 × 350	Text	4	CGA, MDA
		640 × 350	Graphics	16	CGA, MDA
		320 × 200	Graphics	16	CGA, MDA
		640 × 200	Graphics	16	CGA, MDA
		640 × 350	Graphics	16	CGA, MDA
1987	Video Graphics Array (VGA)	720 × 400	Text	16	CGA, EGA
		360 × 400	Text	16	CGA, EGA
		640 × 480	Graphics	16	CGA, EGA
		320 × 200	Graphics	256	CGA, EGA
1990	Extended Graphics Array (XGA)	640 × 480	Graphics	256	VGA
		1024 × 768	Graphics	256	VGA
		640 × 480	Graphics	65536	VGA
		1056 × 400	Text	16	VGA

Generally, the newer PC standards provide graphic and text displays with more colors and dot resolution than older systems. However, as video standards improve, the capabilities of the microcomputer must also increase to obtain an appropriate balance between resolution and computer performance. In general, improved resolution and color require faster CPU speeds and added RAM support. The significant exceptions to this rule are computers that include graphics coprocessors. Graphics coprocessors relieve the CPU of intensive graphics processing tasks. Two popular graphics coprocessor boards for MS-DOS computers are IBM's *8514—A* and Texas Instruments' *TMS34010*.

Print Output

Computers can provide **hard copy** output, such as paper, to provide users with text, number, or graphic information. The printer is a peripheral designed to produce hard copy output. There are a number of major categories of printer systems. These peripherals connect to the computer through the system unit's I/O bus slots or printer ports. The printing speed and quality of output from these different printers can vary significantly. Printing speed can be measured in characters per second (cps) or pages per minute.

Impact dot-matrix printers are a popular and widely available print technology. Dot-matrix printers use impact print technology to produce images by printing single dots on paper. **Impact print** technology produces characters by using a hammer or pins to strike an ink ribbon that in turn impacts the sheet of paper producing the character. Dot-matrix printers use 9- and 24-pin print heads. These printers are inexpensive and provide users with the flexibility to create both text and graphics. In addition, dot-matrix printers can print in color using multicolored ribbons. Dot-matrix print quality can vary from draft to near-letter quality. Speeds can vary from 50 cps in near-letter quality mode to over 300 cps in draft mode. Examples of dot-matrix systems include the Apple Computer's *ImageWriter II*, Epson's *FX 850*, Okidata's *Okidata 320*, IBM's *Proprinter*, and Panasonic's *KX-P1695* systems.

The second impact print technology is the daisy-wheel printer, named because its print head resembles a daisy; at the end of each "petal" is a molded character (Church & Bender, 1989). The character is then struck by a hammer which produces very high quality text. These printers can print many different typefaces (character styles). Daisy-wheel printer speed varies from 30 cps to over 150 cps. Qume's *Qume LQP* is an example of a daisy-wheel printer.

Nonimpact printers do not strike the page to produce output on paper, instead, these printers use ink-jet, thermal-transfer, or laser technologies to produce hard copy. These printer technologies are much quieter than impact print systems.

Ink-jet printer technology, as the name implies, produces output by spraying ink from tiny nozzles directly onto paper. The timing of each ink droplet ejection is controlled by the printer's electronics. The major attraction of ink-jet systems is their quiet operation. For example, laptops are often used with small, portable ink-jet systems involving assistive technology solutions for written communication in classroom situations (Church & Bender, 1989). Examples of commercial ink jet systems include Kodak's *Diconix 150 Plus,* Canon's *BJ-10e* and *130E,* Hewlett-Packard's *PaintJet* and *PaintJet XL,* and Howtek's *Pixelmaster.*

Thermal-transfer printers use heat to transfer ink to paper. Thermal printers produce both text and graphics by passing the heated print head over a special ribbon. The production of color text and graphics is one of the most practical applications for these printers. Using a multicolored wax ribbon, thermal printers can produce high-quality color print output very inexpensively. In addition, these printers offer high resolution printing (200–300 dots per inch). These printers usually require special wax ribbons and low-rag bond or polyester-based paper. Two examples of color thermal printers include Mitsubishi's *Thermal Color Printer* and NEC's *Colormate Printer.*

Laser printers are setting new standards for speed and quality of microcomputer printing solutions. Laser printers produce images on paper by directing a laser beam at a mirror which bounces the beam onto a light sensitive drum. The laser leaves a negatively charged image on the drum's surface to which positively charged toner powder will stick. As paper rolls over the drum, the toner is transferred to the paper. A heated roller system melts the toner to the paper to produce the finished page. Laser printers offer high resolution printing (300 dots per inch) and have speed ranges from 4 to 15 pages per minute. Examples of this laser technology include Apple's *LaserWriter II/NTX,* IBM's *4019,* Hewlett-Packard's *LaserJet II* and *LaserJet III,* Epson's *EPL-6000,* Panasonic's *KX-P4420,* and QMS's *PS 410* and *810* laser printers.

Speech Output

Another very popular output method available to assistive technologists is speech output. Computerized speech synthesis can offer individuals with disabilities a variety of alternatives for interacting and participating in home, school, work, and community settings. Individuals with impaired speech may use speech synthesis as a means of learning or improving articulation or voice skills. For nonspeaking individuals, speech synthesis can replace lost speech and provide an augmentative communication system for independence and self-expression (Church & Bender, 1989). Further, for computer users who are visually impaired or blind, speech synthesis can provide the keys to unlock text-based information that was previously difficult to view or simply unreadable. Speech output also has practical applications for special education populations with cognitive and language disabilities.

Three mainstream speech synthesis technologies are now being used successfully in assistive technology applications. These include: (1) text-to-speech synthesis, (2) digitized speech, and (3) linear predictive coding. These hardware and software systems interface with the personal computer using a variety of input methods, including, for example, expansion slots, serial ports, and software drivers. Each of the three speech technologies have clear advantages and limitations in different technology applications.

TEXT-TO-SPEECH SYNTHESIS. Text-to-speech synthesis currently is the most popular technology in speech communications aids, educational software, and related rehabilitation environments. The reason for its popularity is that the system does not store or contain speech units, such as words or sentences; instead, it defines and stores the phonemes or sounds of the English language as a set of mathematical rules and procedures. These compact algorithms account for the minimal memory requirements of text-to-speech synthesis. Each phoneme is stored separately as a mathematical variation of the formant frequencies of the sound. Formant frequencies for whole words can also be stored. Typically, text-to-speech systems include hundreds of such pronunciation rules to describe the English language.

Text-to-speech synthesis has two distinct advantages in assistive technology applications. First, because the system stores only pronunciation rules, not actual speech recordings, it is extremely compact, requiring minimal computer memory. In addition, because the system includes a comprehensive set of pronunciation codes, it has the potential to speak any word encountered. This makes text-to-speech synthesis very flexible.

The major limitation of text-to-speech synthesis relates to its sound quality. Robotic sounding voice output is common with the use of this speech approach and listeners may find it difficult to understand. Comprehension difficulties may put distinct limits on the applicability of this computerized speech.

Microcomputers produce text-to-speech synthesis with their own built-in hardware or with the addition of a speech synthesizer expansion board. A wide variety of speech peripherals are available for Apple and DOS personal computers. Examples include Street Electronics' *Echo 1000* (Tandy), *Echo IIb* (Apple II series), *Echo PC2* (IBM PC,XT), and *Echo MC* (IBM PS/2s). Other popular text-to-speech synthesizers include AICOM Corporation's *Accent* series, Jostens Learning System's *Ufonic Voice System*, Votrax's *Votalker*, and Artic Technologies *SynPhonix*. These text-to-speech products generate speech through the use of mathematical models that analyze a word and translate it into the appropriate phonemes. After analyzing the phonemes, the hardware and software system generates sound and pitch codes so that the speech synthesizer can pronounce the word.

DIGITIZED SPEECH. Digitized speech is very different from text-to-speech approaches. Digitized speech does not use phoneme rules to speak. Instead, it stores a real person's actual words and sentences in the form of "digitized" sounds. These sounds are recorded by a peripheral device that converts sound input from a stereo system, an instrument, or a microphone into a form that the computer can process, store, and play back. This speech technique requires large amounts of RAM and storage space to sample and convert words and phrases into digitized speech.

To produce digitized speech a microcomputer system must include a peripheral device that is capable of recording and playing the speech. Examples of peripheral speech systems include Farallon Computing's *MacRecorder* (Apple Macintosh) and MDIdeas' *SuperSonic Digitizer* (Apple II series). In addition, some microcomputer systems provide built-in recording circuitry and a small microphone. Therefore, clients using Apple's *Macintosh LC, IISI* or Tandy's *1000 SL* and *TL* series microcomputers have direct access to digitized speech. Lastly, some newer dedicated speech aids are utilizing digitized speech technology. Prentke Romich's *Intro Talker*, Sentient System's *DynaVox*, and Zygo Industries' *Parrot* are a few examples of portable augmentative communication aids that incorporate digitized speech.

Digitized speech technology can produce very realistic sounding speech. Currently, the major reason for its limited use in assistive technology devices is that the technology is extremely memory-intensive. Digitizing hardware can record voices or sounds at sampling rates between 5 kHz and 44 kHz. For example, the 44 kHz rate provides the best sound quality, but sounds recorded at this rate use more memory and disk space. Speech-compression schemes, methods that allow voice and sounds to be compacted by 3:1 or higher ratios, require less memory and disk space, but they lack the fidelity of uncompressed voices or sounds. Even with compression techniques, the storage requirements of digitized speech can quickly exceed the capabilities of many microcomputer systems. However, as the price of memory decreases and the use of mass-storage devices become more prevalent, the use of digitized speech in assistive technology solutions will become more practical.

LINEAR PREDICTIVE CODING. The third approach to speech output, linear predictive coding (LPC), which many professionals refer to as custom-encoded speech, spans the gap between text-to-speech and digitized speech techniques. LPC speech technology utilizes a combination of speech digitizing and mathematical modeling to reconstruct and produce high-quality voice. The resulting blend of speech technologies greatly reduces memory and storage requirements for creating voice output.

To create LPC speech, microcomputers must have specialized digitizing hardware and a speech-synthesis chip. These systems usually are integrated with an add-on speech expansion board. The digitizing hardware records the real human speech and converts each word or phrase into digital data. In addition, LPC techniques compress the digital signal and break it down into small LPC units. Then, using support software and/or hardware, the LPC units are extracted and reconstructed using the speech-synthesis chip into an appropriate voice. The speech chip uses mathematical models of the human voice to reconstruct and simulate the original speech signal.

A variety of educational software publishers take advantage of LPC's minimal memory requirements and include custom-encoded words and phrases in their instructional software. LPC speech is commonly used in reading and language arts software. The speech produced by LPC is of better quality than text-to-speech techniques. However, it does not have the fidelity of digitized speech. Still, LPC software programs are limited to speaking only words that have been prerecorded and digitized for unique applications. Hence, the technology is not nearly as flexible as text-to-speech methods.

Microcomputer Storage

The last major hardware component of a microcomputer system is the storage device. These hardware components are used for both the retrieval (input) and storage (output) of information. Microcomputers utilize two very broad categories of storage systems: magnetic storage and optical storage.

Magnetic Storage

The disk drive is the most common magnetic storage device used with microcomputers. A **disk drive** is a peripheral device that holds a disk, retrieves information from it, and saves information on it. Disk drives provide storage for data, documents, and software programs that need to be kept for an extended period of time. Without disk drives, a computer's only storage medium is RAM, and the contents of RAM are volatile — all data is lost when the computer's power is turned off.

DISK DRIVES AND DISKETTES. The magnetic medium used to store information is called a **floppy disk** or **diskette** (see Figure 2–6). The diskette is a circular sheet of mylar that has a ferrous oxide coating capable of holding a magnetic charge. The diskette is covered in a plastic jacket to protect the surface from damage as a result of fingerprints, dust, smoke, liquids, or other contaminants. At the bottom of the protective jacket is an elongated elliptical opening that allows the disk drive to read and write magnetic data on the disk. Floppy diskettes come in a number of different sizes, the 5¼-inch and 3½-inch size formats being the most common sizes.

Before the computer can use a diskette, the floppy disk must first be **formatted** or **initialized**. This process prepares the diskette's magnetic surface for data storage by dividing it into concentric circles (one within the other) called **tracks**. The formatting process then subdivides all tracks into **sectors** (see Figure 2–6). Tracks and sectors are the storage bins for data bits. The computer's disk operating system gives each track and sector a unique number, much like mailbox addresses. These numbers help identify specific locations on the diskette, so that the computer can find the proper information requested by the software program.

As with most other microcomputer components, a number of different standards exist for disk drive systems. For example, Apple II series computers use 140K and 800K disk drives; Apple Macintosh computers use 400K, 800K, and 1.4MB disk drives; and MS-DOS personal computers use 360K, 720K, 1.2MB, and 1.44MB systems. However, market trends are moving toward the higher capacity 3½-inch diskettes. These include double-sided, double-density (2DD) diskettes that can store 720K of data and double-sided, high-density (2HD) diskettes that can store 1.44MB of data, and new 2.8 MB diskettes.

HARD-DISK DRIVES. The hard disk is the second member of the magnetic storage family. Hard-disk drives are available in various sizes and are configured as fixed disk or removable cartridge systems. Fixed hard disks are self-contained units that have permanently mounted disks inside the disk drive unit. Removable hard disks allow the user to insert and remove the disk from the drive system. In general, hard disks have three distinct features that separate them from floppy disk drive technology.

First, hard-disk drives have all their magnetic media permanently encased in a hard disk unit. No floppy diskettes are used in the disk unit. The actual hard disk is made of an inflexible aluminum substance instead of mylar. In addition, the hard-disk drive contains a stack of one or more rigid disk platters that magnetically store information.

The storage capacity of the hard-disk drive is another feature that makes hard disks unique. Hard-disk drives can store millions of bytes

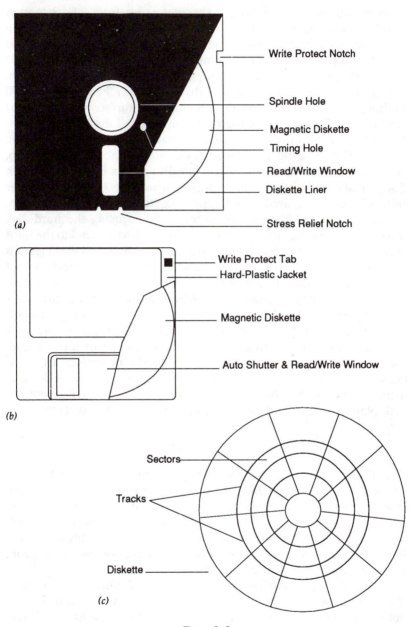

Figure 2–6
Magnetic storage media: floppy diskettes. (a) 5¼-inch floppy disk. (b) 3½-inch floppy disk.
(c) Diskette formatting scheme.

of information. Typical storage capacities range from 20MB to over 300MB of data. In relation to floppy disks, hard disks, depending on their storage capacity, can hold the equivalent of twenty to over several hundred floppy disks' worth of information.

Finally, hard-disk drives incorporate high speed disk operation. The read-write head of a hard-disk drive floats at a height of about 50 millionths of an inch above the rotating disk surface retrieving and storing data. Because of the high rotation speed of the hard disk platter, information on the disk is almost instantly accessible. In contrast, a floppy-disk drive must wait several seconds for the drive to light up, start spinning and attain the right speed to access information on a floppy diskette. The hard disk spins at nearly 3,600 revolutions per minute (rpm) compared to a floppy diskette that spins at 350 rpm.

Some precautions must be observed when using the hard-disk drive. Because of the close proximity of the read-write head to the hard disk surface during operation, contaminants such as dust particles can cause the read-write head to bounce and come into physical contact with the disk platter, resulting in "head crash." These accidents can cause severe damage to the read-write head or the hard-disk drive, destroying the data stored there. The sealed environments of fixed hard-disk drives almost eliminate the problem, but it can occur with removable hard disk cartridges. In addition, sudden or harsh movements to the hard-disk drive during read-write operations can also cause head crashes. Hard-disk users can "park" the read-write head to avoid head crashes. This method withdraws the read-write from the disk platter surface and parks it away from the disk surface.

Optical Storage

Recent advances in storage technology have provided microcomputer users with new storage options. Optical storage technology is emerging as a new alternative to more traditional floppy disk and hard disk systems. Optical technology utilizes precisely focused beams of light, called "lasers," to read and write data. This technology has the potential to give users access to huge volumes of encyclopedia information, video, text, graphics, voice, and music.

Optical storage devices have a number of inherent advantages over traditional magnetic storage systems. First, optical storage technology can hold considerable more data than floppy or hard disk systems. For example, optical systems can hold approximately 600 MB of information. This is equivalent to a 10-million-word or 20-volume encyclopedia. In addition, the disk surface of optical media is protected from physical damage, as from finger prints, spilled liquids, magnetic fields, and scratches, by a transparent plastic coating. Finally, optical storage is a better distribution media than magnetic media because optical disks can be stamped out in mass, whereas magnetic disks must be duplicated one by one, byte by byte electronically. Optical systems fall into three categories, each having distinct applications with microcomputers. These categories are: CD-ROM, WORM, and Erasable Optical Storage.

COMPACT DISK READ-ONLY MEMORY (CD-ROM). The CD-ROM is fast becoming the most common type of optical medium. These 4.72-inch silvery disks are physically identical to the popular audio compact disk (CD). Unlike the many tracks on a floppy or hard disk, a CD carries a single spiral track that starts at the center of the disk and winds its way outward. Much like the grooves on old phonograph records, the turns in the spiral are so densely packed together that over 15,500 can fit in 1 inch. The spiral track is located on the disk's surface, called the "land." The data on a CD-ROM is organized on the single track as billions of microscopic grooves. These grooves, which are sunk into the CD-ROM's land, are called "pits." These pits represent individual data bits. A laser shoots a finely focused beam of light at the pits. The light beam, which is then reflected off the pits, is read by the optical drive and converted into data the computer can use.

The major drawback of current CD-ROM applications involves its slow rate of data access. The speed of data retrieval is much slower on CD-ROMs than on more conventional hard-disk drive systems. In addition, CD-ROMs are a "read-only" optical medium. As such, microcomputer users cannot save data to CD-ROMs, they may only retrieve information. As a result, most current applications for CD-ROMs involve distribution of software containing libraries of music, sounds, graphics, and encyclopedia reference material. Examples include Denon's *DRD-253,* Toshiba *XM-3201,* CD-Technology's *Porta Drive,* and NEC's *Intersect CDR-35.*

Grolier Electronic Publishing's *New Grolier Electronic Encyclopedia* is a CD-ROM that includes 33,000 articles; 2,000 color images; 250 color maps; and a broad range of audio selections, including speeches, music, and sounds. All information is searched through a boolean search method. Britannica Software, Inc.'s *Compton's Multimedia Encyclopedia* CD-ROM features 15,000 color pictures, maps, graphics, and digitized voice in its reference work. *Compton's Multimedia Encyclopedia* also provides an on-line dictionary, audio glossary, and search and retrieval methods. Discis Knowledge Research's *Discis Books* is an interactive series of children's books. The series includes high-quality illustrations, sound effects, digitized voice, and music. The stories can be read aloud by the computer; children can request pronunciations, explanations, and syllabication of words and objects. Trace Center's

Hyper-ABLEDATA-Plus is a CD-ROM database of rehabilitation and assistive technology products. The CD-ROM includes information on more than 16,000 individual products from over 2,200 companies. The system allows users to search by company name, product name, and product type.

WRITE ONCE READ MOSTLY (WORM). WORM technology is a second form of optical storage. Like CD-ROM, it stores information in the form of pits on the disk's land. However, unlike CD-ROMs, the WORM drive is capable of writing and reading information. Because the creation of pits on the disk surface is irreversible, written data pits cannot be altered, although they can be read as often as desired.

Some advantages of WORM technology are its ability to write and read information to the disk, combined with its large storage capacity. In addition, WORM technology does not suffer the same inherent speed problems in accessing data as CD-ROM recording schemes. The WORM drive uses the same concentric tracks as the more traditional magnetic storage media. A laser reads and writes information to and from tracks and sectors on the disk.

Unfortunately, WORM storage systems are considerably less standardized than the CD-ROM class of optical storage devices. There are no recognized file format standards for storing data on WORM disks. As a result, there are many compatibility problems among different vendor products. In addition, because data can be written on disks only once, they are not a practical storage solution for daily personal computer use. The most common applications of WORM are high-level data security applications and large document archiving activities. Examples include the Panasonic *WORM,* Mitsubishi *WORM,* and Pioneer's *LaserMemory DE-U7001* systems.

ERASABLE OPTICAL STORAGE. The third class of optical storage devices are erasable optical storage systems. This storage medium can read and write data as often as magnetic disks. These drives use erasable, removable 5¼-inch disks that store approximately 300 megabytes of data per side. The erasable disk looks like an audio CD and is packaged in a hard plastic cartridge, with a metal door and write protect switch. Unlike CD-ROM disks, which you can remove from the drive case, erasable optical disks always stay in the case, even when inserted into the drive.

The storage medium is patterned after magnetic storage formats, utilizing tracks and sectors that hold millions of pits. A read-write laser is used to store and retrieve data on the polycarbonate and metallic-film disks. The data transfer rate and file retrieval of erasable optical systems are not as fast as hard disk systems but further refinements are improving performance.

The major advantages of erasable technology include:

1. The ability to read and write innumerable times;
2. The disks are very portable and durable;
3. Erasable disks have very large storage capacities (300–600 MB).
4. Erasable opticals do not suffer from head crashes because the read-write head is far from the disk surface.

Examples include Ricoh's *9GB,* Pinnacle's *REO-600,* Microtech's *OR650,* and Quantum's *Quantum 80* drive systems.

SUMMARY

Microcomputers can be configured as desktop, portable, laptop, notebook, or tablet systems. However, microcomputers all contain the same basic system components: (1) processing, (2) input, (3) output, and (4) storage. Microcomputer processing includes the CPU, memory, and I/O interface. Microcomputers also have different input and output configurations. Microcomputers can employ LCD displays, CRTs, speech synthesizers, floppy and hard disks, optical storage, and printers, to name a few. The reader should realize, however, that this chapter provides a general overview of microcomputer technology. If more background information on any of the subjects that follow is required, some of the more specific books listed in the references at the end of each chapter may be consulted. Chapter 5 builds on the concepts presented in this chapter, exploring practical methods and procedures for implementing assistive technology aids with microcomputers.

REFERENCES

Church, G., & Bender, M. (1989). *Teaching with computers: A curriculum for special Educators.* Boston: College-Hill Press.

3

Positioning and Power Mobility

■ Susan E. Harrymann, MS, RPT ■
■ Lana R. Warren, MS, OTR/L, FAOTA ■

The most sophisticated technology in the world is useless if it is not accessible to the person in need of assistance. Although many factors need to be considered to ensure that recommendations for a technology system are realistic, this chapter specifically addresses an individual's ability to directly access the system from the viewpoint of physical ability.

The initial section of this chapter will review common problems that may interfere with the maintenance of a stable sitting position. Specific postural problems and potential solutions related to positioning in a wheelchair and accessing assistive technology will be discussed. This section of the chapter is arranged in the sequence that positioning problems are usually assessed. The latter section of this chapter will review indications for power mobility, mobility bases, methods of control, and compatibility of technology systems.

Individuals in need of assistive technology usually are severely physically handicapped and have complex physical needs. They frequently have difficulty maintaining a stable sitting posture and may have problems with directed voluntary movement. Orthopedic problems, including joint limitations, muscle shortening, and musculoskeletal deformities, are numerous. Individuals with upper motor neuron lesions, such as cerebral palsy or head injury, have significant alteration in muscle tone; whereas individuals with muscular or lower motor neuron lesions, such as Duchenne's muscular dystrophy, spinal muscular atrophy, osteogenesis imperfecta, or arthrogryposis, may have significant muscular weakness. Either of these neuromotor problems affect proximal (neck, trunk, pelvic girdle, shoulder girdle) musculature, which leads to difficulty with maintenance of postural alignment. In individuals with cerebral palsy, the presence of retained primitive reflexes may cause stereotyped postures and movements. These reflexes may also influence body position and muscle tone depending upon the client's head position in space. Individuals with multiple physical problems may also have other medical problems such as frequent changes in medications, seizure disorders, problems with skin integrity, intercurrent illnesses, and decreased endurance.

The multitude of problems experienced by individuals in need of assistive technology points to the need for comprehensive and detailed assessment methods. Decisions related to choice of a seating and mobility system should be made by professionals with expertise in positioning individuals with significant neuromotor and musculoskeletal disorders in conjunction with the individual and his or her caregivers.

POSTURAL ASSESSMENT

Because the majority of human functions are executed in the seated position, it is important to provide each person with a secure and stable sitting position to maximize function. Important components of normal stable seating include an erect spine over a pelvis perpendicular to the support surface, a chin tuck with neck elongation, and the ability to maintain the arms free and forward for function (see Figure 3-1). As many candidates for assistive technology are unable to independently achieve or maintain such a posture, it is mandatory that a seating assessment be an initial and integral part of the evaluation and selection process. An optimal seating system should provide sufficient support, stability, and comfort to promote functional improvement and optimize motor control. The system should decrease abnormal muscle tone and movement while facilitating components of more normal movement patterns and maximizing upper limb function.

The purpose of a technology assessment is to attain varied functional goals in a system that will allow for personal and system changes in the future. To best address postural needs related to these important goals, consideration should be given to consultations with

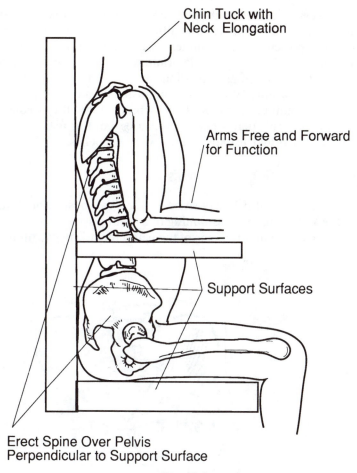

Chin Tuck with
Neck Elongation

Arms Free and Forward
for Function

Support Surfaces

Erect Spine Over Pelvis
Perpendicular to Support Surface

Figure 3–1
Components of normal seating.

orthopedics for present and potential musculoskeletal problems;
therapists for functional assessments; orthotists for deformity management; durable medical equipment specialists who may be able to customize standard wheelchair components for individuals; biomedical
and rehabilitation engineers; and perhaps a specialist in ergonomics
to assess efficient use of energy for specified tasks.

Adjustments and refittings to a seating system that is not optimal
consume considerable time and finances. Every effort should be made
to address all the needs of the individual and team prior to ordering
specific equipment. Assessment of problems should be addressed in a
variety of situations using a problem-solving approach. Individuals

must be assessed in an upright position, because the effect of gravity on muscle tone and posture is quite different from that in a recumbent position. The presence of deformities must be recognized. Fixed musculoskeletal (muscle and bone) deformities cannot be corrected with chair adaptations, although adaptations may have the potential to prevent further deformity. When assessing distal (hand, foot) problems and potential solutions, it should be remembered that they frequently have proximal (trunk, pelvis, shoulder) causes. For this reason, assessment of an individual usually begins with the pelvis.

Pelvis

Maintaining a neutral pelvic position is often the most difficult task, yet it is the key to optimal positioning in a seating system (see Figures 3–2 and 3–3). Common problems of the pelvis include pelvic tilt in the

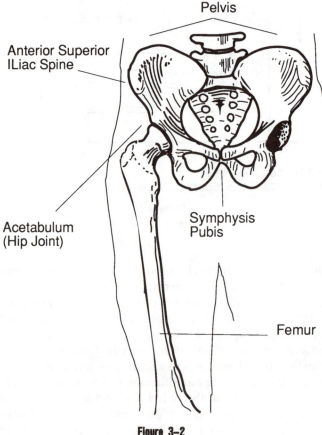

Figure 3–2
Pelvis.

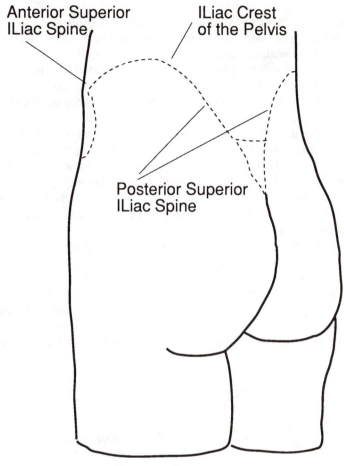

Figure 3-3
Surface features of the pelvis.

anterior/posterior plane, pelvic obliquity in which one side of the pelvis is higher than the other, pelvic rotation in which one side of the pelvis is more forward than the other, increased extensor tone, and asymmetrical deformities from contractures around the hips and/or trunk.

When the person is placed in a seated position with the hips flexed to 90 degrees, a frequent occurrence is posterior pelvic tilt in which the pelvis deviates so that the posterior superior iliac spine moves posterior and inferior (see Figure 3-4). Causes of this deviation include decreased tone, increased extensor tone, and shortening of the hamstrings. If an individual's hamstrings are short, this problem must be addressed to allow seating of the pelvis in a neutral position prior to

determining a means of stabilizing the pelvis. If surgical hamstring release is not considered, shortening the seat depth to allow the knees to
flex under the seat, or adjusting the foot rests to allow increased knee
flexion will potentially allow the pelvis to be seated in a neutral position. Pelvic obliquity or rotation often is found in conjunction with
scoliosis (spine curvature) or hip dislocation. If there are fixed deformities, the seating system must be adapted to the deformity, most often
through the use of a chair insert molded to the individual.

Once the pelvis is seated in neutral, or in the optimal position for
a specific individual, a stabilizing system must be chosen to maintain
the position. Pelvic stabilizers include seat belts, lap belts, pelvic
straps, and subASIS bars, which may or may not be used in combination with anterior rolls or wedges on the chair, contoured seats, or
biangular backs.

A seat belt is the simplest means of stabilizing the pelvis and may
be effective if the individual has a posterior-pelvic tilt without obliquity or rotation and does not have significant tone or movement disorder. The line of pull of the seat belt should be in a posterior inferior
direction, approximately 45 degrees, and inferior to the anterior
superior iliac spine (see Figure 3–5). If the line of pull is superior to the
anterior superior iliac spine, there is danger of increasing deformity of

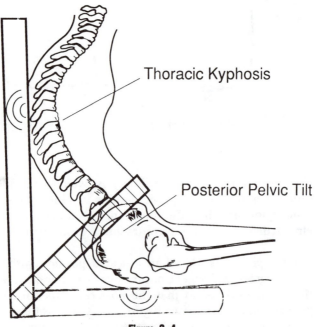

Figure 3–4
Posterior pelvic tilt.

the spine. The belt must be securely fastened with the back insert of the chair providing a support to counterbalance the posterior directed force of the belt. If the individual exhibits the tendency for hip extension while seated in the chair, a lap belt at a 90-degree angle across the thighs may be added to assist in maintaining the hips at 90 degrees and the pelvis in the neutral position (see Figure 3–5). A seat belt is not sufficient for control of pelvic rotation, because the webbing is flexible. In the presence of a significant tone or movement disorder a seat belt may cause skin discomfort if an individual repeatedly thrusts against the belt. In these situations an alternative means of stabilizing the pelvis should be considered.

Pelvic straps can provide effective stabilization of the pelvis in younger children. To provide optimal control, straps should be attached to the chair in a manner that provides a posterior-directed force, lateral to the midline and inferior to the anterior superior iliac spine. As with seat belts, pelvic straps must be fastened securely and used consistently to be effective.

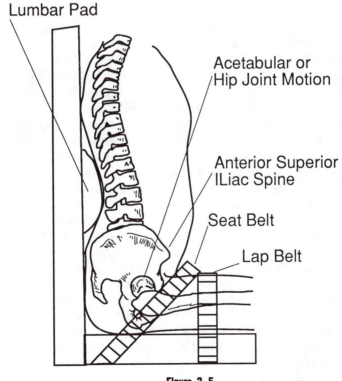

Lumbar Pad

Acetabular or Hip Joint Motion

Anterior Superior ILiac Spine

Seat Belt

Lap Belt

Figure 3–5
Seat or lap belt.

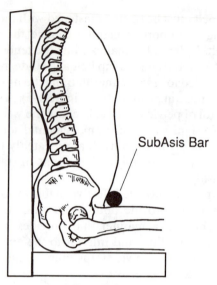

SubAsis Bar

Figure 3-6
SubASIS bar.

A subASIS bar is designed to be used with individuals who need pelvic control in an anterior/posterior plane as well as control of pelvic rotation (see Figure 3-6). The subASIS bar is a closely fitting padded aluminum bar attached to lateral seat brackets of a positioning system, and is usually used in combination with a biangular back. The goals for use of a subASIS bar include reducing posterior pelvic tilt, maintaining pelvic stability in the presence of increased extensor tone, preventing pelvic rotation, and providing consistent objective positioning by varied caregivers. The subASIS bar should be attached to the chair so that it fits in the area of the femoral triangle, an anatomical area bordered by the sartorius muscle, the inguinal ligament, and the adductor tendon. Because the adductor tendon is relaxed in a seated position, the femoral triangle is a viable area to provide force. The subASIS bar must fit snugly and be used with a well-designed, firmly padded seating system. The pelvis should be perpendicular to the seating surface and parallel to the back surface. Hip flexion to 90 degrees and pelvic tilt to neutral is desirable, but some success may be experienced in moderately fixed deformities using an asymmetrically attached subASIS bar. Potential problems which may preclude use of the subASIS bar include deformities that decrease the area of the femoral triangle, insufficient clearance in small children, and diaper distribution in incontinent persons. In climates requiring heavy outdoor clothing there may not be sufficient space for the bar, and an alternative seat

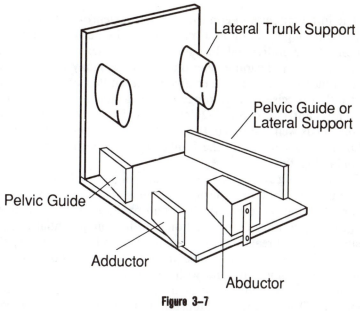

Figure 3–7
Chair adaptations.

belt should be provided (Margolis, Jones, & Brown, 1985; Margolis & Wengert, 1988).

In some individuals, due to asymmetrical muscle tone, the pelvis will tend to shift laterally in the chair, either immediately when placed in the chair or over a period of time. To correct the lateral shift and maintain the pelvis midline in relation to the edges of the chair, lateral supports or guides may be built into the insert or attached to the armrests (see Figure 3–7).

Hips

Once decisions are made regarding the optimal position of the pelvis, problems of the lower extremities can be addressed. Common concerns include increased extensor tone, limited range of passive movement, the presence of involuntary movement, asymmetry of the hip musculature, and fixed musculoskeletal deformity, such as hip dislocation. The presence of increased extensor tone at the hips is a frequent finding and may be intermittent or constant, symmetrical or with a rotation component. Intermittent symmetrical thrusting is usually accompanied by minimal deformity whereas a rotation component, either intermittent or constant, usually is accompanied by or leads to fixed musculoskeletal deformity of the spine and/or hips.

The initial attempt to control increased extensor tone at the hips should be through seating and maintaining the pelvis in an optimal position. If the individual has adequate hip flexion, wedging the seat to provide hip flexion greater than 90 degrees may also be considered as a means of decreasing extensor tone. In this situation it is imperative that precise passive range of hip flexion at the acetabulum (actual hip joint) (see Figure 3–2) be measured, one extremity at a time, with the pelvis well stabilized. If the pelvis is not stabilized, flexion at the lumbosacral joint or in the lumbar spine may first appear to be acetabular hip flexion.

In any seating system, the seat-to-back angle should allow for any limitation of acetabular hip flexion. Attempts to place an individual in a chair requiring more hip flexion than available will result in the pelvis rotating to a posterior position, and has the potential to cause pressure and skin breakdown over the bony prominences of the pelvis and spine. With the pelvis seated in a posterior tilt, compensatory kyphosis of the spine will occur with a resultant decrease in head control and upper extremity control against gravity (see Figure 3–4). Nwaobi (1987) and Nwaobi, Hobson, and Taylor (1988) have compared the mechanical hip flexion angle or seat-to-back angle of the seating system to the anatomical hip flexion angle which is the angle of the vertical plane of the pelvis to the long axis of the femur. This comparison reveals that these angles are not equal in most seating positions, with the anatomical hip flexion angle larger than the mechanical hip flexion angle when the seat-to-back seating system angle is 90 degrees or more.

Problems with increased, decreased, or asymmetrical hip abduction are common in individuals who need assistive technology. Before attempting to stabilize the hips in a symmetrical neutral position, it is necessary to determine that sufficient passive range of hip movement is available when the pelvis is maintained in optimal alignment. An abduction wedge or pommel is one option to maintain the hips in a neutral or abducted position (see Figure 3–7). The wedge should extend from between the knees approximately one-third of the way up the thigh and be well-padded. The abduction wedge must be used in combination with a pelvic stabilizer. The wedge itself should be viewed only as a means of maintaining hip abduction and not as a means of stabilizing the pelvis. Attempts at placing the wedge further up the medial thigh may result in weight bearing through the groin or at the symphysis pubis, neither of which is appropriate (see Figure 3–2). Although this may prevent the individual from sliding forward in the chair, it does not prevent a posterior pelvic tilt nor can it control problems with pelvic rotation.

If the decision is made to use an abduction wedge, a system must be devised for secure attachment and the ability to remove the wedge during transfers to and from the chair. The wedge is most functional when attached with a system that allows, it to be flipped under the chair. A wedge that remains attached to the chair reduces opportunities for misplacement or loss. The means of activating removal and repositioning must be assessed with a view toward client and caregiver accessibility.

For individuals presenting with the hips in significant abduction/external rotation, lateral thigh supports to maintain hip adduction may be added to the chair (see Figure 3–7). These supports must be firmly attached to the seat insert or armrests to provide adequate support and prevent loss or misplacement of loose pieces. Transfers to and from the chair will be facilitated if the supports are attached to the armrest rather than seat, but such an attachment will require the armrests to be removed in order to fold the chair.

Individuals presenting with tonic asymmetry at the hips may be supplied with a combination of medial and lateral thigh supports to maintain optimal position of the lower extremities. Again, in this situation, it is necessary to be sure that passive range of hip motion allows optimal positioning of the pelvis prior to making the final decision to attempt symmetrical positioning of the hips.

In the presence of fixed musculoskeletal deformity at the hips, the best decision for optimal seating may be a custom-molded contour seating system which will allow maximum contact with body surface area. This system, which is designed for a specific individual by making a mold of the trunk and pelvis, increases postural stability and decreases potential skin integrity problems from pressure (see Figure 3–8).

Knees

Problems at the knee usually center around increased muscle tone, muscle shortening, and limitations in range of motion of the joint. Knee extension problems frequently are only one part of a more general tonic extensor pattern and may be best addressed through optimizing the position of the pelvis and hips, as previously discussed. If tonic knee extension is intermittent and relatively mild, a distal extremity strapping system may be sufficient to assist with lower extremity control and prevent injury. However, distal straps have the potential to cause injury in the presence of significant tone or movement disorders. If there is a fixed knee extension deformity that does not allow knee flexion to 90 degrees, total support to the lower leg, compatible with the limited range, must be provided by the seating system (see Figure 3–9).

Individuals who need assistive technology frequently present with involvement of the hamstring muscles, resulting in muscle short-

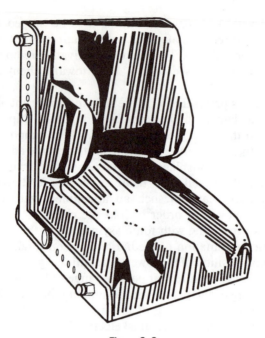

Figure 3–8
Custom-molded contour seating system

ening and limitation of extension at the knee joint. Because the hamstrings cross both the hip and knee joints, problems can occur with tonic hip extension, limited hip flexion, tonic knee flexion, and limited knee extension. In turn, tonic hip extension will result in posterior pelvic tilt.

For many of the problems at the hip and pelvis, the methods previously discussed will assist in alleviating the problem. If hip flexion is limited due to hamstring shortening, providing the option to allow increased knee flexion in the chair has the potential to allow increased hip flexion. If passive range of knee extension does not allow the lower leg to rest comfortably on the leg and foot rests, it may be necessary to adjust the angle of the leg rest to the chair to allow 90 degrees or more of knee flexion to preserve optimal position of the pelvis and prevent skin breakdown behind the knees (see Figure 3–10).

Feet

Increased extensor tone at the ankles, involuntary movements of the feet and ankles, or fixed musculoskeletal deformity of the feet may re-

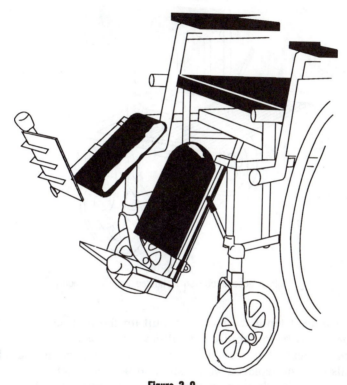

Figure 3–9
Wheelchair accommodation to limited right knee flexion.

quire adaptations to the foot support of the chair. Heel loops, toe
straps, ankle straps at a 45-degree angle, or figure-eight straps may be
sufficient to stabilize the feet and can at least be used as a starting
point if significant tone or deformity is present. In the presence of
marked extensor tone of the lower extremities, 45-degree ankle straps
in conjunction with a slightly dorsiflexed position of the foot may shift
the weight-bearing position toward the heel and assist in reducing extensor tone. If there are fixed plantar flexion contractures, the footplate
should be angled to accommodate the position of the foot. If involun-

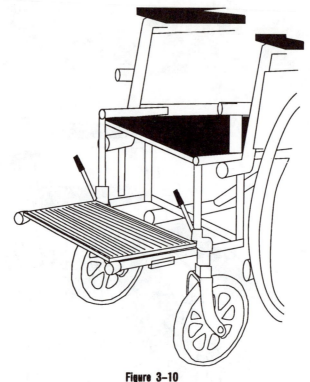

Figure 3–10
Footrest accommodation to limited knee extension.

tary movement tends to repeatedly pull up the foot pedals, the best approach may be to stabilize the pull-up mechanism and use only the swing-away feature as needed for transfers to and from the chair. Foot rests also can be replaced with a single flip-up footplate. In the presence of severe involuntary movement or fixed musculoskeletal deformity, it may be necessary to replace the footrest mechanism of the wheelchair with a well-padded, cradle-type support for the lower legs and feet.

Spine and Trunk

The ability to maintain an erect trunk is essential to optimal function in a seated position. Once the position of the pelvis is optimized and stabilized, problems of trunk control can be assessed. Abnormalities of muscle tone may have a profound effect on a person's ability to maintain trunk extension. Decreased muscle tone or weakness of trunk musculature will result primarily in collapse of the trunk and spine into gravity. Individuals with hypotonia may attempt to compromise with voluntary stabilization patterns of shoulder elevation and neck fixation, which in turn further limit functional use of the head and upper extremities. Increased muscle tone may be in the symmetrical distribution of extension or flexion or, more frequently, result in an asymmetrical involvement of trunk musculature with accompanying rotation deformities of the trunk. Variable or fluctuating muscle tone, usually accompanied by involuntary movement, produces instability and an inability to control the trunk.

The back of the chair insert that provides posterior support to the trunk may be flat or contoured, depending upon the needs of the individual. The insert may be adjustable in height, hinged to the seat, or a rigid piece attached to the seat with brackets. Anterior and lateral trunk supports as well as a system to provide forward control are often necessary. All attempts should be made to provide the necessary control with the least possible bulk.

In general, the natural alignment of the spine with lumbar and cervical lordoses, sacral and thoracic kyphoses (see Figure 3–11), should be preserved or restored, if possible, for optimal function. A lumbar pad or roll (see Figure 3–5) is often considered as a means of inducing a lumbar curve. In the presence of decreased tone or weakness, such an adaptation will maintain a lumbar and lower thoracic curve by locking the vertebral facet joints in some extension which provides increased stability. However, in the presence of increased tone, compensatory flexion of the thoracic spine and hips may be induced, thus compounding problems with maintaining the trunk against gravity.

Nwaobi (1987) feels that the natural alignment for the seated position may facilitate abnormal extensor patterns in clients who present with increased tone. Adjustment of the normal spine and pelvis in sitting includes psoas muscle relaxation, tightening of the hamstrings and hips extensors, and posterior tilting of the pelvis, thus reversing the lumbar lordosis. When the lumbar spine reverses to a more flexed alignment, the center of gravity moves anterior to the vertebral joints, and there is increased activity in the lumbar extensor muscles to maintain equilibrium in the spine. Therefore, the kyphotic position of the lumbar spine may not be the optimal seated position for clients with increased extensor tone. In contrast, the maintenance of lumbar lordosis will alter the line of gravity and decrease the extensor muscle activity needed to maintain equilibrium in the spine.

A two-section, or biangular back (see Figure 3–12) has been proposed by Wengert, Margolis, and Kolar (1987) to address the need to maintain an extended lumbar spine. The lower section of the biangular back is attached to the seating surface at a 75- to 85-degree angle, as

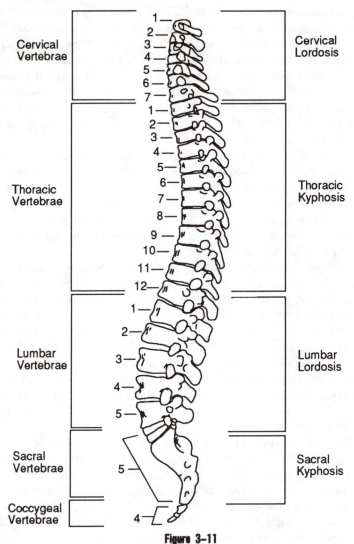

Cervical Vertebrae — 1, 2, 3, 4, 5, 6, 7 — Cervical Lordosis

Thoracic Vertebrae — 1, 2, 3, 4, 5, 6, 7, 8, 9, 10, 11, 12 — Thoracic Kyphosis

Lumbar Vertebrae — 1, 2, 3, 4, 5 — Lumbar Lordosis

Sacral Vertebrae — 5 — Sacral Kyphosis

Coccygeal Vertebrae — 4

Figure 3–11
Natural alignment of the spine.

allowed by passive range of hip flexion of the individual, and extends to the level of the posterior superior iliac spine (see Figure 3–3). The upper back is rigidly attached to the lower back at an angle that complements the seat-to-back angle plus 5 degrees. The incline of the upper section is such that the anterior/posterior position of the head is set just posterior to the midline of the pelvis. The seat belt or subASIS bar should be positioned inferior to the anterior superior iliac spine

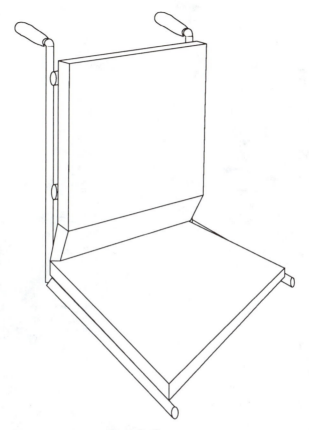

Figure 3–12
Wheelchair biangular back.

(see Figures 3–5 and 3–6) and exert a counterforce to the anterior directed force at the posterior superior iliac spine. Increased extensor tone is
thus decreased by putting the extensor muscles on stretch and decreasing the mechanical advantage of the hip extensors. Pathological hip
extensor patterns are interrupted, the lumbar spine is allowed to
extend, and the back extensors can be used to increase stability and
function. If trunk extension is not sufficient, a posterior force must be
provided to the upper thoracic spine in the form of anterior trunk support or shoulder stabilizers (see Figure 3–13).

Kyphosis of the spine is a frequent finding. A flexible kyphosis
may be compensatory for a posterior pelvic tilt (see Figure 3–4), a
result of flexing into gravity in the presence of low muscle tone or
weakness, or due to the pull of increased flexor tone in individuals

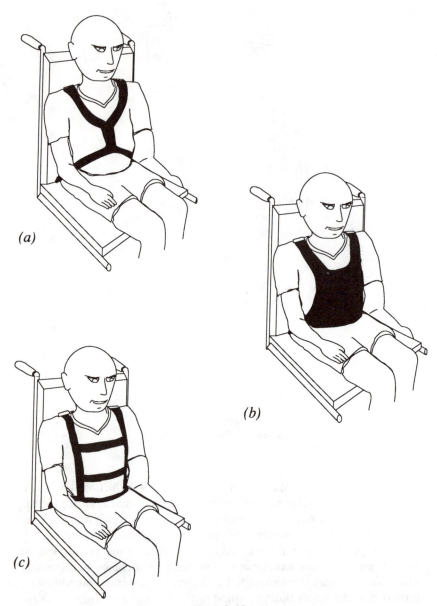

Figure 3–13
Anterior trunk supports. (a) Butterfly support. (b) Vest plate support. (c) H-strap support.

with increased tone. A kyphosis that can be reduced in recumbent positions, or with therapeutic handling, cannot necessarily be reduced in a seated position against gravity. This must be considered when addressing trunk alignment for function. Specific molding of the back insert may be required for optimal positioning.

To maintain midline position of the trunk, lateral trunk supports are usually necessary (see Figure 3-7). The supports should be firmly attached to the chair and fit close to the body to provide optimal positioning. When viewed from the side, lateral trunk supports should extend past the midline. If scoliosis, functional or fixed, is present (see Figure 3-14), a three-point system of lateral trunk support should be used for optimal support. One support should be attached on the convex side of the curve opposite the rib that is attached to the apical vertebra, which may be slightly below the observable apex of the curve. The remaining two lateral supports should be placed on the concave side of the curve, inferior and superior to the apical support, in a position to provide optimal alignment of the spine. If the spine has significant curvature, multiple curves, or a curve in the lumbar area, the use of lateral trunk supports alone will not be sufficient. In this situation, if surgery is not considered, the use of a spinal orthosis or contoured client-specific molded seat insert should be considered.

Candidates for adaptive technology commonly need anterior support to provide forward control in the seating system (see Figure 3-13). Butterfly, vest support, H-strap, or other supports frequently are used to

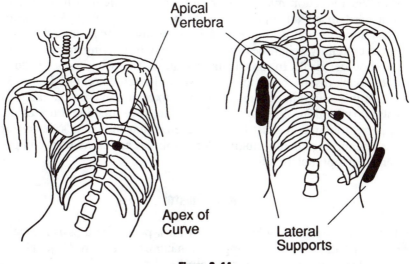

Figure 3-14
Scoliosis.

provide control over the sternal area. Anterior trunk supports that include shoulder straps should have a separate bottom strap for attachment and should not be attached to the seat belt. Attempts to use the seat belt for this attachment result in either the seat belt or shoulder straps not being firmly secured. This compromises the seating system and function of the individual. If the client does not need anterior support for forward control, the use of a horizontal strap at the level of the xiphoid process should be considered as a minimal support during transport.

Upper Extremities

The shoulder girdle/scapulae needs to be depressed downward to elongate the neck muscles and thus optimize head position. The attachment of shoulder straps to the anterior chest supports previously mentioned is commonly used to facilitate shoulder girdle depression. The straps should be inserted at shoulder level, or slightly below, and pull down behind the person. If the person tends to pull forward or roll the shoulders inward, there must be both backward pull and downward pressure to depress the shoulders. Padding to the shoulder straps and/or extra padding in the back support may be necessary for comfort.

Rigid shoulder supports may be used to hold the shoulder girdle back against the chair when there is a significant problem with shoulder protraction. Such rigid supports must be attached with care to preserve voluntary movement in flexion of the shoulder. A position of shoulder retraction may result from increased tone or a fixation pattern used in an attempt to increase proximal stability. An anterior chest support that optimizes the head position, or a tray added for upper extremity weight-bearing may assist in improving the position of the shoulder girdle. In some instances supports or wings may be added to the back insert or tray to control shoulder retraction (see Figure 3–15). In this situation care must be taken to maintain a usable range of voluntary motion. When attempting to improve functional use of the upper extremities it must be remembered that the client's desire for control and the client's motor control abilities are mandatory components for optimal function.

Head Control

The goal of optimizing head control for a person with assistive technology needs is to provide support to maximize function. Although the individual may be able to maintain head control with less support, decisions should be made to provide the support necessary to allow

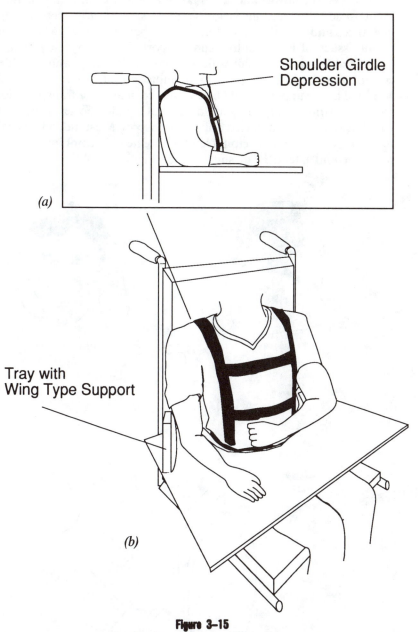

Figure 3–15

Upper extremity supports. (a) Shoulder straps should be inserted at shoulder level or slightly below and pulled down behind the person to support the shoulder girdle and optimize head position. (b) Tray with wing-type support.

easy access to controls and to enhance interaction with the environment. In addition, feeding, vision, comfort, skin integrity, personal appearance, and social interaction should be considered when evaluating issues of head control and support.

A stable seating system with optimal pelvic, trunk, and shoulder control must be in place prior to attempts to optimize head control. Minimal head support should be considered at least for transportation purposes. Minimal support should be a flat, padded posterior support, which is removable and used only for transport. Most individuals will need support to the suboccipital ledge of the head in combination with posterior and lateral head support (see Figure 3–16).

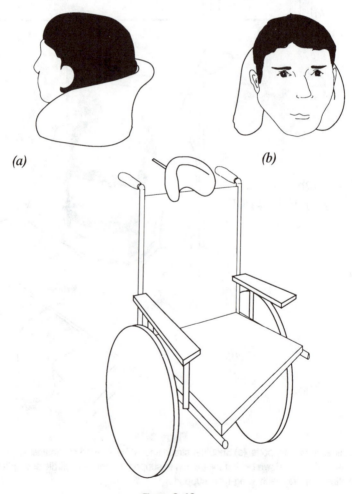

(a)   *(b)*

Figure 3–16
Combination head occipital support. (a) Side view. (b) Front view.

Hyperextension of the neck occurs frequently. Hyperextension is usually best controlled through optimal spinal alignment, anterior trunk support, shoulder girdle depression without protraction, and posterior occipital head support. Correction of uncontrolled forward flexion of the neck will require a slight recline in the chair to correct. As maintenance of a completely erect posture is tiring over time, this option should be considered for all individuals who need even minimal head support. If adequate head control cannot be provided with a combination of posterior and lateral support, consideration should be given to total cervical support, such as a neck collar, to maintain the head in an erect supported position. Because the head is frequently used to access assistive technology, consideration must be given to potential switch placement on the posterior or lateral aspects of the headrest, use of a head stick, and freedom to access other controls. To maintain adequate range of vision and voluntary movement, an occipital headrest with switches mounted separately on the back of the chair might be considered.

The option of providing a mechanism to tilt the chair in space 10 to 15 degrees is often considered to provide optimal orientation for individual activities (see Figure 3–17). This option allows the chair and insert to recline without changing the seat-to-back angle. For individuals who spend extended periods of time in their chairs, a tilt in space will shift the anatomical weight-bearing surface, decrease dependence on anterior supports, and has the potential to increase safety of the individual during transport by improving trunk stability and head control.

Figure 3–18 provides a sample wheelchair prescription form that is helpful in matching client measurements with vendor specifications for wheelchair systems.

POWER MOBILITY SYSTEMS AND ASSESSMENT

Once positioning needs have been determined, the next priority is choosing the type of mobility base that will be used on the seating system. The most basic question is whether to use a manual or power mobility system. Historically, power mobility has been provided primarily to adults, particularly when it enabled them to get to and from work independently. Exceptions to this were children with muscular dystrophy, spinal cord injuries, and birth defects. Use of power mobility systems by children has steadily increased over the past 10 years as has the quality and reliability of the technology. Today, it is increasingly common for preschool children to have power mobility systems.

The emerging philosophy regarding power mobility systems for young children is that children, as well as adults, have a right to be

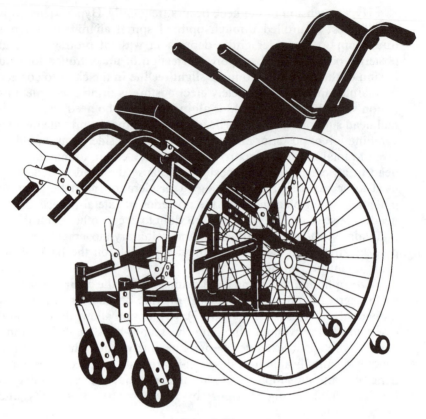

Figure 3–17
Wheelchair tilt in space feature.

mobile. Research has indicated that 18- to 24-month-old children with motor impairments who have normal or near-normal cognitive abilities can control a power mobility system with a joystick (Butler, Okamoto, & McKey, 1983). Using a power mobility system also has a positive impact on the child's self-esteem, motivation, and sense of control over the environment (Butler et al., 1983; Paulsson & Christofferson, 1984). Two of the most common "fears" of parents and therapists are: (1) the provision of a power mobility system will discourage ambulation; and (2) young children are not responsible enough to have a power mobility system. Research has not supported these fears (Paulsson & Christofferson, 1984). It should be noted, however, that the existing studies in this area have very small sample sizes.

If the assumption is made that all wheelchair users are candidates for power mobility, the following is a short list of the most common reasons for not considering power mobility:

Wheelchair Prescription

Name: _____   Date: _____

D.O.B.: _____   Therapist: _____

Parents: _____   Funding: MA #: _____

Address: _____   Exp.: _____

_____   Priv. Ins. _____

Phone: _____

Diagnosis: _____   _____

_____

Vendor Specifications: Actual Measurements:

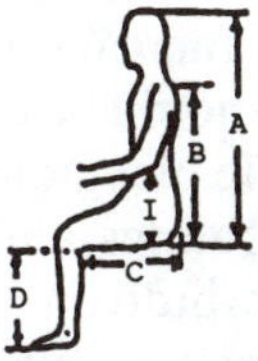

A____   F____   A____   F____

B____   G____   B____   G____

C____   HR____   C____   HR____

D____   HL____   D____   HL____

E____   I____   E____   I____

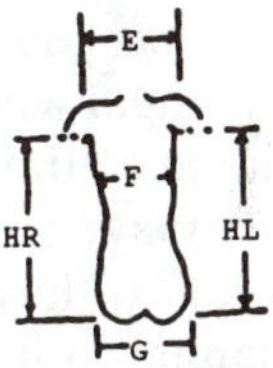

CHAIR SPECIFICATIONS:

Type of Chair: _____

Color: Frame: _____ Upholstery: _____

Solid Seat Insert: W_____ D(R)_____ D(L)_____

Solid Back Insert: W_____ H_____ Biangular: Angle_____ Height to Angle____

Armrests: _____   Lateral Supports:

Foot Supports: _____   Trunk: D_____ H_____

Foot Straps: _____   Tapered_____

Head Support: _____   Hip: W_____ H____

Shoulder Support: _____   Adductors: W_____ H____

Grommet Placement: 1st____ 2nd____ 3rd____   Abductor: Fixed____

Pelvic Stabilization: Flip Down_____

    Pelvic Straps:_____ SUB ASIS Bar_____   Size:_____

    Hip Belt:_____ Lap Belt:_____   Tray: Wood_____ Lexan_____

    Buckle:_____ Velcro_____ Velcro-D_____   Hardware_____

Power Specifications: Joystick R_____ L____   Edge____ Dowel____

                      Other:_____   Easel____ Wings_____

Other Specifications:_____

Figure 3–18
Wheelchair prescription form.

1. The individual is too young (under 20 months) or too limited cognitively to use power mobility.
2. A functional control mechanism cannot be found for the individual.
3. The individual's primary environments do not physically support power mobility.
4. The child and his or her family are unable to provide appropriate maintenance of the system.
5. The child and his or her family does not want power mobility.

Issues such as funding and bus transportation are not felt to be adequate reasons to avoid power mobility unless all resources are exhausted.

One other situation that needs to be discussed is the individual who has good upper extremity control and can functionally maneuver a manual wheelchair. Power mobility should be considered if the individual cannot keep up with peers on the playground during spontaneous play or cannot manage family outings and field trips, such as going to the zoo, park, or mall. Some individuals may require both manual and power wheelchair systems for different environments.

It is critical for an individual with severe motor disabilities or deformities to be positioned optimally before evaluating power mobility systems. Without optimal positioning, a means of control, or the most efficient means of control, may be overlooked. It is usually far wiser to postpone the assistive technology assessment until positioning can be optimized, rather than making an educated guess about what the individual might use. A relationship with a durable medical equipment specialist knowledgeable in power mobility can be invaluable. Ideally these specialists can provide modular seating and access systems that can be used in the evaluation process.

Types of Power Mobility Bases

For the purpose of this text, only power mobility bases will be addressed. Four major categories of power mobility systems will be discussed: scooters, modular bases, standard power chairs, and add-on systems. The emphasis of this chapter will be on the first three. In determining which system is most appropriate for a given individual, the following factors must be considered: degree of motor involvement; cognitive level, including perceptual deficits and problems with judgment; environments where the chair will be used; ability to transport the chair; and the individual's and family's commitment to using and maintaining a power system. Although funding is certainly a factor, this should not determine which is the most appropriate system. In general, an individual should be given the simplest system that best meets his or her needs.

Scooters/Three-Wheelers

In general scooters are the power mobility system of choice (see Figure 3–19). Scooters look less handicapping, are lighter in weight, often are narrower than a wheelchair, are easier to transport, and are considerably less expensive than other systems. However, although some

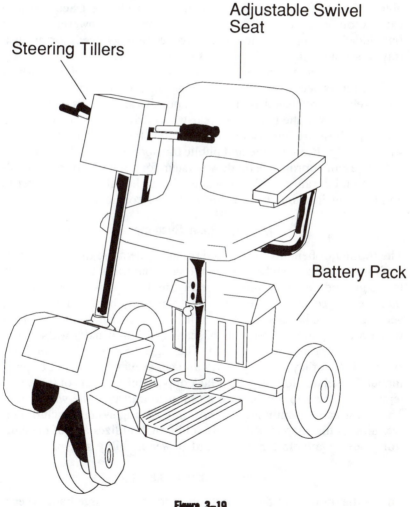

Adjustable Swivel Seat

Steering Tillers

Battery Pack

Figure 3–19
Scooter or three-wheeler

scooter seats can be adapted for users, they often cannot adequately support an individual who is severely physically handicapped. Scooters also require more arm and hand function to drive than a system with a joystick control. With scooters, the individual typically is required to squeeze a lever for forward or backward movement, while steering at the same time. Steering tillers can usually be ordered "bent" so that they can be positioned closer to the user. This is particularly useful for individuals with limited range in their shoulders or arms. Scooters have a lever under the seat that allows the user to swivel the seat for transfers and for positioning purposes. Seat heights are adjustable so that the floor of the scooter can serve as a footrest. Scooters also can accomodate crutch holders and baskets. However, for an individual who has significant assistive technology needs, or needs a tray, a scooter may not be the system of choice.

Several scooters come with the option of front- or rear-wheel drive. Front-wheel drive systems are lighter and traverse curbs more effectively. Rear-wheel drive is more expensive and results in a heavier system. However, the benefits of rear-wheel drive are more power and stability. These are important considerations for the outdoor user. It is wise to verify ahead of time that public transportation used by the individual has an appropriate tie-down system for a scooter. If the individual cannot be transported in a scooter, his or her ability to transfer to another seat in a bus or van must also be considered.

Modular Base Systems

The two major benefits of a modular base system are that a variety of seats and seat sizes can be used on the same base, and that they are low to the ground and very sturdy (see Figure 3–20) This allows them to manage rugged terrain well. The seat-flexibility benefit may not be very significant, because the typical life of a power mobility system is under 5 years, and a given type of seating system usually will accommodate at least 3 years of growth. The biggest drawback to modular systems is that they are very heavy and consequently difficult to push manually. Related to this is their lack of portability. Users of these systems need access to a vans with a ramps to transport the wheelchair. This chair can accommodate almost any seating system, including a reclining or tilt-in-space system. In addition, it utilizes any of the control modes available for a standard power mobility system.

Standard Base Systems

This is the traditional power mobility system with large back wheels and smaller front wheels (see Figure 3–21). This system would be used when the features of either of the other types of chairs are not appro-

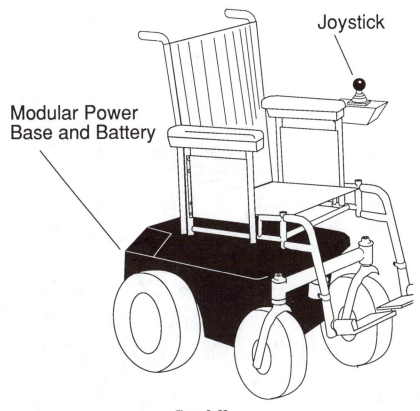

Figure 3–20
Power wheelchair with modular base.

priate. Any type of seating system or control mechanism can be accommodated in this chair. When considering tires, semi-pneumatic tires have the advantage of providing a smooth ride, yet are flat-free. This chair usually weighs less than a modular base but more than a scooter. Costs can range from $5,500 to $15,000, depending on the complexity of the control and positioning system. This system also can accommodate a reclining or tilt-in-space mechanism.

Add-On Power Systems

Several manufacturers make power systems that can be used to convert a manual wheelchair to a power wheelchair (see Figure 3–22). In general, these systems tend to be less durable and functional than a dedi-

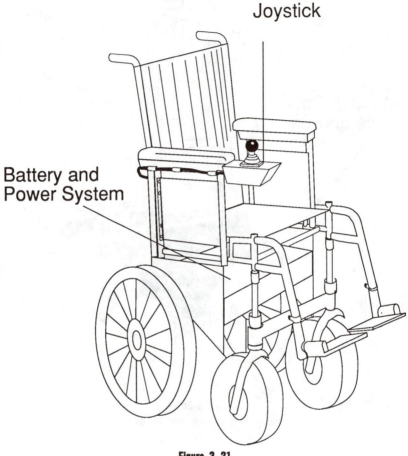

Joystick

Battery and Power System

Figure 3-21
Standard power wheelchair.

cated power mobility system, and they are not easily transported without a van. Add-on power may be considered for an individual who has limited funds, needs power mobility, and has a relatively new manual wheelchair.

Power Mobility Control Methods

For individuals who are power mobility candidates but cannot use a scooter, the next question to examine is method of control. There are

Add-On
Power Drive System

Add-On
Proportional Joystick

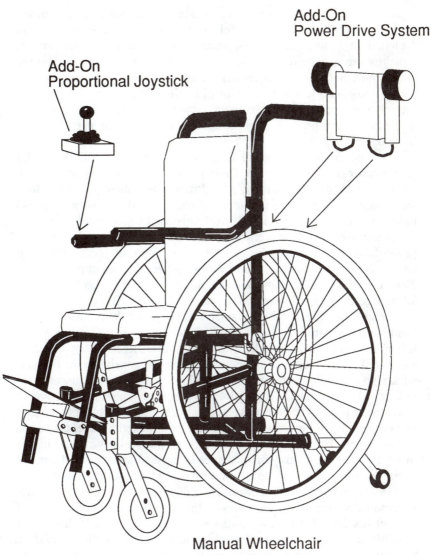

Manual Wheelchair

Figure 3–22
Add-on wheelchair system.

many different ways to control wheelchair movements. The selection of a power control method should be based on the individual's motor abilities. Body parts that offer accurate, reliable movements that are not overly effortful should be considered first. If the user does not have sufficient arm or hand control, a chin- or head-pointer controlled joystick typically is the next choice, as this still allows maximal directional control. If this is not possible, some type of single-switch system for left, right, forward, and reverse needs to be considered. Single switches typically are activated by hands, head, feet, or knees. The individual, family members, and teachers can be good resources for determining which body parts to assess for control methods. Body symmetry, involuntary movements, and overflow movement also must be considered in the evaluation process. In general, using existing asymmetries should be avoided.

A hand-controlled joystick is the method of choice for operating a power chair (see Figure 3–23). There are two types: proportional drive joysticks and microswitch joysticks. **Proportional drive** joysticks allow gradations in speed and angle of movement. **Microswitch** joysticks have simple on-off directional mechanisms. Proportional drive joysticks are used most frequently. Several adjustments can be made to proportional drive joysticks to customize them to meet individual user's needs. For example, a **short throw feature** requires approximately 50 percent less joystick movement than the standard proportional drive joystick setting. This is particularly useful for individuals with limited movement. Another method of customizing joysticks is called **tremor damping**. This feature assists individuals who have significant involuntary movement controlling the wheelchair more effectively by reducing unwanted short, jerky movements. The overall sensitivity of the joystick also can be adjusted to make a wheelchair less responsive to an individual with strong, forceful movements or more responsive to someone with weak motor movements. Further, the turning speed and reverse speed of a power wheelchair can be adjusted to meet the needs of the user. These control features are particularly valuable for individuals using a slow forward speed, because the standard control setting is often too slow to allow turns and reverse movement.

In general, a hand-controlled, variable speed joystick is the method of choice, because it goes in the direction the stick is pushed and allows for all directions and speeds of movement. If this is not possible, use of a remote joystick with a head pointer or chin usually is the next consideration. **Remote** joysticks are similar to regular joysticks, except that they are smaller and can be used in multiple locations on the wheelchair. Remote joysticks often are center-mounted and operated by head-stick or chin control. For individuals using a head-stick or chin for access, the standard joystick handle is replaced with a chin cup or hollow cylinder (see Figure 3–23). The individual can place his or her chin or the tip of the head-stick inside the cup or cylinder to control the joystick. If control with a head-stick is being assessed, it is critical that the head-stick be stable. This usually requires custom fabrication.

When the individual cannot use a joystick for control, microswitch

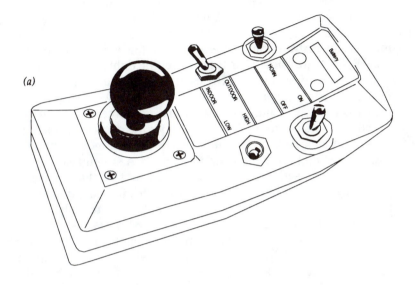

(a)

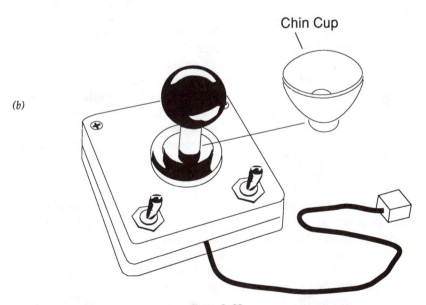

(b)

Chin Cup

Figure 3–23
Joystick systems. (a) Standard joystick. (b) Remote joystick with optional chin cup.

control schemes are available as power control options. Control efficiency is greatly reduced when an individual has to use a switch-activated control method that only goes in four directions or combinations thereof (see Figure 3–24). A chair typically will start to drift to the left or right after going approximately 10 feet due to uneven surfaces, unequal weight distribution in the chair, or the adjustment of the motors. As the chair starts to drift to the left or right, the user has to constantly correct direction, which results in continually going in a zigzag pattern. Some single-switch control systems allow two switches to be activated at once, allowing a 45-degree movement between the two directions. This is helpful, but it is still not nearly as functional as a full-range joystick. Any switch can be **latched**, which means hitting it once turns it on, and hitting it again turns it off. A switch also can be configured so that it activates for a specific time interval then turns off. This is particularly helpful for individuals with minimal strength or endurance. However, they must be able to quickly and reliably hit the switch to turn off the chair to avoid unexpected obstacles.

A wide variety of switch-activated methods can be used for power mobility control. One method is pneumatic switches, which require sip-and-puff breath controls to operate. These usually are used by individuals with no functional movement, typically high-level quadriplegics. For example, forward is a hard puff, reverse is a hard sip, left is a soft sip, and right is a soft puff. Proportional head control switches provide proportional speed and direction. The harder the switch is pushed, the greater the wheelchair's speed. Additional side-mounted switches control on-off and reverse-forward functions.

Another method of control is to use a switch interface box with multiple single switches (see Figure 3–24). The box may interface with a variety of single-switch systems: including: wafer boards (five directional circle switches in a single horizontal array), separate single switches, an array of head switches, and arm-slot switch controllers. Usually five switches are used; one for on-off and the other four for forward, backward, left, and right.

Single-switch scanning systems for power mobility control can be used as a last resort. Scanning systems are very slow, effortful, and frustrating to use. The individual has to scan for the desired direction, activate the switch, and then scan and activate the switch again to change directions. The previously mentioned "zigzag" directional problem is extremely frustrating with this system.

When evaluating various control methods it is wise to have an individual initially use a chair in a wide open space or relatively clear hallway with minimal environmental distractions. Begin by having them go forward. The individual should practice going relatively straight, starting, and stopping. Wide corners can then be assessed,

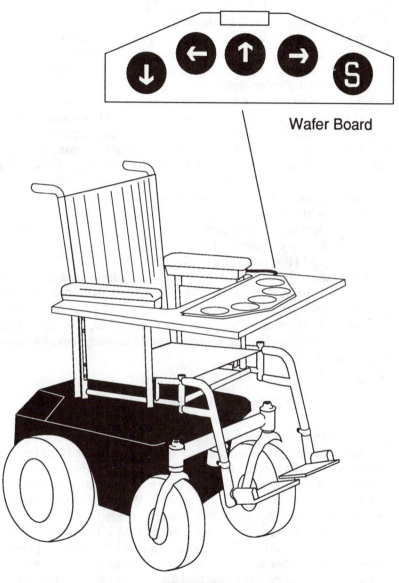

Wafer Board

Figure 3–24
Power wheelchair accessed by a wafer board.

followed by going through doorways, and navigating an obstacle course. Young children initially may delight in going in circles. In general, it is best to let them enjoy this movement sensation before embarking on a rigid training program. As the individual is mastering basic controls, introduce surprise variables into the environment, such as someone entering a hallway or a box on the floor. The individual must be able to respond quickly enough to avoid people or objects in his or her environment by stopping or changing direction. Some individuals who are easily visually or auditorily distracted may not be able to safely maneuver the wheelchair in typical daily environments.

Although some software packages are available for power wheelchair assessment and training (Taplin, 1989), actual experience in the wheelchair appears to be the most effective means of assessment and training. The potential user must be assessed not only in regard to physical control, but also in regard to judgment, visual-perceptual abilities, and safety. The latter three areas are definitely more accurately assessed while in an actual power mobility system.

For readers who are interested in wheelchair assessment software, Technical Resource Centre's *Wheelchair Control Evaluation Program* (Amiga 500 and IBM and compatibles) provides 2-D and 3-D simulations that allow the trainee to move through customized floor plans with walls, doors, and furniture. Other software-based evaluation systems for joystick training include R. J. Cooper and Associates' *Joystick Trainer* (Apple II series), Computability, Inc.'s *Joystick Mastery* (Apple II series), and Technology for Language and Learning's *Joystick Games* (Apple II series).

MISCELLANEOUS CONSIDERATIONS

Once the seating components, type of mobility base, and controls have been determined, other client needs must be considered. If the individual needs a tray, its specific features need to be determined. These may include an easel, a mounting system for an augmentative communication device, and/or a cutout for a joystick. When mounting a device, consideration must be given to the angle needed by the user, and whether the device should be recessed so that it is mounted at the height of the tray surface. Environmental control units often can be integrated with either a power mobility system or augmentative communication system. Making sure that the various systems are compatible is critical. If the individual is going to drive a power wheelchair when an augmentative communication system is in place, the ability to see around the augmentative device needs to be carefully considered.

Equally important is having a training plan for the client and any others who will assist in the mobility system's use and care. Improper use of the positioning system can result in a user who is unable to access technological aids. Interestingly, the majority of problems with power mobility bases are related to routine battery care and charging.

Bus Transportation

There are many factors to consider when transporting power mobility systems in vans and buses. These include the battery powering the system and the tie-down system used to hold the chair in place. Individuals who are being transported to and from school should power their wheelchairs with gel rather than acid batteries. Many states will transport only gel batteries. Currently, the average life of gel batteries is 6 to 9 months. They are significantly more costly than acid batteries. Gel batteries with longer life spans have been developed; however, they are still not widely available commercially.

It is also critical that the chair tie-down on any public transportation system is adequate (Wevers, 1983). It should be a four-point tie-down system, preferably with all four points originating from the floor and securing the chair in a forward-facing direction. The chair should be secured only at the frame. The footrests and armrests should never be used to secure the chair. The individual should also have a three-point seat belt system, as in a car, to hold the user in place, separate from the chair-tie down system.

SUMMARY

Proper seating is critical for individuals with technology needs who have physical disabilities. Only when proper seating has been established can an accurate assessment be made of how to access technology. This includes accessing augmentative communication and computer writing devices, environmental controls, and power mobility. Physical and occupational therapists are the technology team members who are usually responsible for determining proper seating.

Pelvic stabilization is the key to functional, safe, and optimal postural seating. Only after the pelvis has been stabilized can other seating needs be determined. An individual's need for head and trunk support also must be carefully evaluated to ensure that the client has optimal function without undue effort. Once this support has been provided, the most efficient and least effortful means of technology access can be determined.

Assessment of power mobility potential begins after seating has been determined, along with an appreciation for the individual's cognitive abilities. A hand-operated, variable-speed joystick is the method of choice because it provides multi-directional control and graded speed control. The use of multiple single switches or scanning generally is avoided because these systems are much less efficient.

Providing an optimal seating and mobility system for a client is complex and time-consuming. Numerous decisions regarding physical problems, motor control, financial resources, and appearance of the seating system need to be finalized. Ongoing access to facilities and professionals with expertise in positioning and adaptive technology should be ensured. Clients are likely to have numerous caregivers and may have limited ability to instruct them. Therefore, all aspects of positioning should be easily reproducible and documented in writing. Finally, the needs, goals, and wishes of clients and caregivers must be included throughout the decision-making process. This will ensure optimal use and function of the client in the seating and mobility system.

REFERENCES

Butler, C., Okamoto, G., & McKey, T. (1983). Powered mobility for very young disabled children. *Developmental Medicine and Child Neurology, 25,* 472–474.

Margolis, S., Jones, R., & Brown, B. (1985). The subASIS bar: An effective approach to pelvic stabilization in seated positioning. *RESNA 8th Annual Conference Proceedings, 5,* 45–47.

Margolis, S., & Wengert, M. E. (1988). The subASIS bar: No component is an island. *Proceedings of the Fourth International Seating Symposium,* 1–4.

Nwaobi, O. (1987). The relationship between the mechanical and anatomical hip angle in adaptive seating. *The Proceedings of the Third International Seating Symposium,* 116–119.

Nwaobi, O., Hobson, D., & Taylor, S. (1988). Mechanical and anatomic hip flexion angles on seating children with cerebral palsy. *Archives of Physical Medicine and Rehabilitation, 69,* 265–267.

Paulson, K., & Christofferson, M. (1984). Psychosocial aspects of technical aids — How does independent mobility affect the psychosocial and intellectual development of children with physical disabilities. *Proceedings from the Second International Conferences on Rehabilitation Engineering,* 282–286.

Taplin, C. S. (1989). Powered wheelchair control, assessment, and training. *RESNA '89, Proceedings of the 12th Annual Conference, 9,* 45–46.

Wengert, M. E., Margolis, S., & Kolar, K. (1987). A design for the back of seated positioning orthoses that controls pelvic positioning and increases head control. *Proceedings of the RESNA 10th Annual Conference, 7,* 216–218.

Wevers, H. W., Jr. (1983). Wheelchair and occupant restraint system for transportation of handicapped passengers. *Archives of Physical and Medical Rehabilitation, 64,* 374–377.

4

Augmentative and Alternative Communication

■ Sharon Glennen, PhD ■

Communication occurs when people come together to exchange information, socialize, and interact with one another. These interactions form the social networks that bind people to each other, their communities, and the world. People normally conduct these interactions using speech as their primary mode of communication. Augmentative and alternative communication occurs when one of the interaction partners relies primarily on other modes of communication. These modes can range from gestures, facial expressions, and sign languages, which are **unaided modes** of augmentative communication, to the use of augmentative communication aids. This chapter will focus on the use of **aided augmentative modes** of communication. Aided communication methods can range from using paper and pencil, typewriters, and alphabet letter boards to the use of sophisticated microcomputer systems.

Aided augmentative communication systems are a relatively new modality of communication. The first documented use of communication aids as a primary mode of communication occurred in 1973 (McDonald & Schultz). At that time, most communication aids were simple home-made, low-technology **communication boards** without written or spoken output. Messages were spelled letter by letter or created by pointing to picture symbols. With the dawn of the microcomputer revolution in the late 1970s, high technology electronic communication aids with spoken and written output were developed. In 1978, Phonic Ear's *HandiVoice 110* became the first commercially available communication aid with **synthesized speech** produced in the United States. Since that time, communication aid technology has changed rapidly with improvements in memory, system storage and accessing methods, speech output, size, and software flexibility.

AUGMENTATIVE COMMUNICATION AIDS AND THEIR COMPONENTS

Augmentative communication aids are classified as low-technology or high-technology systems. Within each of these two categories, a wide range of communication aids with varying features is available. These features include accessing methods, symbol systems, message storage and retrieval systems, and output methods.

Low-Technology Aids

Low-technology communication aids are simple devices that do not have printed or speech output. Although these systems can be electronic, they are not microcomputers, therefore they have no vocabulary storage or programming capabilities. Messages must be spelled letter by letter, or identified through picture or word symbols. Low-technology communication aids range from simple alphabet communication boards and picture boards to electronic scanning systems such as the Prentke Romich *VersaScan*.

High-Technology Aids

High-technology communication aids are computerized systems that are operated through special software. The software can be specifically designed to operate on a device which can only be used as a communication aid, or it can be designed to operate on a standard microcomputer. Microcomputers that can be operated only as communication aids are known as **dedicated** systems. Prentke Romich's *Touch Talker, Light Talker,* and *Liberator,* Adamlab's *MegaWolf,* and Adaptive Communication System's *Dynavox,* and *Digital Augmentative Communicator (DAC)* are examples of dedicated communication aids. Many portable microcomputers are being adapted for use as augmentative communication aids. The Epson *HX-20* microcomputer has been adapted for use as a communication aid by Adaptive Communication Systems in the *Real Voice* communication aid. Some software applications give users the ability to program frequently used messages for storage in the system. By **prestoring messages**, a user can quickly communicate lengthy messages with a minimum number of keystrokes. The *Touch Talker, Light Talker, Liberator, Dynavox,* and *Real Voice* have options for prestoring messages. Other software programs rely on **message prediction** techniques to predict what a user is going to say next. Words Plus Company has developed several software programs, such as *Scanning WSKE II,* that rely on message prediction. High technology communication aids have speech output, printed output, or sometimes both output modes. On some systems, the size, location, and type of symbols displayed on the communication aid overlay can be completely customized for the user. Finally, some of these communication systems can be attached to a computer to operate as a keyboard for running standard computer programs (Vanderheiden & Lloyd, 1986).

Accessing Methods

Augmentative communication aids can be accessed through **direct selection** or **scanning** methods (see Figure 4–1). With direct selection methods, a user points directly to communication aid symbols. Scanning methods present communication aid symbols to a user until the user indicates that the selected symbol is the correct choice. With scanning communication systems, a user must wait until the system finds the desired communication aid symbol.

Use of direct selection methods ranges from pointing with a finger to pointing with the help of sophisticated technology. At the simplest level, a user can point directly using a part of the body. Fingers, hands, elbows, toes, noses, and eyes are but a few of the body parts that can be imaginatively used for direct selection with an augmentative communication system. Sometimes the user requires a simple aid to improve the pointing process. Pointing aids include **head sticks**, **hand splints**, and **mouthsticks**. A user also can use indirect methods of direct selection. These include use of **light beam pointers**, **joysticks**, and **ocular eye-gaze monitors**, which electronically measure eye movements (Vanderheiden & Lloyd, 1986).

Many different kinds of scanning methods are available for operating communication aids. Most of these methods can be categorized as **automatic scanning** or **step scanning**. In automatic scanning, the augmentative communication aid does all of the work in the scanning process. Symbol choices are presented to the user who presses a switch

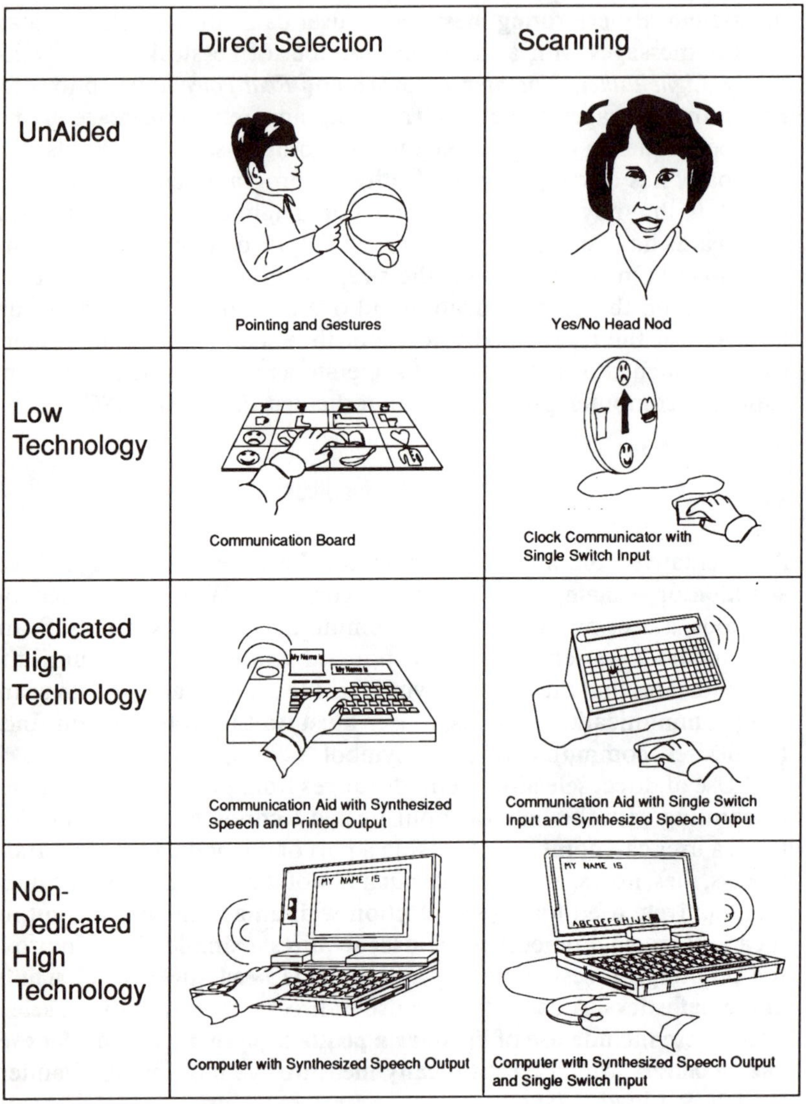

	Direct Selection	Scanning
UnAided	Pointing and Gestures	Yes/No Head Nod
Low Technology	Communication Board	Clock Communicator with Single Switch Input
Dedicated High Technology	Communication Aid with Synthesized Speech and Printed Output	Communication Aid with Single Switch Input and Synthesized Speech Output
Non-Dedicated High Technology	Computer with Synthesized Speech Output	Computer with Synthesized Speech Output and Single Switch Input

Figure 4–1

Augmentative communication classification system.

when the desired choice is reached. In contrast, step scanning requires the user to push a switch repeatedly to move the scanning cursor from selection to selection. Once the desired symbol choice is reached, the user either waits for a time delay, or pushes a second switch to activate the symbol choice.

Item-by-Item scanning is the simplest method of automatic or step scanning for communication aids. All possible symbol choices are reviewed one at a time in the same linear order. If a communication aid has 36 symbol choices, the device would scan repeatedly through all 36 items. Adamlab's *ScanWolf* and *WhisperWolf* use item-by-item automatic scanning. The Prentke Romich *Light Talker* and *Scanning Intro Talker* can be configured to use item-by-item step scanning in the eight-symbol mode. Item-by-item scanning methods are simple but slow, since the communication aid must always scan through all possible choices. Because of its slow speed, this type of scanning is not feasible for devices with more than a few symbol choices (Vanderheiden & Lloyd, 1986).

Scanning speeds can be increased when multidimensional scanning methods are used. Multidimensional techniques include **row-column scanning** and **group-item scanning**. These techniques can be developed for automatic scanning systems or step scanning systems. With row-column scanning the communication aid first scans through each row of symbols until the user pushes a switch, then each symbol in the selected row is scanned until the switch is pushed again. Group-item scanning involves presenting large groups of choices in multidimensional layers until the desired symbol is reached. For example, a group-item scanning array might first present a choice between four quadrants of symbols on the communication aid, then choices between four rows of symbols within the quadrant, then choices between the beginning half or end half of the selected row, then choices between individual symbols in the final section of the selected row. Group-item scanning is recommended for communication aids with vocabularies of over 200 symbols (Vanderheiden & Lloyd, 1986). Most sophisticated high-technology communication aids offer multidimensional scanning options. These include Prentke Romich's *Light Talker,* and *Liberator,* Adaptive Communication System's *Scanning Real Voice* and *Dynavox,* and Words Plus' *Scanning WSKE II.*

A final scanning strategy is based on frequency of use. **Frequency of use scanning** can involve **static** or **dynamic communication aid displays**. The order and placement of the symbols never changes in a static display. A static communication aid display might have letters of the alphabet listed in order from the most frequently used to the least frequently used. Sophisticated communication aids can now produce dynamic picture symbol displays with constantly changing arrays.

These devices present symbol choices based upon a user's previous choices. For example when spelling, the letter *t* at the beginning of a word can only be followed by the letters *a, e, i, o, u, r, w,* and *h*. After selecting the letter *t*, a dynamic scanning display would then present the user with these eight choices ordered by frequency of use. The Words Plus *Scanning WSKE II* software uses a dynamic frequency of use strategy to present written word and letter choices to a user. Adaptive Communication System's *Dynavox* also has a dynamic display with constantly changing picture arrays arranged in category groupings. Finally, Prentke Romich's *Liberator* has scanning options that predict picture symbol choices and automatically scan through those options.

Whenever possible, direct selection techniques should be used to access communication aids because they are cognitively easier to learn than scanning. Young children learn to reach and point to get what they want as early as 9 months of age (Owens, 1988). Scanning requires waiting for a communication aid to reach the desired symbol choice. Children who function below a 4-year-old age level have difficulty learning to use scanning systems because they are unable to attend to the communication aid throughout the scanning process. Row-column and group-item scanning methods are even more difficult for children to learn. Another reason to choose direct selection techniques over scanning is because they are faster. Users of direct selection letter spelling devices have communication speeds ranging from 6 to 25 words per minute. Users of letter-based item-by-item scanning communication aids have communication speeds of only 2 to 4 words per minute (Foulds, 1980). For these reasons, scanning methods should only be used after direct selection methods have been ruled out.

Symbol Systems

Augmentative communication aids can be developed using a wide variety of symbol systems that range from concrete to abstract. Table 4–1 lists general symbol systems in order from symbolically easiest to most abstract.

At the easiest level, actual objects and miniature objects can be used to represent concrete concepts. Children who function as young as 7 months developmentally can be taught to reach toward a desired object. Objects can be glued onto communication boards, hooked onto belts, attached with velcro to vests, or carried in a backpack or purse by a user. While objects are useful symbols they cannot be used to represent abstract concepts such as feelings, size, or actions. Even simple word concepts that develop early, such as *more, no,* and *want* cannot be depicted with objects.

Table 4–1. Augmentative communication symbol hierarchy.

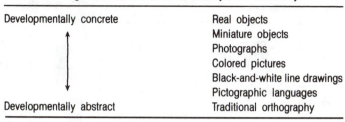

Developmentally concrete	Real objects
↑	Miniature objects
	Photographs
	Colored pictures
↓	Black-and-white line drawings
	Pictographic languages
Developmentally abstract	Traditional orthography

Photographs, colored line drawings, and black-and-white line drawings also can be used as symbols on communication aids. Young children are able to begin identifying realistic colored pictures of objects at 18 months of age. Communication boards can be developed using photographs of favorite toys and persons and places in the child's environment. Action words can be conveyed by photographing the user or others performing the action. Colored line drawings and black-and-white line drawings can be obtained commercially or from magazines and picture books. Children's dictionaries are excellent resources for colorful small pictures to use on communication boards.

The next category of symbols are those that belong to pictographic sets. Unlike simple line drawings, **pictographic symbols** are designed to convey most language concepts including abstract terms such as *more, again,* and *no.* Pictographic symbol sets include *Core Picture Vocabulary* (Johnston, 1985), *Picture Communication Symbols* (Johnson, 1985), *Oakland Picture Dictionary* (Kirstein & Bernstein, 1981), *Talking Pictures* (Leff & Leff, 1978) and *Picsyms* (Carlson, 1984) among others (see Figure 4–2). Each pictographic set varies in the total number of vocabulary items in the set and the manner of depicting vocabulary items. Most sets depict concrete concepts similarly, but vary widely in their depiction of abstract symbols. Some sets such as *Talking Pictures* do not contain any abstract symbol concepts.

Blissymbols are among the most sophisticated pictographic language systems. They were developed by Charles Bliss as a graphic visual language that could be used by people who spoke different languages (Bliss, 1965). In the early 1970s they began to be used with nonspeaking persons in Canada at the Ontario Crippled Children's Center (McNaughton, 1976). Blissymbols were designed to represent concrete and abstract symbol concepts using consistent linguistic rules. The Blissymbol system consists of 100 basic symbols which are combined to create thousands of vocabulary items. For example, the Blissymbol for *cookie* consists of the Blissymbols for *food, nose,* and *positive feeling* (something you can eat that smells good). New sym-

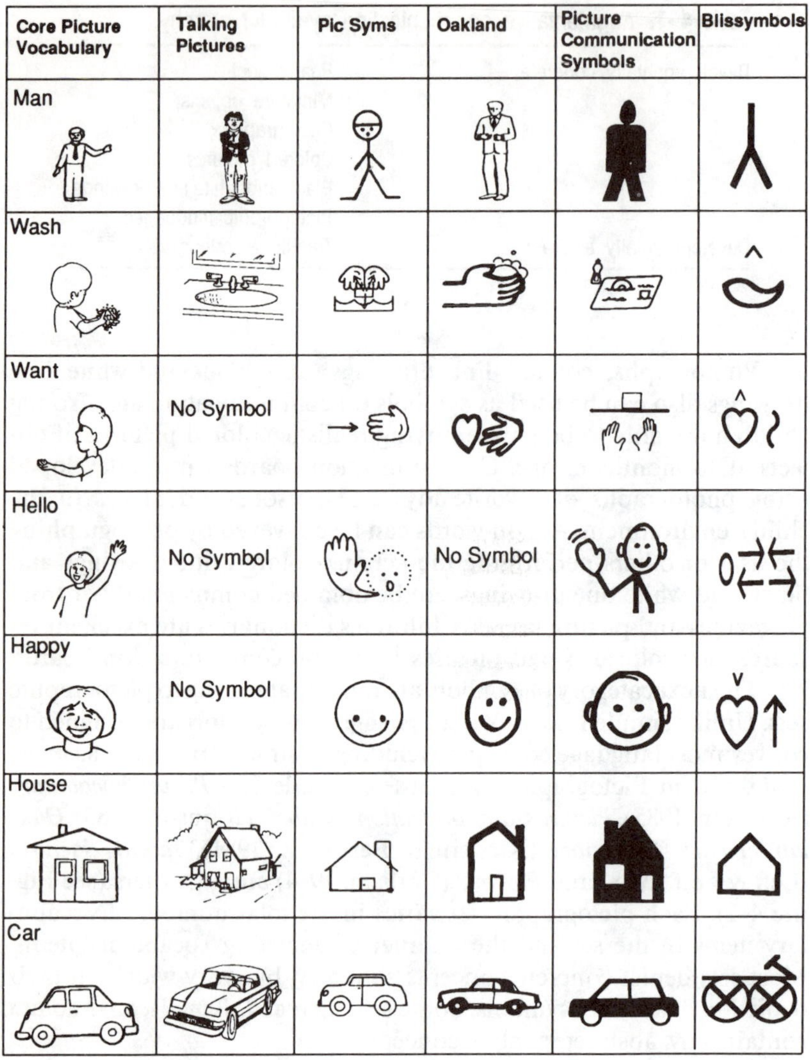

Core Picture Vocabulary	Talking Pictures	Pic Syms	Oakland	Picture Communication Symbols	Blissymbols
Man					
Wash					
Want	No Symbol				
Hello	No Symbol		No Symbol		
Happy	No Symbol				
House					
Car					

Figure 4–2

Pictrographic symbol systems. From left to right the systems are: Core Picture Vocabulary, Talking Pictures, PicSyms, Oakland Picture Dictionary, Picture Communication Symbols, and Blissymbols. Not all symbol sets have picture representations for every word.

bols can be created at any time by combining the basic symbol concepts. Blissymbols are not as immediately transparent when compared to symbols from other pictographic languages; however, once the linguistic patterns of Bliss are learned, the system allows greater flexibility for communication than other pictographic systems (Vanderheiden & Lloyd, 1986).

Nonspeaking persons who use printed alphabet letters as symbols are using a **traditional orthography** system. Learning to use written letters for communication is difficult for many nonspeaking persons (Vanderheiden & Lloyd, 1986). Traditional orthography can be modified to make it easier to learn and use. Young children who are first learning the alphabet can use picture cues or color coding to enhance learning. Those who have some literacy skills can use whole printed words and sentences on communication aids. Finally, written symbols that are partial words can be used as communication aid symbols (Goodenough-Trepagnier & Prather, 1981). For example, a communication aid might have the symbols *thr, pl, gr,* and *ow.* By combining the symbols together the user can easily communicate *throw, plow,* and *grow* with only two keystrokes per word. Other orthographic systems also can be used with communication aids. These include braille, graphic pictures of manual fingerspelling signs, and Morse code.

When choosing a symbol system for a communication aid it is important to consider the transparency of the individual symbols and the openness or flexibility of the entire symbol system (Vanderheiden & Lloyd, 1986). Concrete picture symbols that look like the objects they portray are easy to learn, but limit the user's communication options. A picture communication board with 20 concrete symbols allows the user to communicate only 20 thoughts. Blissymbols and traditional orthography are more abstract and difficult to learn but have the advantage of being more flexible. A user who can use a simple alphabet communication board can communicate any thought at any time to any person.

Message Storage and Retrieval Systems

One of the factors that separates high technology from low-technology communication aids is the use of **prestored messages** and **message prediction** techniques. Both methods are called **acceleration techniques** because their purpose is to increase the speed of communication. Using prestored messages involves storing language units, such as words, phrases, or sentences, into a communication aid for later recall. Instead of spelling *Hello how are you?* letter by letter, a user can push one or two keys on the communication aid to communicate the entire prestored message. Communication aids with message prediction capabilities use complex software to predict a user's next letter or word. For example, after a user types *Hello,* the software automatically generates a list of words that could follow. If the first choice presented by the software was *how,* the user pushes a single key to select the word.

Prestored Message Techniques

Communication aids that use prestored messages vary in the length of the language unit stored and retrieved by the system. Letters, words, phrases, and sentences can be stored in communication aids. In theory, systems that store and retrieve phrases or sentences are faster than systems that store letters and words. However, accessing these large language units limits message flexibility (Glennen, 1989). Prestored sentences are useful for communicating general routine thoughts such as *Hello, my name is, What's that,* and *I like that.* They become less useful when more specific or unusual topics of communication are encountered. Prestored words are more flexible than sentences. A basic vocabulary of 700 words will meet 80 percent of most users' communicative needs (Yorkston, Dowden, Honsinger, Marriner, & Smith, 1988). Minspeak Corporation has developed several software programs that have large prestored vocabularies for use in *Touch Talker, Light Talker,* and *Liberator* communication aids. Adaptive Communication System's *Dynavox* also has software programs on *Dynacards* with large single-word vocabularies.

Communication aids vary in the amount of fixed and open memory available for message storage. **Fixed memory** is not user-programmable. Messages are stored in fixed memory by the manufacturer and cannot be changed by the user. The *Scan-Wolf* is an example of a communication aid with only fixed memory. **Open memory** is user programmable. A user can develop and store novel messages within the software and memory constraints of the system. Communication aids may have only fixed memory or various combinations of fixed and open memory. The more open memory a communication aid contains, the more flexible the system is for customized message storage. Most sophisticated high-technology communication aids such as Prentke Romich's *Touch Talker,* Adaptive Communication System's *Real Voice,* Phonic Ear's *VOIS,* and Words Plus' *Scanning WSKE II* contain large amounts of open memory. Prestored messages can be individually developed based on the needs of a communication aid user. As communication needs change, new messages can be stored at any time.

Open memory systems allow a user to select individualized message **retrieval codes**. Retrieval codes are sequences of symbols that are used to recall the stored messages from computer memory. The previous discussion of symbols in this chapter focused on using a single symbol to convey a single thought. For example, a picture of *frog* represented the language concept of *frog.* Computerized communication aids that use sequences of symbols to recall prestored messages use symbols in a very different way. Symbol sequencing allows a user to communicate a large number of prestored messages with a limited symbol set. A 30-symbol communication aid that does not sequence symbols can only communicate 30 messages. A 30-symbol communication aid that allows two-symbol sequencing theoretically can communicate 900 different messages if every symbol combination is used.

Currently *Minspeak* (Baker, 1982), and *abbreviation expansion* are two methods of symbol sequencing commonly used in communication aids.

Minspeak is a method of using semantically meaningful picture symbols to store and recall prestored messages (Baker, 1982). The message *Hello, how are you?* might be stored using the meaningful picture sequence of *waving hand* plus *question mark*. To gain maximum use from a limited number of pictures, the user has to assign more than one meaning to each picture symbol (Baker, 1986). For example, a picture of *frog* might be used in sequences for messages that have concepts associated with frogs, jumping, water, green, wet, throats, and dying (croaking). *Minspeak* systems can be used to store sentences, phrases, and words. *Minspeak* is currently available only on communication aids manufactured by Prentke Romich Company.

Abbreviation expansion uses alphabet letter symbols as sequences for prestored messages (Vanderheiden & Lloyd, 1986). The message *Hello, how are you?* might be stored using the letter sequence of *H* plus *Y*. Many computerized communication aids such as the *Real Voice* offer some form of abbreviation expansion. Each system varies in the number of letters that can be sequenced in an abbreviation and in the amount of memory available for storing messages. Abbreviation expansion also can be used as a storage technique for sentences, phrases, and words.

A final technique, which is currently available on the *VOIS Shapes* communication aid manufactured by Phonic Ear, involves using manual sign handshapes as symbols for sequencing (Shane & Wilbur, 1989). This technique uses 60 symbols based on manual sign handshapes, locations, and movements. Theoretically, the system can generate up to 5,700 words using three symbol sequences for each manual sign.

Message Prediction Techniques

The development of portable computers with large memory storage capabilities has made the use of message prediction techniques more prevalent in communication systems. Message prediction techniques can be used for letter spelling and whole words. Message prediction for letter spelling does not require much computer memory. The software only needs to predict between 26 letters, a blank space, and a few punctuation markers. Message prediction techniques that use words need massive amounts of computer memory. Most of the word-based techniques use a frequency of use formula for prediction. The software presents word choices based on previously written words. For example, in this paragraph I have used the word *message* four times, and the word *memory* three times. If this chapter was being typed with word prediction software, the next time *me* was typed, the computer would present choices based on the frequency of using previous words. The word *message* would be at the top of the choice listings because it had been used more frequently. The word *memory* would follow since it was used less frequently.

Recently message prediction systems have been developed that use frequency of use information and syntactic word ordering rules for prediction. For example the word *with* is almost always followed by an article (*the, a*) or pronoun (*their, my*). Software with syntactic word ordering rules would limit word choices to these two categories, then order the words by frequency of previous use. Message prediction systems place a high cognitive load on the user. A user has to think about the next desired word, then scan a message prediction array to look for it. Message prediction systems work best when a user does not have to look back and forth between the current work area and the message prediction array. The message prediction array should be positioned near the current work area on the system's display screen (Vanderheiden & Lloyd, 1986). Message prediction techniques slow down communication for users who are able to use direct selection methods with good accuracy and speed. This technique should be limited to persons who need to use slow accessing methods such as scanning (Vanderheiden & Lloyd, 1986), or persons whose orthographic spelling skills could be significantly enhanced with message-prediction assistance.

Combination Techniques

Some augmentative communication aids combine the benefits of prestored messages with prediction capabilities to create unique acceleration techniques. A variation on message prediction techniques is called **symbol prediction**. Users prestore messages using sequenced symbol retrieval codes. When the user presses the first symbol in the sequence, the software predicts what the next symbol in the sequence will be. Prentke Romich's *Liberator* gives symbol prediction information in both direct selection and scanning modes. In direct selection, the system highlights predicted symbols with **light emitting diodes** beside each symbol choice. In scanning modes, the system reduces scanning choices to the predicted symbols.

Output Methods

Communication aids can have one of the following four output methods: (a) no output, (b) spoken output, (c) printed output, and (d) both spoken and printed output. Low-technology communication aids do not have any message output. These systems require listeners to be present and actively watching symbols being selected while a user is communicating. Listeners must then remember all of the symbols that were selected and mentally put the message together. Low technology communication aids rely heavily on the attention span and language skills of the listener. If a listener momentarily looks away from the system and misses a symbol selection, the user typically must start the message over again (Glennen, 1989).

Adding intelligible output to a communication aid can significantly change the communicative interactions of both the user and listener. In a study that compared various output methods, nonspeaking persons were placed into a responding conversational role more frequently when no communication aid output was available. When intelligible output was available, nonspeaking persons initiated conversation more frequently and had fewer conversational breakdowns (Glennen, 1989). Having either spoken or printed output frees a listener from having to closely attend to the communication aid during interactions. It also lets the listener watch the communication aid user, instead of the communication aid itself.

Spoken output currently is available on many high-technology commmunication aids. The quality of speech varies widely depending on the type of spoken output used. Three basic types of spoken output can be used in communication aids: taped, synthesized, and digitized (Gunderson, 1985).

Communication aids with **taped speech** use cassette tapes with prerecorded words, phrases, and sentences. The system uses software to find tape locations for message retrieval. SciTronic's *Form-a-Phrase*, which is no longer available commercially, is an example of a dedicated communication aid that used taped output.

Of the three types of spoken output used in communication aids **synthesized speech** is the most common. Synthesized speech systems store part of the numerical waveform parameters representing the formant frequencies of speech. When recalled, the stored numerical coordinates are retrieved and assembled to generate spoken language. Approximately 300 phrases of synthesized numerical waveform data can be stored in 32 kilobytes of computer memory (Gunderson, 1985).

There are three basic types of speech synthesizers: encoded, phonetic, and phonetic systems that use linear predictive coding. Encoded speech synthesizers store waveform parameters for entire words and phrases. These synthesizers are used in communication aids with limited fixed memory vocabularies, such as Texas Instrument's *VoCaid,* or in talking toys. Speech synthesizers in communication aids with open programmable memory need to be more flexible. This requires using phonetic speech synthesizers which store waveform patterns for individual sounds (Gunderson, 1985). Phonetic speech synthesizers are also known as text-to-speech synthesizers. Software is used to translate written alphabet text into spoken messages. The software uses standard rules of pronunciation to decide which sound to retrieve from memory for each letter or group of letters. For example, the letter *G* can be pronounced soft or hard (e.g., giraffe or girl). These are stored as two different sounds. The software uses rules to decide which sound to use in a given word. The quality of a phonetic speech synthesizer is related to the complexity and quality of the software that operates the system and the synthesizer hardware. Some phonetic synthesizers recognize commonly used words and automatically retrieve all of the correct sounds necessary for production of the entire word. Typically, a software program that recognizes individual words produces more intelligible speech than software without this capability (Gunderson, 1985). Communication aids that use Street Electronic's *Echo II* synthesizers are examples of systems with phonetic text-to-speech synthesizers.

Phonetic systems that have **linear predictive coding** capabilities provide synthesized speech output with the quality of digitized speech. These systems use text-to-speech translation rules to initially decode a word, then match the word to stored digitized representations of the word. *DecTalk* by Digital Equipment is the best known synthesizer with linear predictive coding capabilities. *DecTalk* gives a user the option of choosing between 10 different male or female voices or creating a novel voice. *DecTalk* is currently available in Prentke Romich's *Touch Talker, Light Talker,* and *Liberator,* and Adaptive Communication System's *DynaVox. RealVoice,* which is also made by Adaptive Communication Systems, is another eample of a synthesizer that utilizes linear predictive coding.

Digitized speech is becoming more widely used in communication aids as the availability of cheap computer memory improves. Digitized systems operate much like synthesized speech systems. However, sythesized speech systems store only part of the numerical speech waveform pattern, whereas digitized systems store the numerical waveform parameters for the entire speech signal. When recalled, the stored numerical coordinates are retrieved and assembled to generate spoken output. Storing numerical waveform information requires large amounts of memory. Each second of stored digitized speech requires several kilobytes of memory (Gunderson, 1985). Most augmentative communication aids with digitized speech capabilities record spoken messages directly into memory through an attached microphone. The digitized speech output then sounds like the person who did the recording. Zygo's *Parrot* and *Macaw* use digitized speech along with Adaptive Communication System's *DAC* and Prentke Romich's *IntroTalker* and *Scanning IntroTalker.*

Two major types of printed output are available for communication aids. These are temporary print displays and paper printers. Temporary print displays show messages on **liquid crystal** (LCD) or **light emitting diode** (LED) displays. As new messages are formed, the display erases previous messages. A listener must be present and attend to each message as it is printed on a temporary print display. Some communication aids such as Adaptive Communication System's *Real Voice* and the *Liberator* by Prentke Romich, have built-in paper printers. These are usually small and print on adding machine tape or paper strips. Other communication aids can produce paper copy when attached to peripheral printers. This allows users to print on standard size paper but decreases the portability of the communication system. Paper printers let a listener leave the communication aid while messages are being prepared and return later to read messages. The major advantage of paper copy is for lengthy written language tasks.

Some communication aids offer both spoken and printed output options. Adding printed output to devices with synthesized speech improves the overall intelligibility of the system for listeners who can read. Adding synthesized speech to devices with printed output allows the user to communicate with listeners who cannot read. Glennen (1989) found that nonspeaking persons who used communication aids with both spoken and printed output were placed into a respondant role in conversation less frequently than when they used systems with either spoken or printed output alone.

Summary of Augmentative Communication Aid Options

Augmentative communication aid accessing methods, symbol systems, message encoding and retrieval systems, and output combine in different ways to create augmentative communication systems customized for each user. Before attempting to prescribe a communication system, the nonspeaking person should be carefully evaluated for his or her ability to access a communication aid, cognitive abilities to understand symbols and message retrieval systems, and needs for printed and spoken output. The next section of this chapter outlines assessment methods that can be used during the evaluation process.

AUGMENTATIVE COMMUNICATION EVALUATION PROCEDURES

Evaluating a nonspeaking person for an augmentative communication system is a methodical step-by-step process. Areas to be evaluated include expressive language skills, receptive language skills, augmentative communication symbol use skills, and motor accessing skills. The first three assessment areas can be evaluated without the use of sophisticated technology. These three areas will determine if a non-speaking person has the necessary linguistic skills to use a particular communication system before evaluating motor skills necessary for using the system. By assessing linguistic skills first, an evaluator will know whether a nonspeaking person's difficulty in operating a communication aid is caused by not understanding how the system works or motor control difficulties (Glennen, 1990). A careful evaluator will assess each area and use the information from each section to develop a final prescription for an augmentative communication system.

Evaluating Expressive Language Skills

Evaluating the **expressive language** skills of nonspeaking persons may seem like an oxymoron. However, just because a person cannot speak does not mean that they are not communicating. The expressive language evaluation assesses a nonspeaking person's need for communication and his or her current communication abilities. The first part of an expressive language assessment includes an interview with those who interact regularly with the nonspeaking person, and for older nonspeaking persons, a direct interview (see Figure 4–3). The interview should review current methods of communication and the success or lack of success of each method. In addition, the interview should include a needs assessment (Yorkston & Karlan, 1986). The needs assessment evaluates a nonspeaking person's environment to determine when, where, and with whom an augmentative communication system would be used.

The second part of an expressive language evaluation involves directly observing a nonspeaking person's communication skills. Spontaneous interactions or structured interactions designed to elicit communicative behaviors can be used. For young children, spontaneous interactions during play activities usually work best. For older children and adults, **barrier game** activities are often successful methods of evaluating communication skills (Farrier, Yorkston, Marriner, & Beukelman, 1985; Glennen, 1989). One type of barrier game involves showing an individual an interesting picture, then asking them to describe it to a listener who has not seen the picture. The listener then attempts to draw the picture as it is described.

The communication skills of nonspeaking persons can be analyzed in many different ways. For research purposes, detailed interaction procedures have been developed that evaluate interaction skills (Buzolich, 1983; Glennen, 1989; Light, Collier, & Parnes, 1985). More realistically, an evaluator should be able to assess interaction skills through direct on-line observation. Several checklist procedures have

Augmentative Communication Evaluation

Needs Assessment and Interview

Client Name:_____ _____   Date of Evaluation:_____

Date of Birth:_____   Age:_____   Informant:_____

---

1) Describe any methods of communication currently used by the client (List below).

2) Which method is used most frequently? How well do others understand this method? (Record below).

3) Which method is used next frequently? How well do others understand this method?
   Continue ranking communication methods until all have been completed.

Description of Method   Frequency Ranking   Intelligibility

_____   _____   _____

_____   _____   _____

_____   _____   _____

_____   _____   _____

_____   _____   _____

_____   _____   _____

4) Does the client use any assistive technology or adaptive equipment? (Describe below).

5) Where is this technology or equipment used? (List below).

6) How successful is this technology or equipment? (Record below).

Technology Description   Location   Successful?

_____   _____   _____

_____   _____

_____   _____   _____

_____   _____   _____

7) Describe the locations where the client spends time each day (List below).

8) How much time is spent in each location? (Record below).

9) How is he/she positioned in each of these locations? (Record below).

(continued)

10) Are there any locations or positions that an augmentative communication system is not needed, or would be difficult to use? (Record below).

Location   Time Spent   Positioning   Need Communication?

_____

_____

_____

_____

11) During a typical day, who does the client interact with? (List below).

12) What relationship does this person have with the client? (Record below).

13) List some communicative messages that the client might need to say to this person. (Record below).

Person   Relationship   Messages

_____

_____

_____

_____

_____

_____

_____

_____

_____

14) What type of augmentative communication system, or systems will best meet this client's needs?

_____

_____

Figure 4–3

Augmentative Communication Needs Assessment and Interview Form.

been developed for this purpose (Bolton & Dashiell, 1984; Calculator & Luchko, 1983). Most checklist procedures assess **communication modes**, pragmatic **communicative acts**, and **communication breakdowns** by mode and communicative act. Figure 4–4 is a sample checklist that can be used for evaluation purposes.

At the end of the expressive language portion of the evaluation, an examiner should have determined if a nonspeaking person has the desire to communicate with others. Nonspeaking persons who are not

Augmentative Communication Interaction Checklist

Instructions: List the communication modes to be analyzed in the blank spaces across the top of the grid. Observe the individual interacting with other persons while participating in a fun activity for 30 minutes. Check the communication act categories that occur spontaneously by marking an "S" in the appropriate grid. Check communication act categories that can be elicited after using specific cues by marking "E" in the appropriate grid. Communication act categories not observed should be left blank.

Communication Act Categories	Communication Mode Categories				
(Examples in Parentheses)					
Request Objects (Want ball)					
Request Actions (Throw ball)					
Request Other (Where's ball?)					
Statement (Pretty ball)					
Yes/No Response (Want ball? Yes.)					
Wh Question Response (Where's ball? There.)					
Acknowledgement (It's round. Uh-huh.)					
Other Response (Do you want this? This.)					
No Response					

Figure 4–4
Augmentative Communication Interaction Checklist.

motivated to communicate need preliminary training before a final aided communication system can be prescribed. The examiner should also be able to evaluate the success, or lack of success, of current modes of communication. Many nonspeaking persons are extremely successful using their current modes of communication and would not significantly benefit from having a new aided communication system. Conversely, if a new aided communication system is needed, information on the lack of success of current modes of communication will be needed to obtain funding for the equipment.

An examiner will also determine when and where the augmentative communication system will be used. A nonspeaking person who spends most of the day in a wheelchair has different system needs than an individual who spends a few hours in an electric wheelchair, a few hours in a regular wheelchair, and a few hours in bed. These system needs should be taken into consideration when the final device prescription is made.

Evaluating Receptive Language Skills

This portion of the evaluation will determine if an individual has the basic **receptive language** ability to begin considering use of an aided augmentative communication system. In addition, it will determine an approximate receptive language age level that can be compared to chronological age to determine a gross rate of development. Rate of development is important when considering an augmentative communication prescription. A nonspeaking person who is developing receptive language skills at a normal rate might quickly outgrow a communication system designed for his or her current skill level. Conversely, an individual developing at a slower rate might be able to use a simple communication system for many years before considering the purchase of a sophisticated system with expensive options.

Any standardized or nonstandardized test that requires direct multiple choice pointing responses can be used for the receptive language portion of the evaluation. Tests that meet this requirement include: *Peabody Picture Vocabulary Test—Revised* (Dunn & Dunn, 1982) and the *Test of Auditory Comprehension of Language—Revised* (Carrow-Woolfolk, 1985). The following tests have subtests that require pointing responses: *Test of Language Development—Primary* (Newcomer & Hammill, 1988); *Test of Adolescent Language* (Hammill, Brown, Larsen, & Wiederholt, 1980); and *Clinical Evaluation of Language Functions—Revised* (Semel, Wiig, & Secord 1987). Whenever possible, standardized testing should be given using a direct selection format. This is especially important when an individual's cognitive skills are unknown, or

Before giving any test to a physically handicapped person, the examiner should first assess the motor skills necessary for accurate pointing to test items. With very young children or older clients with severe cognitive delays, motor skills should first be examined in play using simple objects. Range of motion can be grossly evaluated by having a child reach for an interesting toy. As the child reaches, the toy should be moved around so that the child has to go after the toy. By moving the toy from one side across midline to the other side and from locations near the child to locations that require full arm extension, the evaluator can determine where to place test materials. Once range of motion is determined, the examiner then needs to assess if the child can accurately point to pictures within the range. The examiner should place a set of test materials within the child's range, and point to the desired stimulus picture while simultaneously telling the child, *Point here* or *You do it.* Note that the examiner does not name the picture nor expect the child to find the picture by name during this part of the assessment.

If the individual is able to point to all necessary stimulus pictures, the test can then be administered. If the person has difficulty pointing accurately, the following remedies can be tried:

1. Cut the stimulus items apart and spread them further or closer together as needed.
2. Using the cut stimulus pictures, see if eyegaze or another direct selection method can be used for responding.
3. Using the cut stimulus items, reduce the number of choices required for the pointing response.

If the final option is used, each test item will need to be given more than once to keep from totally invalidating the test norms. For example, if a test requires pointing between four pictures but the individual is only able to accurately point to two pictures, the correct picture will need to be paired with each of the three incorrect pictures across three testing trials. If the correct picture is selected all three times, the individual can be credited with a correct response. If an incorrect picture is selected during any of the three trials, the response is credited as being incorrect. To prevent learning which picture to select across repeated trials, the three trials for a single test item should be intermixed with trials for other test items.

For older nonspeaking persons who are known to have good cognitive skills a **yes/no scanning** method of testing can be used. Most older nonspeaking persons have established yes/no responses that can be used for assessment. These might include eyeblinks, head nods, facial expressions, vocalizations, or arm movements. The examiner should be able to reliably read the nonspeaking person's responses before beginning the assessment. Testing consists of pointing to each stimulus item and asking: *Is it this one?* The individual then answers yes or no. It is important to always point to every stimulus item in the same order across all test pages and to maintain the same intonation patterns and facial expressions so that the correct response is not given away. In addition, some examiners make the mistake of looking directly at a nonspeaking person whenever the correct answer is reached. These examiner cues should be avoided at all costs.

Receptive language assessment results should not be used as the only criterion for determining a nonspeaking person's ability to use an augmentative communication system. The relationship between receptive language skills and augmentative communication skills is currently unknown. A nonspeaking person who cannot identify pictures by name may be able to match pictures to objects and learn to request objects on a communication board through this matching process. Therefore, the ability to identify and expressively use symbols should always be included in the augmentative communication evaluation process.

Augmentative Communication Symbol Use

To use an augmentative communication system, an individual must know how to use graphic symbols communicatively. Glennen (1990) developed an assessment hierarchy to evaluate a nonspeaking person's symbol use skills. The hierarchy is listed in Table 4–2.

At the simplest level, a nonspeaking person should be able to understand that pointing to a picture can be communicative. An array of pictures representing enticing objects are placed where the nonspeak-

Table 4–2. Augmentative communication symbol assessment hierarchy.

---

1. Picture symbol understanding and use
2. Picture symbol sequencing
3. Picture symbol association skills
4. Picture symbol encoding sequences
5. Memory for encoded picture symbol sequences
6. Alphabet letter recognition
7. Sight word recognition
8. Letter spelling
9. Letter encoding sequences
10. Memory for encoded letter sequences

---

ing person can point to them. Corresponding objects are placed within sight but out of reach. The nonspeaking person is encouraged to point to the pictures to request the objects. If necessary, the examiner should model picture-pointing skills and provide manual prompting when appropriate.

If a nonspeaking person understands that pointing to pictures is communicative, the next stage is the ability to sequence picture symbols. An array of pictures relating to a simple play activity is placed in front of the nonspeaking person. The pictures represent persons, actions, and objects associated with the activity (Glennen, 1990). The examiner first models symbol sequencing for the nonspeaking person by pointing to a picture sequence while verbally describing the sequence. For example, the examiner might point to *baby* plus *eat,* verbally say "baby is hungry," then proceed to feed a baby doll. Initially, the nonspeaking person may require physical guidance or verbal prompts to complete a picture sequence. Over time, prompts should be faded until the nonspeaking person is able to sequence pictures spontaneously.

The next stage of assessment evaluates an individual's ability to make concrete and abstract associations with picture symbols (Elder, 1987; Glennen, 1990). This skill is necessary for using high-technology communication aids that allow picture sequencing with a limited number of picture symbols. For this stage of the evaluation, a limited set of picture symbols is placed in front of the nonspeaking person. The individual is asked to point to a picture when given the correct object name and when given associated concept words such as actions, colors, shapes, and category names. For example, the picture of *apple* might be associated with apple, eating, red, round, fruit or food, tree, outside, bible, and banana. Very young children may only be able to make concrete associations based on action names, categories, and colors. Older nonspeaking persons should be able to make increasingly more abstract associations. The nonspeaking person's performance on this part of the evaluation will give the examiner information needed to develop appropriate picture sequences on a high-technology communication system.

The final two stages of evaluating picture symbol communication skills are the ability to create novel picture sequences for storing messages and the ability to remember the picture sequences once they are created. The nonspeaking person is given a limited set of picture symbols and asked to point to two pictures to describe a message (Glennen, 1990). For example, the sentence *I love to eat apple pie* might be depicted with the pictures *eat* plus *apple.* Following a limited time lapse, the nonspeaking person is asked to remember the original sequences and point to them again after each sentence is read.

The next stage of the assessment process is to evaluate symbol skills necessary for operating communication aids with letter-spelling capabilities. At the earliest level an individual needs to identify letters and have a sight word-reading vocabulary (Glennen, 1990). To evaluate these skills, individual alphabet letter cards are placed where the nonspeaking person can reach them. The client is then asked to point to letters when named. Cards with printed words are used similarly for assessment. The words should be developmentally ordered from those that are learned early in the reading process to those that are learned later.

If the nonspeaking person is able to identify alphabet orthographic letters and has basic sight word-reading skills, letter-spelling abilities should be evaluated. A limited set of letter cards is placed in front of the nonspeaking person who is then asked to spell words using the cards (Glennen, 1990). The words should again be developmentally ordered from easy to difficult.

Nonspeaking persons who have basic orthographic letter-spelling skills should be tested for letter encoding skills. This skill is necessary for communication aids that use abbreviation expansion strategies for encoding prestored messages. A limited set of letter cards is again placed where the nonspeaking person can reach them. The examiner reads a message aloud, then asks the nonspeaking person to point to two or three letters which represent the message (Glennen, 1990). For example, the sentence *I like to eat apple pie* can be represented with the letters *E* and *A*. After a brief time lapse the nonspeaking person is asked to remember the letter sequences used for each message.

At the end of this portion of the augmentative communication evaluation, the examiner will know a nonspeaking person's ability to use symbols for communication. Nonspeaking persons who do not understand that symbols are communicative need to be taught this skill using one or two highly motivating symbols and objects. Nonspeaking persons who can point to picture symbols communicatively but are unable to sequence picture symbols are candidates for simple communication boards, or inexpensive high technology communication aids that do not require picture symbol sequencing capabilities, such as Adamlab's *Mega Wolf* or Innocomp's *Say it Simply Plus*. Nonspeaking persons who can sequence picture symbols but cannot make complex associations with symbols should be able to use high-technology communication aids such as Prentke Romich's *Intro Talker* and *Scanning Intro Talker* with limited symbol sequencing memory. If the nonspeaking person is able to make complex associations and remember picture symbol sequences, a high-technology communication system that uses *Minspeak* software or Adaptive Communication System's *Dynavox* should be considered.

Nonspeaking persons who have orthographic symbol skills should have alphabet symbols incorporated into their communication systems. Individuals who are only able to identify letters and read simple sight words should have written orthography combined with picture symbols. Nonspeaking persons who are able to spell words need written alphabet symbols on their communication systems. The addition of picture symbols will depend on the person's ability to spell at a level commensurate with their receptive language level. If the individual is only able to communicate with a limited spelling vocabulary, picture symbols or whole written words should be added to the system.

Nonspeaking persons who can develop and remember encoded orthographic letter sequences are candidates for high-technology systems with alphabet abbreviation expansion capabilities. A dilemma occurs with individuals who are able to create and remember abstract picture symbol sequences and alphabet abbreviation expansion codes. The examiner and nonspeaking person will need to choose between these two symbol sequencing systems when selecting a communication aid. Information from this portion of the assessment can assist the examiner in making this decision. Some nonspeaking persons are able to develop and remember picture-encoding sequences better than letter-encoding sequences, and vice versa. If the nonspeaking person is equally adept at both strategies, a device with alphabet abbreviation expansion capabilities such as Adaptive Communication System's *RealVoice* should be given higher consideration. Light, Lindsey, Siegel, and Parnes (1990) compared use of picture-encoding strategies against letter-encoding strategies with 12 nonspeaking subjects. They found that 11 of the 12 subjects learned letter codes better than picture codes. In addition to these considerations, the final decision in selecting a communication aid symbol system rests with the nonspeaking person being evaluated. Nonspeaking persons functioning at this level should be given a choice in deciding which symbol system will best meet their needs.

Motor Accessing Skills

Prior to this stage of the evaluation the examiner has been collecting data to help determine what type of augmentative communication system will best meet a nonspeaking person's needs. By using that data, the examiner should be able to narrow the field of potential communication systems to one or two devices for final testing. The nonspeaking person's ability to motorically access the selected communication aids is then evaluated. This evaluation should always be done in conjunction with a professional trained to evaluate motor skills; usually a physical or occupational therapist. If a physically handicapped, nonspeaking person is not optimally positioned in a seating system, this portion of the assessment may need to be delayed until seating has improved. Chapter 3 in this book gives more information on optimizing seating and positioning for individuals who are physically handicapped.

When evaluating specific motor skills for accessing communication aids, direct selection methods of accessing should be considered before scanning methods. As mentioned previously, these methods are cognitively easier and motorically faster for most communication aid users. Direct selection methods that do not require accessing tools, such as a head stick or hand splint, should be considered first. Extra equipment adds an additional source of breakdown and repair to a communication system.

Direct Selection Evaluation Methods

Before using an augmentative communication system, the nonspeaking person should be given a brief demonstration of the device and accessing method. The individual should then be given time to try out the communication device and any accessing tools before formal evaluation occurs. Minor changes in positioning the communication aid and adjustments to accessing tools can be made at this time.

Once the nonspeaking person is familiar with the communication aid, the actual motor assessment can begin. The following motor components need to be assessed: **range of motion** with the communication aid, **pointing accuracy**, and **speed of pointing**. These motor components are evaluated across multiple trials that compare communication aid positioning, symbol size, and accessing methods. Individuals with high function can be asked to point to letters in alphabetical order as quickly and accurately as possible. Young nonspeaking persons can be asked to point to letters or pictures as they are dictated aloud. Nonspeaking persons who are unable to follow verbal directions can be shown where to point by the examiner. Timed trials are given and errors are recorded. In addition to noting accessing speed, the examiner should notice error patterns. Some individuals are accurate with symbols on one side of a communication aid but have difficulty reaching symbols on the other side. Others may fatigue and show more errors near the end of the trial, or show a practice effect with fewer errors as the trial progresses. Individuals who fatigue easily should be given adequate time to rest between trials.

Single Switch Evaluation Methods

Single switch skills need to be assessed if a scanning system is being considered. Several different switches should be evaluated as well as several different anatomical placement sites. Staff at Hugh Macmillan

Medical Center have developed the MSIP model of switch evaluation (Single Input Control Assessment, 1983). This model records data on movement necessary for switch activation (M), site of switch placement (S), interface or name of the switch being evaluated (I), and position of the nonspeaking person and switch (P).

Because operating a communication aid through a switch is cognitively difficult, the initial stages of switch assessment should be completed by attaching the switch to a simple cause–effect toy or to simple computer-based cause–effect switch games such as *Fire Organ* or *Interaction Games*. The individual should first be shown how the switch operates and told where the switch will be placed. The switch is then positioned and a brief trial period using the switch is given. If needed, physical guidance initially should be provided to assist in learning how to operate the switch. Once the nonspeaking person has had a chance to become comfortable with the switch, the evaluation can begin. For each switch that is evaluated, the examiner should record MSIP information. The examiner then assesses the user's ability to activate and release the switch across multiple trials. This can be done by simply asking the individual to activate and release the switch on command. Timing between commands should be varied so that the nonspeaking person cannot anticipate when the switch will need to be activated. The trials should continue for several minutes so that the effect of fatigue on switch performance can be evaluated.

Once a promising switch and anatomical site is found, further switch assessment is needed. Small changes in switch placement often produce major changes in performance. For example, a hand-operated Zygo *Tread Switch* can be placed on the surface of a wheelchair tray, recessed into the surface of the tray, mounted at a 45-degree angle, mounted sideways, or positioned above the surface of the tray. These options should be assessed to determine the ideal switch and switch placement.

The final step is attaching the switch to an augmentative communication aid. The nonspeaking person again should be shown how to use the switch to operate the communication aid. As in the direct selection evaluation, the user's ability to use the switch to indicate letter or picture symbols on command should be assessed. Timed trials should be given and error patterns recorded.

Summary of Evaluation Methods

A methodical evaluation process should result in an appropriate prescription for an augmentative communication system. The expressive language portion of the evaluation gives the examiner information on an individual's current communication methods and communication needs. The receptive language assessment gives information on his or her developmental level and rate of development. The augmentative communication symbol evaluation gives information on the specific symbolic skills necessary for using various communication aids. Information from these three assessment areas is used to select the augmentative communication systems with the best potential to meet a nonspeaking person's needs. Finally, the individual's ability to motorically operate the chosen communication system is evaluated. Individuals who are not severely physically handicapped often can complete the evaluation process in a few hours. Individuals with physical limitations may require several days to complete a thorough evaluation. If an individual is not adequately positioned, a seating evaluation should be completed before developing the final prescription for an augmentative communication system.

The final step in the evaluation process is assessing a nonspeaking person's ability to use the prescribed augmentative communication system in the real world through a series of performance trials (Yorkston & Karlan, 1986). If possible, augmentative communication aids should be loaned to a potential user for short-term use until performance trials are completed. Assessment methods used in the expressive language portion of the evaluation can be used for the performance evaluation. Performance trials are needed because they give the user an opportunity to show improvement on the communication system over time. In addition they allow the examiner to make adjustments in the communication system before seeking funding and finally purchasing the device.

SUMMARY

The components of augmentative communication aids and methods for evaluating their potential use by nonspeaking persons were reviewed in this chapter. Knowing what communication equipment is available and determining which system will work best for an individual nonspeaking person is only the beginning step of the augmentative communication process. In addition to considering aided modes of communication, the individual's ability to use unaided modes of communication such as gestures and head nods should also be considered. Most nonspeaking persons use aided communication modes less than 15 percent of the time (Glennen, 1989). This is partially due to the slow communication speeds of aided augmentative communication systems. It is always faster to point to an object than to spell out a message requesting the object. For most nonspeaking persons, aided modes of communication are used only to introduce new topics of conversation and to convey specific detailed information. Unaided modes are used to respond to old topics of conversation and to convey nonspecific information (Glennen, 1989).

No matter which mode of communication is used, nonspeaking persons need intensive augmentative communication training. They need to learn the mechanics of operating communication aids, memory strategies for recalling communication aid messages, and the pragmatic skills for interacting with others using the communication aid in conjunction with unaided modes of communication. Chapter 7 reviews guidelines and suggestions for training in school settings.

REFERENCES

Baker, B. (1982). Minspeak: A semantic compaction system that makes self-expression easier for communicatively disabled individuals. *Byte, 2,* 186–202.

Baker, B. (1986). Using images to generate speech. *Byte, 6,* 160–168.

Bliss, C. (1965). *Semantography.* Sydney, Australia: Semantography Publications.

Bolton S., & Dashiell, S. (1984). *Interaction checklist for augmentative communication (INCH).* Huntington Beach, CA: INCH Associates.

Buzolich, M. J. (1983). *Interaction analysis of augmented and normal adult communicators.* Unpublished doctoral dissertation, University of California at San Francisco.

Calculator, S., & Luchko, C. (1983). Evaluating the effectiveness of a communication board training program. *Journal of Speech and Hearing Disorders, 48,* 185–199.

Carlson, F. (1984). *Picsyms categorical dictionary.* Lawrence, KS: Baggeboda Press.

Carrow–Woolfolk, E. (1985). *Test of Auditory Comprehension of Language—Revised Edition.* Allen, TX: DLM Teaching Resources.

Dunn L., & Dunn, L. (1982). *Peabody Picture Vocabulary Test—Revised.* Circle Pines, MN: American Guidance Service.

Elder, P. (1987). Semantic compaction assessment. In *Proceedings Minspeak 1987.* Wooster, OH: Prentke Romich Company.

Farrier, L. M., Yorkston, K. M., Marriner, N. A., & Beukelman, D. R. (1985). Conversational control in non-impaired speakers using an augmentative communication system. *Augmentative and Alternative Communication, 1,* 65–73.

Foulds, R. (1980). Communication rates for nonspeech expression as a function of manual tasks and linguistic constraints. *Proceedings of the Third International Conference on Rehabilitation Engineering.* Washington, DC: RESNA.

Glennen, S. (1989). *The effect of communication aid characteristics on the interaction skills of nonspeaking persons and their adult speaking partners.* Unpublished doctoral dissertation, Pennsylvania State University, State College.

Glennen, S. (1990). *Augmentative communication assessment for children.* Unpublished paper, The Kennedy Institute, Baltimore, MD.

Goodenough–Trepagnier, C., & Prather, P. (1981). Communication systems for the non-vocal based on frequent phoneme sequences. *Journal of Speech and Hearing Research, 24,* 322–329.

Gunderson, J. R. (1985). Conversation aids for nonspeaking physically impaired persons. In J. G. Webster, A. M. Cook, W. J. Tompkins, & G. C. Vanderheiden (Eds.), *Electronic devices for rehabilitation.* New York: John Wiley.

Hammill, D., Brown, V., Larsen, S., & Wiederholt, J. (1980). *Test of Adolescent Language.* Austin, TX: Pro-Ed.

Johnson, R. (1985). *The picture communication symbols: Book II.* Solana Beach, CA: Mayer-Johnson.

Johnston, D. (1985). *Core picture vocabulary.* Wauconda, IL: Don Johnston Developmental Equipment.

Kirstein, I., & Bernstein, C. (1981). *Oakland schools picture dictionary.* Pontiac, MI: Oakland Schools Communication Enhancement Center.

Leff, S., & Leff, R. (1978). *Talking pictures.* Milwaukee, IL: Crestwood Company.

Light, J., Collier, B., & Parnes, P. (1985). Communicative interaction between young nonspeaking physically disabled children and their primary caregivers: Part I. Discourse patterns. *Augmentative and Alternative Communication, 1,* 98–107.

Light, J., Lindsay, P., Siegel, L., & Parnes, P. (1990). The effects of message encoding techniques on recall by literate adults using AAC systems. *Augmentative and Alternative Communication, 6,* 184–201.

McDonald E. T., & Schultz, A. R. (1973). Communication boards for cerebral palsied children. *Journal of Speech and Hearing Disorders, 38,* 223–228.

McNaughton, S. (1976). Bliss symbols: An alternate symbol system for the non-vocal pre-reading child. In G. Vanderheiden & K. Grilley (Eds.), *Non-vocal communication techniques and aids for the severely physically handicapped.* Baltimore, MD: University Press.

Newcomer, P., & Hammill, D. (1988). *Test of Language Development–2 Primary.* Austin, TX: Pro-Ed.

Owens, R. E. (1988). *Language development: An introduction.* Columbus, OH: Merrill.

Semel, E., Wiig, E., & Secord, W. (1987). *Clinical Evaluation of Language Functions—Revised.* San Antonio, TX: The Psychological Corporation.

Shane, H., & Wilbur, R. (1989, November). *Conceptual framework for AAC strategy based on sign language parameters.* Paper presented at The American Speech-Language-Hearing Association Convention, St. Louis, MO.

Single-Input Control Assessment. (1983). *Microcomputer applications programme. The Hugh MacMillan Medical Centre.* Wauconda, IL: Don Johnston Developmental Equipment.

Vanderheiden, G., & Lloyd, L. L. (1986). Communication systems and their components. In S. Blackstone & D. Ruskin, *Augmentative communication: An introduction.* Rockville, MD: ASHA Press.

Yorkston, K., Dowden, P., Honsinger, M., Marriner, N., & Smith, K. (1988). A comparison of standard and user vocabulary lists. *Augmentative and Alternative Communication, 4,* 189–210.

Yorkston, K., & Karlan, G. (1986). Assessment procedures. In S. Blackstone & D. Ruskin, *Augmentative communication: An introduction.* Rockville, MD: ASHA Press.

5

Adaptive Access for Microcomputers

■ Gregory Church, MS, MAS ■

Only a few decades after personal computers were first introduced, they have become an integral part of many people's lives, helping them to work, learn, communicate, and play. Until very recently, however, handicapped individuals whose impairments made it difficult or impossible to use standard computer keyboards and related equipment had few options for computer access. Over the past few years computers have become more affordable, easy to use, mainstreamed, and their potential benefits to disabled populations more widespread.

Children and adults with physical, sensory, speech, cognitive, behavior, and multiple impairments can now access microcomputer systems as a result of new and innovative assistive technology aids. These systems provide access to the vast majority of computer hardware and software already being used by nondisabled populations in home, school, and work settings. Microcomputers with appropriate adaptations can empower disabled individuals, provide them with independence, and offer tools with which they can realize their full potential.

To service providers, clients, and their families, microcomputers often seem incomprehensible as the result of constantly changing computer technologies and standards. The quantity and variety of these systems can often lead to confusion over the dynamics of emerging technologies, the associated technical jargon, and, most importantly, understanding what capabilities and advantages various technologies may hold for clients and service providers.

This chapter's intent is to provide readers with a general introduction to the wide array of microcomputer-based assistive technology systems available to disabled users. This introduction will encompass concepts and terminology associated with the function, adaptability, and integration of assistive devices with microcomputers. The reader also will be introduced to the assistive technology assessment process. The chapter will continue with the exploration of cognitive, sensory, motor, and related factors that have the potential to influence the design of technology solutions. After discussing these unique variables, the reader will then examine a diversity of computer access methods including, alternative keyboards, touch windows, voice recognition systems, and switch systems among others. A variety of adaptive output systems including screen magnification, braille, and speech output also will be discussed. A number of case histories are included to illustrate issues associated with the design and implementation of assistive technology solutions with disabled users. Finally, to make these technology systems easy to operate, readers will be provided with helpful methods for improving the design of the user interface.

THE TECHNOLOGY ASSESSMENT PROCESS

There are many complexities involved in implementing assistive microcomputer technology with disabled individuals. Gaining access to standard hardware, for example, is only one of a number of issues related to the assimilation of technology in the individual's life. Decisions about integration of microcomputer technology must be made by clinicians who are proficient with hardware devices, knowledgeable about software, and capable of making equipment adaptations as transparent to the user as possible.

Designing optimal assistive technology solutions begins with the identification of the user's needs. This is often done through informal or formal referrals, client observations, or client/family interviews. By detailing the individual's needs, clinicians can clarify the level of performance desired. As an example, a person with limited vision, or no usable vision, may have no way of independently taking notes and producing written copy for sighted peers or co-workers. Hence, they may need to gain access to auditory information from lectures, speeches, and meetings.

After identifying the client's needs, clinicians then determine the individual's present level of ability. Determining the person's existing strengths may be accomplished through informal and formal clinical testing, client and family interviews, patient observations, or by analysis by qualified related service staff. For example, the low-vision individual may require clinical testing for vision loss, testing for compensatory sensorimotor strengths, and educational testing for academic functioning. Depending on the complexity of the person's needs and the comprehensive nature of the service provider, technology services may involve a variety of assessments.

After testing determines actual patient performance, the clinician can evaluate the discrepancies between desired and actual performance. This discrepancy analysis provides the clinician with a fairly accurate picture of the client's "performance gap." The performance gap can then be refined into a problem statement. For instance, from the above example, the problem statement might be defined as: "As the result of a vision impairment the individual is unable to independently transcribe, store, and reproduce written output." The problem statement does not describe what technology intervention may be required to solve the client's problem. Instead, it simply helps the technologist focus attention on the specific characteristics of the problem itself.

Because the difference between the client's *desired performance* and *actual performance* can be significant, clinicians often must make pragmatic decisions regarding the viability of the client's performance gap. Specifically, professionals must use clinical experience and judgments to set realistic treatment goals. These pragmatic treatment goals should be discussed with the client and members of the client's support network. The practical examination of the client's problems and review of what solutions technology can offer will help to integrate caregiver goals with patient expectations. In addition, service providers, patients, and families must recognize that, although a performance gap might exist, it does not imply that the problem is a priority in the client's continuum of treatment, or that a "cure" or solution is possible, given certain technology confines, equipment costs, time restrictions, funding limitations, or other constraints.

After defining and identifying specific patient performance gaps, clinicians must determine if assistive technology can be an appropriate treatment approach. If applicable, service providers must identify which solution meets the individual's needs in a cost-effective manner. Equipment prescriptions often are based on functional tasks that the disabled user needs to perform on a regular basis. Too often, clients can be prescribed high-technology solutions when low-technology solutions can be more practical. A well-designed and integrated technology solution contributes to user comfort, motivation, productivity, and independence. A poorly conceived system may cause unnecessary fatigue, discomfort, and ultimately fall short of expected treatment goals. Before technology prescriptions are formulated, consideration should be given to how the client's individual profile affects the use of assistive technology devices.

ASSISTIVE TECHNOLOGY: ACCOMMODATING THE USER

Implicit in the design of technology solutions is recognition that one must first identify client factors that influence successful technology integration. These factors, in the broadest sense, refer to the interaction of the user, hardware, and software elements necessary to achieve a particular functionality. The breadth and exact nature of these factors will vary among different client populations. In fact, clear lines of demarcation are inevitably blurred; and, more importantly, the human and machine elements of a technology solution interact dynamically. Accordingly, the reader will be presented with broad, illustrative factors that can affect the client's use of assistive technology. Successful technology integration is most readily achieved with a team approach that includes an interdisciplinary perspective on client factors related to alternative technology solutions.

Assistive technology specialists are encouraged to request the neuropsychological, educational, and medical records of the person they intend to serve. It is wise to contact these disciplines for pragmatic interpretation of formal findings and recommendations for further treatment. This collection of medical, rehabilitative, and psychometric data will provide the necessary background and baseline for subsequent technology evaluations and treatment.

Cognitive Skills

Generally, cognition refers to the acquisition and use of knowledge. With regard to the use of technology devices, it is useful to address those cognitive factors that are important in assessing an individual's ability to interact successfully with hardware and software systems. To use adapted computers well, the user must first understand the procedural and cognitive skills associated with operating the adaptive computer interface. Human factors research has established that users vary in the efficiency of control across various computer access methods, and that some of this variation is related to cognitive demands of the interface and task (Cress & French, 1991; Karat, McDonald, & Anderson, 1985). For this reason, clinicians must carefully consider the patient's cognitive profile. The need for interdisciplinary programming is supported by the fact that cognitive problems can manifest themselves in a variety of handicapping conditions. The elements of cognition are not only important to special educators, but also to speech pathologists and occupational therapists, to name a few. For example, cognitive problems associated with memory and learning processes may hinder the mastery of computers that demand multi-step commands to operate. Cognitive problems related to organization and perceptual processing also can have a direct impact on the individual's abilities to use a computer-based speech aid.

There are many important interrelationships among the cognitive processes listed in Table 5-1. Because problems in one area of functioning often have implications in other cognitive areas, technology assessments must be thorough and systematic. In addition, because individual cognitive profiles in various handicapped populations can vary significantly, clinicians need to make careful, flexible interpretations of assessment results. Further, tests may need to be modified to examine cognitive and academic processing, particularly if perceptual or motor problems are present. Cognitive assessment modifications may include allowing different response modes, making directions more precise, enlarging print, reducing visual stimuli, or providing timed and untimed responses.

Whether the technology assessment is based on standardized cognitive tests, observations, or informal diagnostic probes, technologists must identify the individual's learning style, knowledge base, and related strengths. This information will identify the strategies persons will use to understand and discern the relationships between the access method, computer operation, and use of application software. By matching cognitive profiles with appropriate access methods, technologists can promote efficient operation and independent use of technology interventions.

Sensory Skills

In addition to cognitive factors, sensory problems also can affect an individual's ability to use technology. Most information is processed through visual and auditory channels (Batshaw & Perret, 1987). Therefore, the problems in any of these areas can seriously affect the client's ability to access and use microcomputers. For example, sensory difficulties can impede the client's ability to see, hear, or discriminate

Table 5-1. Cognitive and motor factors that affect assistive technology interventions.

Factors	Impact on Use of Technology
Cognitive Factors	
Attention deficits	Failure to follow screen prompts and directions
	Inability to consistently perform multi-step procedures
	Inability to filter information on busy screens
	Difficulty with large amounts of computer speech
Sensory deficits	Inability to separate command menus from other screen data
	Inability to track user information on rapidly changing screens
	Slow visual–motor dexterity
	Difficulty understanding computer speech
Memory deficits	Unable to complete multistep operations or device commands
	Unable to follow set-up directions
	Unable to locate and recall disk files
	Difficulty recalling knowledge of computer symbols and commands
Abstract reasoning and thinking deficits	Unable to analyze equipment procedures and generalize operations
	Unable to understand scanning methods
	Unable to build abstract symbol sets to infer selections or choices
	Unable to reproduce a sequence of operational tasks
Problem-solving deficits	Unable to operate device because of a hardware or software procedure problem
	Unable to use software or hardware rules to back out of an operation
	Unable to use device prompts or cues to accomplish task
	Unable to sequence steps to complete computer commands
Motor Factors	
Voluntary motor deficits	Inability to make deliberate switch and keyboard selections
	Limited control of trunk and extremities during movement

(continued)

Factors	Impact on Use of Technology
Motor Factors (continued)	
Voluntary motor deficits	Eye twitching resulting in overshooting the mark when reaching for objects Limits the ability to produce speech communication
Fixed-posture and positioning deficits	Limited hand positioning and stabilization for access to assistive devices & peripherals
Recurring purposeless motion	Accidental triggering of switches and keys Limited fine motor control in isolating symbol, key and button selections
Motor paralysis	Changes in muscle tone interfere with motor movements Spastic movements result in poor control and accidental selections Limited movement of arm, face, and leg Inhibits movement of arm, face, and leg
Low muscle tone	Loss of balanced muscle control in extremity for selection and stability
Rigidity	Inhibits arm and leg movements and good positioning
Spasticity	Limits full range of motion Reduces accurate and consistent motor movements for switch, key, and button selection
Tremors	Inhibits the precision of fine and gross motor precision selection tasks

sounds associated with a speech synthesizer, computer, keyboard, or switch.

Vision

Operating a standard personal computer is essentially a visual task, and vision impairments can cause significant difficulties in microcomputer access.

Blind users must augment the loss of vision with other sensory inputs. Users who have lost their vision later in life may tend to rely on speech as their information access strategy rather than braille. Individuals with congenital blindness, having more exposure to braille, may prefer to compose and review information in braille form or combinations of braille and speech. To use these sophisticated transcription aids, users who are visually impaired must have good short-term memory because letters are perceived one at a time and the blind person must mentally form the individual letters into words. Blindness may be an isolated disability or part of a multiply handicapping condition. The incidence of blindness in children with multiple handicaps is more than 200 times that found in the normal population (Warburg, Frederiksen, & Rattleff, 1979). With a multihandicapping condition, the technology approach must consider a more pervasive set of cognitive, sensory, and motor factors. In addition to a visual impairment, individuals may also experience problems in learning, mobility, language development, and functional independence.

Hearing

Assistive technology applications should consider the auditory information needs of users relative to one-to-one and group communications, telephone calls, meetings, lectures, and functional school- or job-related requirements. A hearing impairment can affect the individual's ability to interpret and operate home, school, and office equipment. For example, individuals who are hearing impaired may have difficulty determining the status of some computer operations, auditory prompts from application software, or auditory feedback from keyboard or switch input.

Because many children who are hearing impaired have additional handicaps, assistive technology applications must include provisions for dealing with related problems. Approximately one third of all children who are hearing impaired have multiple handicaps, and the rate is even higher among certain groups of children, such as those having hearing loss secondary to rubella (Meadow, 1980).

Motor Skills

In addition to cognitive and sensory factors, the patient's motor profile also profoundly affects the use of technology (see Table 5-1). Motor impairments influence independent movements and locomotion, reducing the individual's ability to control his or her environment. Motor deficits may range from mild impairment of fine volitional movements to severe paralysis causing a complete loss of functional ability. The variability of motor deficits can affect the reliability and efficiency of motor movements. The reliability of motor movement will affect the user's voluntary ability to operate a standard computer keyboard. In conjunction with the reliability of the motor movement, the efficiency of motor movement will also affect the individual's overall performance in the speed and endurance of computer operation.

Assistive technology is regularly prescribed for individuals with many types of developmental and acquired motor disabilities. Although a wide variety of disabilities can cause motor dysfunction and paralysis, positioning can make a critical difference in the individual's ability to use technology aids. In addition to providing comfort and stability, proper seating and positioning can influence the quality of a person's motor movement. For specific strategies on improving patient seating and positioning, readers are encouraged to consult Chapter 3.

The severity of an individual's motor problems can dictate the use of a wide variety of assistive technology options. If motor dysfunction is permanent, technology strategies may focus on helping the individual compensate for lost functions. For example, the transfer of handwriting requirements to a nondominant or noninvolved hand may be a time-consuming and fatiguing process for the disabled student. Instead, the implementation of a laptop computer with word processing may be considered when impaired motor functions negatively affect the student's writing and academic progress.

Mild motor deficits may be augmented with systems that support existing functions. An occupational therapist may provide a hand splint so that the user's thumb is held in an abducted position and the wrist in a neutral position, increasing the functional use of the hand for keyboard selection activities.

Related User Factors

In addition to cognitive, sensory, and motor variables, a number of other related factors also affect the design of technology solutions. These factors include the knowledge and experience of the user's support network, the complexity of the technology system, and the individual's operational environment.

The existing technical knowledge base of the user's support network is of prime concern when evaluating alternative technology systems. In some instances, a technology solution may require the assistance of the user's caregivers or paraprofessionals. In these settings, nurses or teachers' aides are most often the caregivers. These individuals are often asked to work with patients and their equipment in a variety of self-help and instructional situations. Therefore, technology evaluations should also consider the knowledge and skills the client and/or caregiver will require for successful use and maintenance of technology aids. In addition, there may be attitudes that must be dealt with before learning and understanding can take place. For example, some caregivers who are afraid of computers often have difficulty learning to use or accept the technology. Past convictions and biases can affect the acceptance of technology aids.

The research on use of one-shot inservice sessions to train caregivers and paraprofessionals rarely has shown significant effects (Joyce & Showers, 1980). Technology training programs should be designed around skills necessary for proper setup, use, maintenance, and storage of technology equipment. The effectiveness of client and caregiver training has a major impact on the success of technology interventions. Follow-up site visits to the client's school or workplace can help identify training weaknesses, aid in equipment troubleshooting, encourage user feedback, and provide additional practice and coaching for clients and caregivers. Videotaping and developing user summary sheets are also helpful in the training process.

The assimilation of microcomputer components also can influence the design and implementation of technology. Computer systems require the support of both hardware and software to operate. The interaction of these elements often can lead to multiple complexities. The configuration of the computer system unit, disk drives, and peripheral devices, along with other special adaptations, plays an important part in how a technology solution is designed. In general, good technology solutions are made as transparent to the user as possible. By insulating users from irrelevant technical complexities, technology systems can help users perform complex tasks in the simplest, most familiar, and most meaningful way possible. However, simplicity on the outside usually does not translate into a simple internal computer system. Generally, just the opposite is true. Thoughtful advance planning of the user interface can alleviate many potential problems. Incorporating automatic sequences, creating user friendly menus, color coding keys, or creating simplified mnemonics are only a few examples of methods that can improve user interaction with assistive technology devices.

Before technologists design solutions to meet the needs of disabled individuals, they must first know something about the individuals they are designing them for and the environment in which the equipment will be used. Service providers need to know the user's profile: cognitive level, sensory and motor impairments, background in using computers, ability to function as an independent thinker and operator, and interests and attitudes toward computers. Effective clinicians usually try to determine the difference between what a realistic user does not know, what the user should know, and what the user realistically wants to know.

The patient's environment is another factor that influences the design of assistive technology applications. Environmental variables such as space considerations, noise, lighting, acoustics, power sources, transportation regulations, storage, or security may have an impact on technology solutions. For example, glare from ceiling lights may affect an individual's ability to see the computer monitor or may cause undue eye fatigue. The placement and storage of computer equipment may require adjustment to optimize user performance. Integrating appropriate computer peripherals within the client's workspace may require adjustment or redesign to accommodate wheelchairs or related equipment (Church & Bender, 1989; Mandal, 1982).

User Skills and Microcomputer Access

An **access method** is defined as what the user does to send commands or characters to the microcomputer. Pressing a key on the keyboard, for example, is an access method. A wide variety of other access methods are available to disabled children and adults. In general, access methods are organized into two broad catagories: (1) direct and (2) indirect selection methods.

Direct selection methods allow the user to indicate a choice by pointing with a body part or technology aid to make the selection. This may be accomplished, for instance, with the use of a finger, hand, or other body part. Similarly, technology aids such as a light pointer or mouth stick may be used in place of the body part. Direct selection is a very efficient method of entering information into the computer. This strategy provides the user with a straightforward approach to sending commands to the computer, but it also requires accurate and consistent motor control.

Indirect selection techniques include intermediate steps between indicating the choice and actually sending the command or character to the computer. The intermediate step, or steps, generally add to the complexity and time necessary to indicate choices and make selections. As a result, indirect access methods are generally much slower than direct select methods when entering data.

To accomplish indirect selection tasks, users augment their available motor skills with an input device and a supporting selection scheme. A variety of input devices are available to help users make selections. These include switches, light pointers, touch tablets, and joysticks, to name a few. A supporting selection scheme is the "intermediate" step in sending commands to the computer. Basically, these schemes replicate the computer's keyboard characters using visual or auditory formats. A wide variety of selection schemes are available to accommodate different client cognitive and sensorimotor profiles. For example, a selection scheme may appear on the computer monitor as a graphic image of a keyboard, a textual scanning array of keyboard characters, or as talking menus of computer commands.

The selection of an appropriate computer access method for an individual user can be a confusing process, especially when one investigates how the user's cognitive, motor, and related factors interact and influence technology alternatives.

Figure 5–1 provides a general hierarchical listing of direct and indirect access methods available for use with disabled populations. The hierarchy is not a strict interpretation of how access methods should be prescribed. Clearly, an adult may find single switch access very functional for operating a business computer. A young toddler may find a standard keyboard appropriate for learning the alphabet on a computer. Instead, the hierarchy provides a perspective on how computer access methods compare across broad cognitive and motor dimensions. For example, **alternative keyboards** often incorporate simplified keyboard layouts of expanded or reduced sets of letters, numbers, or symbols. This often makes the keyboard less complex and easier for the individual to understand and use. In addition, adaptive keyboard overlays often make these devices more accessible to individuals with motor impairments. At the other end of the adaptive computer access spectrum are various switch input techniques. These indirect selection methods are often used by persons with severe motor impairments who are unable to access the standard keyboard. For example, **switch encoding** is a process by which the user sends commands to the

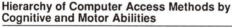

Hierarchy of Computer Access Methods by Cognitive and Motor Abilities

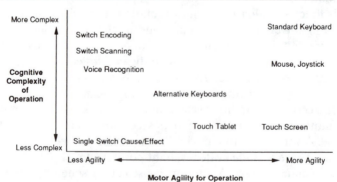

Figure 5–1

Hierarchy of microcomputer access methods by cognitive and motor abilities.

computer through an alternative set of symbols. Morse code is an example of a switch encoding method. Switch encoding methods require just one consistent, controllable body movement to operate. However, a higher level of operational understanding is necessary to utilize the method successfully. The user must have the cognitive ability to understand the symbolic representations associated with the codes as well as the ability to memorize the coding system.

MICROCOMPUTER ACCESS METHODS

The following sections will provide the reader with practical information on the concepts associated with the design and use of specific computer access methods. It is important to understand that all access methods have strengths and weaknesses. In addition, the level of compatibility with standard software and hardware can vary among access alternatives. The term **transparency** is used to describe an access device's level of compatibility with standard computer hardware and software. A device is transparent when it can send information directly to the computer without having to make any modifications to the standard application software. Because the level of transparency varies across assistive technology aids, software and hardware conflicts sometimes result when adaptive devices are used with standard software.

To illustrate ways in which technology solutions are designed and implemented, examples of case histories will be presented at the end of major sections. The individuals selected for inclusion in this chapter are typical of clients using assistive technology in school, vocational, and business settings. The cases, however, are not intended to be viewed as model solutions that can be transferred and applied to other individuals. Rather, they are examples of how various cognitive, sensorimotor, physical, and related factors affect the design and use of technology with disabled children and adults.

Standard Keyboards

Microcomputers usually are configured with standard keyboards for data input. The **keyboard** is a collection of keys and special controls used for typing information into the computer. Two styles of keyboard layout are commonly used with microcomputers: Qwerty, or Sholes, keyboard and Dvorak, or American Simplified keyboard (see Figure 5-2). The Qwerty keyboard, named for the first six letters in the top row of letter keys, is the most commonly used keyboard layout in the United States. The Dvorak keyboard arranges the keys to increase typ-

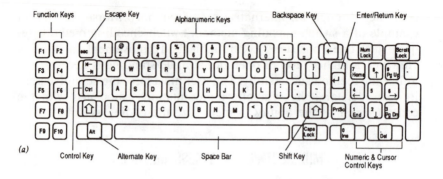

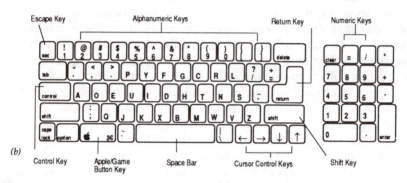

Figure 5-2

(a) IBM keyboard with Qwerty layout. This keyboard layout, the most commonly used system in the United States, is named for the first six letters in the top row of letter keys. (b) Apple IIgs keyboard with Dvorak layout. This layout is designed to increase typing speed and efficiency by locating the keys used most often in the home row.

ing speed and efficiency by locating the most frequently used keys in the home row.

In addition to keyboard layout, the size, number, and function of keys can vary from computer to computer. For example, IBM and compatible desktop computers often use 101-key enhanced keyboards that include 12 function keys on the top of the keyboard. The IBM 5151 keyboard has 10 function keys located on the right side of the keyboard. The AT-style 5060 keyboard is similar to the 5151 but incorporates enlarged Enter and Shift keys. Apple II Plus computers have uppercase-only keys, whereas the Apple IIgs computer includes uppercase and lowercase keys and a numeric keypad. Many laptop and notebook computers also use different types of keyboards. For example, many laptop systems must work in 11- or 12-inch space constraints. The space limitations often require compromises. Some manufacturers do away with separate keyboard function, cursor, numeric, or page-control keys. Some vendors even lower the height of the key caps and shorten the key travel from the standard 3.5 mm to 2 mm to help keep the laptop's case compact.

Effective use of a computer by disabled children and adults may require adaptations to the standard keyboard. The simplest augmentation of the standard keyboard is the use of **alternative stickers** to mark special keys. The stickers' markings can be color-coded, enlarged keyboard letters, alternative symbol sets, or even special tactile stickers. Don Johnston Developmental Equipment's *Large Print Key Labels* allow users to add large letters to standard keyboards for easier key recognition by young children or people with visual impairments.

Moisture guards are clear plastic overlays that protect the standard keyboard's surface and electronic components from excessive dust, liquids, or client drooling. Don Johnston Equipment, TASH, and Computability, Inc., sell clear, flexible moisture guards that protect keyboards from dust, moisture, and liquids. These moisture guards are available for a wide variety of computer systems.

Keyguards can be used to augment a client's motor skills when using a standard keyboard. This hardware device covers the standard keyboard and provides stability and direction for fingers or prods. A keyguard also allows the user to slide a finger or headstick over the surface without accidentally activating keys. Don Johnston Equipment, TASH, Computability, Adaptive Communication Systems, Prentke Romich, and REACH sell keyguards for Apple and IBM systems.

Other modifications to the standard keyboard involve the use of utility software or hardware to change the keystroke responses of the keyboard. For example, **auto-repeat defeat** software eliminates the automatic repeat feature of standard keyboards. For users with limited fine motor control who make frequent, uncontrollable key presses, auto-repeat defeat software eliminates unwanted repetition of keystrokes. Kinetic Design's *Filch,* Ability Systems Corporation's *KeyUp,* and Trace Center's *One-Finger* are auto-repeat defeat software programs designed for use with IBM and compatible computer systems. The Apple *IIgs* and Macintosh computers have built-in facilities to eliminate unintentional key repeats.

One-finger access software is another method to augment the standard keyboard. This utility software supports multiple key-latching for persons who type with a single finger or other pointing device. These utilities lock the Shift, Enter, Command, Alternate, and other keys so users can perform a series of simultaneous keystrokes. Kinetic Design's *Filch,* TASH's *Keylatch,* Trace Center's *One-Finger* and DADA's *PC Assisted Keyboard* are examples of one-finger access software.

Finally, **redefinition** software offers the ability to redefine the functional operation and layout of standard keyboard keys. This class of utility can relocate one or more keys on the standard keyboard to more appropriate locations for users who have a limited range of movement. DADA's *PC Assisted Keyboard* is an example of an **IBM** and compatible redefinition utility software program.

Table 5–2 lists adaptive access considerations involving the design and use of standard computer keyboards.

Tavon: Make It Simple, Make It Work

Tavon sustained a traumatic closed-head injury in a motor vehicle accident during "senior week" of his last year in high school. Tavon spent a total of 38 days in the hospital. Following his discharge from the hospital, Tavon was able to speak and walk, but continued to experience problems with short-term memory and had poor fine-motor control. He had been previously accepted at a four-year college in another state for the fall semester. By the end of the summer, Tavon was still determined to enter a community college. Tavon and his parents pursued assistive technology services to help him keep up with coursework and assignments.

Clinicians used various formal assessments in memory and academic achievement. Tavon was also evaluated by the team's occupational therapist. The various technology assessments identified mild short-term memory problems and residual motor problems in the upper limbs, giving him one good hand for typing activities. In dis-

Table 5–2. Design considerations for standard keyboards.

---

1. What cognitive, sensory, motor, and related factors have an impact on the client's use of the standard keyboard?
2. Does the client have functional range of movements across the standard keyboard?
3. Are the size, spacing, and tactile feel of keys appropriate for access?
4. Is the keyboard layout appropriate?
5. Can keyboard redefinition software remap the keyboard layout?
6. Does the client have a resting position on the keyboard?
7. Does the user accidentally trigger keys?
8. Can a keyguard improve access and reduce accidental key triggering?
9. Can repeat/defeat software improve access and reduce accidental key triggering?
10. Is simultaneous key support (one-finger access software) required for one-finger or headstick users?
11. Can macros, abbreviation-expansion, or word prediction software reduce the number of keystrokes required by the user?

---

cussions with Tavon and his parents, the technology team identified the need for portable written communication with specific software techniques for improving memory. In addition, Tavon and his parents stressed the need for simple solutions that could be easily set up and managed by Tavon while away at college.

In support of Tavon's needs, the team recommended an MS-DOS compatible laptop computer with a standard keyboard for Tavon. His fine motor deficits necessitated augmentation of the laptop's 11-inch Qwerty keyboard. First, a keyguard was added to stabilize his hand and to reduce accidental key selections. Similarly, Tavon's motor deficits required one-finger operation and a method of eliminating unwanted repeat characters when he had difficulty removing his finger from the keyguard. Finally, the laptop's editing keys were located in awkward locations, and Tavon wanted them relocated.

The technology solution called for redefinition, one-finger access, and auto-repeat defeat software. Tavon needed software that had the ability to redefine the functional operation of specific function keys on the keyboard. In addition, Tavon required one-finger access so that he could make multiple key combinations sequentially one at a time. Lastly, auto-repeat defeat software was added so he could only generate keyboard characters on the upstroke of the key, eliminating unwanted repeating keys. DADA Foundation's *PC Assisted Keyboard* software was used to redefine the text editing keys, provide one-finger access to the keyboard, and add auto-repeat defeat features. Because these software utilities operate as TSR programs (memory resident software), Tavon could benefit from their use in word processing, education, and related software applications.

Computer assisted instruction also was included in Tavon's prescription. A series of software programs dedicated to memory treatment also were recommended for Tavon to practice memory development skills. Suggested software applications included Life Science Associates *COGREHAB Volume 3.*

Alternative Keyboards

An **alternative keyboard** is a peripheral that consists of a matrix of keys or switches that replace or supplement the standard microcomputer keyboard. Alternative keyboards address access problems by reducing or enlarging the size of the keys. Expanded and minikeyboards commonly are used as viable options for computer access.

Expanded keyboards are a type of alternative keyboard that provides an enlarged key surface area for the user to input data. These keyboards are usually fabricated with a matrix of touch-sensitive membrane switches. The size of the keyboard's matrix can range from 30 to

128 switches in roughly 1 x 1 inch sizes. The size of the keys is determined by how the user groups the membrane switches. The keyboard can be customized to suit individual needs. In this way, individual membrane switches can be grouped together to form larger keys to assist users with severe motor problems or individuals who are cognitively unable to operate a standard keyboard.

Another type of alternative keyboard is a **minikeyboard.** These keyboards provide a smaller key surface area for the user to enter data. These systems are also manufactured with a matrix of touch-sensitive membrane switches. The matrix of switches can range from 60 to 128 switches in roughly ½ x ½ inch sizes. However, unlike expanded keyboards, minikeyboards are designed for individuals who have limited range of motion as well as limited motor strength. The keyboard also can be used effectively by head- and mouth-stick users, as it reduces the requirements for head and neck movement.

Other alternative keyboards use standard keyboard designs but decrease the activation force required to select keys or alter the physical location of the keys on the keyboard surface (see Figure 5–3). Whatever the design approach, alternative keyboards are versatile and useful access methods that can accomodate users with severe motor impairments or cognitive limitations. Unicorn Engineering, Inc., manufactures three clear acrylic keyguards for its expanded keyboards. The *32-Hole, 64-Hole,* and *128-Hole Keyguards* attach to the expanded keyboard and isolate each key to help the user make more accurate choices.

The operation of alternative keyboards differs somewhat depending on the type of computer and interface the client is using. For example, some alternative keyboards require no additional interface cards to operate the computer. These systems plug straight into the computer's keyboard port and need no special interface or software to operate. As a result, these keyboards are very easy to install on microcomputers. Examples of these alternative keyboards include EKEG Electronics Ltd.'s *Expanded Keyboards* (Apple II series, Macintosh, and IBM PCs and PS/2); In Touch Systems' *Magic Wand Keyboard* (IBM PCs); Parallel System's *Keasyboard* (Apple IIe); and TASH's *PC Mini-Keyboard* and *PC King Keyboard* (IBM PCs and PS/2).

Other alternative keyboards cannot communicate directly with a microcomputer and must rely on the use of an additional interface device to operate. These interfaces are referred to as keyboard emulators. A **keyboard emulator** is a hardware device that connects to the computer and allows input from a source other than the standard keyboard. A keyboard emulator may be configured as an interface card that plugs into an expansion slot or as a box which plugs into a port on the back of the computer. A few examples of alternative keyboards that require keyboard emulators include:

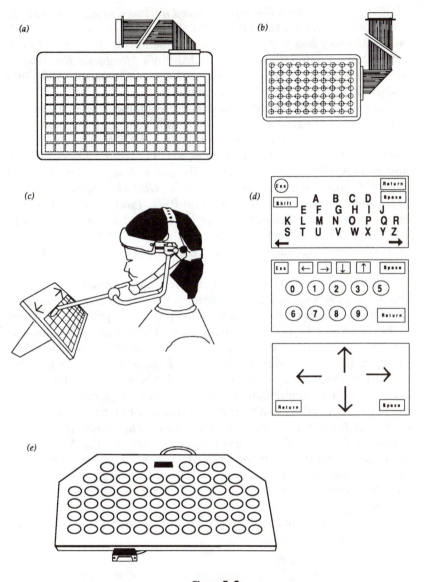

Figure 5–3

Alternative keyboards replace or operate in addition to the standard keyboard. (a) Expanded keyboards have a matrix of touch-sensitive squares that can be grouped together to form larger squares. (b) Minikeyboards are small keyboards with a matrix of closely spaced touch-sensitive squares. (c) The small size of a minikeyboard ensures that a small range of movement is needed to access the entire keyboard. (d) Expanded and minikeyboards use standard or customized keyboard overlays. (e) Some alternative keyboards plug directly into the keyboard jack of the computer, needing no special interface or software.

Unicorn Engineering's *Unicorn Expanded Keyboard Model II* and *Model 510* (Apple II series, Macintosh, IBM, Tandy, MS-DOS compatibles); ACS's *Memkey Board* (Apple II series, Macintosh, IBM PCs, Tandy, MS-DOS compatibles); and ComputAbility's *Membrane Keyboard II* and *Mini-Membrane Keyboard* (Apple II series, Macintosh, IBM PCs and PS/2, Tandy, MS-DOS compatibles).

A number of keyboard emulators are available to operate alternative keyboards. Examples are: Don Johnston's *Adaptive Firmware Card Model G32* and *G32e* (Apple IIgs and IIe) and *KE:NX* (Apple Macintosh); DADA's *PC A.I.D., DADA Entry,* and *PC Serial A.I.D.* (IBM PCs and MS-DOS compatibles); Dunamis, Inc.'s *Power^n* (IBM PCs and MS-DOS compatibles); ComputAbility's *AID+Me* (Apple II series, Macintosh, Commodore,IBM PCs and PS/2, Tandy); Madenta Communications, Inc.'s *ScreenDoors* (Apple Macintosh); Trace Center's *T-TAM* (Apple IIgs, Macintosh, IBM PCs and MS-DOS compatibles); and Words+ *Expanded Keyboard Emulator* (IBM PCs and MS-DOS compatibles).

Alternative keyboards that comprise a programmable matrix of touch-sensitive switches usually require the use of special overlays. **Overlays** are paper representations of the physical layout and function of the alternative keyboard's matrix of keys. The design and creation of custom overlays can be simplified with use of utility software. For example, Unicorn Engineering's *Overlay Express* is an Apple II series software package that allows users to design new overlays by adding color pictures, communication symbols, words, or phrases to custom overlays. The overlays can be printed using a dot matrix or laser printer. Mayer-Johnston Company's *The Communication Board-Builder* and *Boardmaker* are board-making software programs for the Apple Macintosh computer that help construct overlays for communication aids and expanded and minikeyboards. These software programs also include a wide variety of pictures which can be used to build custom overlays.

Table 5–3 lists adaptive access considerations in the design and use of alternative keyboards.

Annette: Developing Expressive Language Skills

Annette is a 4-year-old who has normal gross motor, visual-perceptual, and nonverbal cognitive skills, but whose expressive language is delayed. The classroom teacher was concerned about Annette's difficulty expressing herself despite her adequate oral motor abilities for speech. Assistive technology team members evaluated Annette's psychoeducational skills, receptive language, and expressive language to obtain a profile of her strengths and weaknesses. The team found that

Table 5–3. Design considerations for alternative keyboards.

1. What cognitive, sensory, motor, and related factors have an impact on the client's use of the alternative keyboard?

2. Does the client have functional range of movement for accessing expanded or mini-keyboards?

3. Are the size, spacing, sensitivity, and tactile feel of keys appropriate for access?

4. Does the alternative keyboard require a keyboard emulator? Can the computer accommodate the expansion interface? What cables are necessary for connection?

5. What software can be used with the alternative keyboard? Does the software require a customized or redefined keyboard overlay? Ar commercial overlay setups available?

6. Can customized or redefined keyboard layouts be saved to disk for later use?

7. Can the user avoid accidental key triggering?

8. Can a keyguard improve access?

9. Can repeat-defeat software improve access?

10. Is simultaneous key support (one-finger access software) required for one-finger or wand users?

11. Can macros, abbreviation-expansion, or word prediction software improve keyboard performance?

her receptive language skills were mildly delayed to a 3-year, 6-month-old level. Her expressive language was severely delayed to a 2-year-old level. She was able to produce over 30 single words but was not producing any two-word combinations. All other skill areas were normal for her age.

The technology team implemented a plan for using computers as a supplement to Annette's traditional language-learning play methods. The team felt that the computer was another medium for play activities to stimulate language. An alternative keyboard and keyboard emulator were included in the technology solution, specifically, Unicorn Engineering's *Unicorn Expanded Keyboard Model II* and Don Johnston's *Adaptive Firmware Card Model G32* were used with W. K. Bradford Publishing Co.'s *Explore-a-Story Software Series.* During language-learning play, Annette would have to label objects and actions in the stories and put simple phrases together before she could animate and move objects around the computer screen. A printer was used so that Annette could print out pictures of her stories to take home and label for her mother. The software and keyboard were motivating for Annette and reduced irrelevant key functions.

Mark: Using A Dedicated Communicator
for Written Communication

Mark is a 14-year-old with choreoathetoid cerebral palsy. This form of cerebral palsy is marked by variable muscle tone and involuntary movements of the arms and legs (Batshaw & Perret, 1987). In addition, Mark's cerebral palsy affects his oral motor skills, resulting in a speech motor disability known as dysarthria. Except for a few single words, he is unable to communicate using speech.

Mark currently attends a class for children who are multiply handicapped. The school provides him with a one-to-one aide for note taking; and he uses a *Light Talker* augmentative communication aid for his communication needs. Mark's parents and teachers were interested in having him develop some independence in generating written material such as personal letters, reports, and homework tasks. Testing indicated that Mark has mild mental retardation with scattered reading and math skills.

The technology team, school personnel, teachers, and Mark's parents decided to use Mark's *Light Talker* as both a communication aid and an alternative keyboard. This approach benefits from Mark's understanding and successful use of his *Light Talker*. In addition, prestored messages in the *Light Talker* could produce written output. This approach required a keyboard emulator that would connect to the school's Apple *IIe* microcomputer. Either Don Johnston's *Adaptive Firmware Card* or Prentke Romich's *AKI-IIE* interface card are appropriate for connecting the *Light Talker* to the Apple *IIe* computer. The technology team added various Apple *IIe* specific keyboard commands to Mark's *Light Talker*. These commands would be sent out the *Light Talker's* serial port into the Apple IIe computer, allowing him full access and control of the computer.

In addition, Scholastic's *Bank Street Writer III* word processing software was used for writing assignments. The software's integrated spelling checker and thesaurus supplemented Mark's weak spelling skills. Finally, in order to achieve maximum efficiency and accelerated entry of text, Zygo's Apple II series *Abbreviation Expansion* software was included in the technology solution. This software allows Mark to independently define, edit, and store appropriate words and phrases and then recall them using two- or three-letter abbreviations. Using this method, Mark could rapidly retrieve words and phrases in conjunction with his word processor.

Touch Screens and Touch Tablets

The **touch screen** is a peripheral device that senses the position of a finger or prod on a display screen. The touch screen's intuitive input process makes the technology a very natural and direct method for users to interact with microcomputers (see Figure 5–4). The touch screen's input process requires a contact with the screen's surface. The position is converted into X–Y coordinates (horizontal and vertical positions of the contact point), which are then sent to the computer via an interface. A software program then interprets the coordinates and converts them into movements for the screen's cursor or pointer. The movements can be interpreted to select menus, text, or even draw graphics on the computer screen.

Two common touch screen technologies now in use include **light-emitting diode** (LED) and **capacitive** devices. The light-emitting diode touch screen consists of arrays of LEDs and light-sensing diodes. The LEDs emit a continuous beam of invisible light. The light-sensing di-

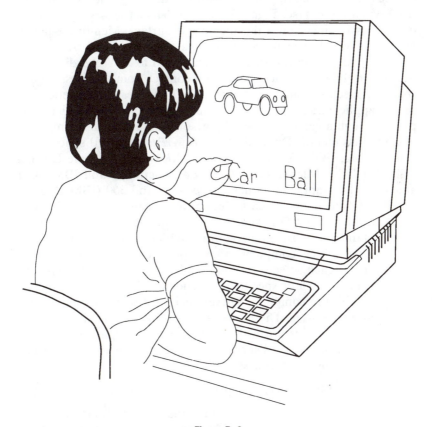

Figure 5–4

Touch windows allow a person to generate input to a computer by pressing on the screen's surface.

odes receive the light beams and complete a circuit. When an object interrupts a pair of invisible light beams, the circuit is broken and X–Y coordinates are computed at the break point. Capacitive touch screens utilize the user's pointer to complete a circuit on the touch screen's surface. The screen contains two or more transparent sheets that have the ability to conduct electricity. When a pointer applies pressure to the sheets, the conductive surfaces contact and complete the circuit. The contact point represents the X–Y coordinates. Touch screens can be connected to the computer through a serial port, game port, interface card, or built into the computer monitor. Examples of touch screens include Edmark Corporation's *TouchWindow* (Apple II, Acorn, Atari, Commodore, IBM PC, and Tandy); Microtouch's *Mac 'n Touch,* and *Clear Tek 1000* (Macintosh, IBM, and Amiga); and IBM's *InfoWindow Display* (IBM PCs and PS/2).

Another popular input device is the touch tablet. This peripheral can be used for operating games, painting, drawing, and even alternative keyboard input (see Figure 5–5). A **touch tablet** senses the positions of a stylus or finger on a flat membrane surface. Membrane tablets consist of two electrically conductive surfaces separated by nonconductive spacers. The two surfaces correspond to X–Y coordinate values. When the two surfaces come into contact from the pressure of a stylus, an electrical circuit is completed. The values are converted and sent to application software. The tablet is connected to the microcomputer through a game port, serial port, or interface card. Examples of touch tablets include Dunamis, Inc.'s *PowerPad* (Apple II series, Atari, Commodore, IBM); Koala Technologies' *Koala Pad* (Apple II series and IBM PCs); MicroTouch's *UnMouse* (Macintosh and IBM PCs); and Polytel Computer Products' *Keyport 60* and *300* (IBM PCs).

Touch screen and touch tablet hardware can operate at different levels of tranparency. For example, some touch tablets are designed to replace standard mouse input, requiring a high degree of transparency between the tablet, computer, and applications software. In other applications, touch screens or touch tablets may require the application software to include specific instructions that enable each to communicate with the computer. These special software instructions are called **software drivers.** These programs manage the details of microcomputer communication with an input or an output device.

Table 5–4 provides a list of adaptive access considerations when evaluating the use of touch screens and tablets.

Shateka: Independence through Control

Shateka is a 7-year-old with mental retardation who functions at a 3-year, 4-month level with an IQ of 52. She currently attends a class for children with moderate retardation. Shateka's teachers suggested the

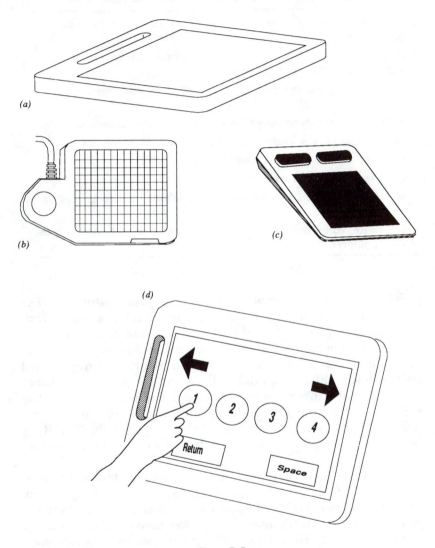

Figure 5-5
Touch tablets are touch-sensitive alternate input devices that replace or operate in addition to the standard keyboard. (a) Some touch tablets are designed with large 12 x 12-inch surfaces so users can define large active areas as buttons or keys. (b) Touch tablets also can replace or emulate standard mouse input. (c) Touch tablets can be designed with small 4 x 4-inch surfaces for individuals with limited range of movement. (d) Touch tablets often use overlays. An overlay defines active button areas on the tablet and assigns a keystroke to each button.

Table 5–4. Design considerations for touch screens and touch tablets.

---

1. What cognitive, sensory, motor, and related factors have an impact on the client's use of the touch screen or touch tablet?

2. Does the client have the motor control and functional range of movements to access a touch screen or touch tablet?

3. Are the size, spacing, sensitivity, and tactile feel of the touch tablet's keys appropriate for access?

4. Is the application software compatible with the touch tablet or touch screen?

5. Can the touch tablet or touch screen be used with keyboard emulators?

6. Can touch tablet users avoid accidental key triggering?

7. Can a keyguard improve access to the touch tablet?

8. Is simultaneous key support (one-finger access software) required for one-finger or wand users?

9. Can macros, abbreviation-expansion, or word prediction software improve touch tablet performance?

---

possibility of using computers during classroom instruction. The school pursued technology services to help formulate an individualized education plan for Shateka. The school was interested in using stimulus discrimination and simple learning in the design of individualized computer-assisted instruction with Shateka. To date, school staff reported that she had difficulties using the standard keyboard and the school's current library of educational software. Teachers were very interested in computer learning activities that could provide her with some independent learning activities. Options that relied on pointing yet simplified the cognitive demands of using the computer were explored.

The technology team and school staff decided to use the classroom's Apple *IIe* computer, a speech synthesizer, and a touch screen. The keyboard was eliminated from Shateka's interaction with the computer. Instead, Edmark's *TouchWindow* was used for direct pointing and selection tasks. The computer also incorporated Street Electronic's *Echo II speech synthesizer* for auditory cuing and feedback. Because of the cognitive difficulties associated with prompting, making selections, and concentrating on instructional tasks, Shateka's software applications needed to have the ability to adjust presentation speed, feedback mechanisms, lesson content, and presentation format. Finally, the software had to be compatible with the *TouchWindow*. Laureate Software's *Creature Chorus* and *First Words* were selected for use with Shateka. The *Creature Chorus* program was a motivating, cause–effect training game for introducing the *TouchWindow*. The games introduced the concepts of cause–effect, visual tracking, and discrete point-ing. The *First Words* program provided instruction in beginning vocab-ulary and categorization.

If Shateka's teachers wish to run Apple II series software not spe-cifically written for the *TouchWindow,* Don Johnston Developmental Equipment's *AFC Access TouchWindow* and *Adaptive Firmware Card Model G32* or *G32e* will allow the software to run with the touch screen.

Mouse and Joystick Systems

The function of the **mouse** is to point and select menu items, text, and graphic objects on the computer screen. The mouse is a small box that is connected to the computer through a serial port or internal expan-sion card (see Figure 5-6). The mouse is designed to move across a flat surface. As the mouse moves, corresponding movement of a pointer appears on the screen. Motion detectors read mouse movements using mechanical or optical methods. For example, a mechanical mouse sys-tem uses a ball bearing on the bottom of the mouse to control two motion detectors. The signals from the motion detectors feed X–Y coordinates to the computer. The X–Y coordinates represent two-dimensional placement of the pointer or cursor on the screen. Alterna-tively, optical mouse systems use light to detect direction and motion. LEDs and light detectors measure changes in the light source. The measurements are then converted into X–Y coordinates that represent direction and motion of the screen's pointer.

If motor problems limit an individual who is physically disabled from using a mouse, assistive technology aids are available to replace the function of the mouse. These aids are referred to as mouse emula-tors (see Figure 5-6). A **mouse emulator** usually consists of an alternate access method which replaces the physical movement tasks associated with the mouse; these can include large or small membrane boards, expanded or minikeyboards, or switches. In addition, the mouse emu-lator provides the user with an alternative selection scheme for pointer or cursor control. Examples of mouse emulators include Don John-ston Developmental Equipment's *KE:NX* (Macintosh); TASH Inc.'s *Mouse Emulator* (Macintosh) and Unicorn Engineering's *Mousing Around* with Don Johnston Developmental Equipment's *Adaptive Firmware Card G32e* (Apple *IIe* and *IIgs*).

The **joystick** is a peripheral designed to provide two-dimensional control of objects on the computer screen. Unlike the mouse, the joy-stick is a stationary box with a movable stick (see Figure 5-6). The stick is connected to two motion detectors, either mechanical or optical, that feed X–Y coordinates to the computer. Any changes in the stick's posi-

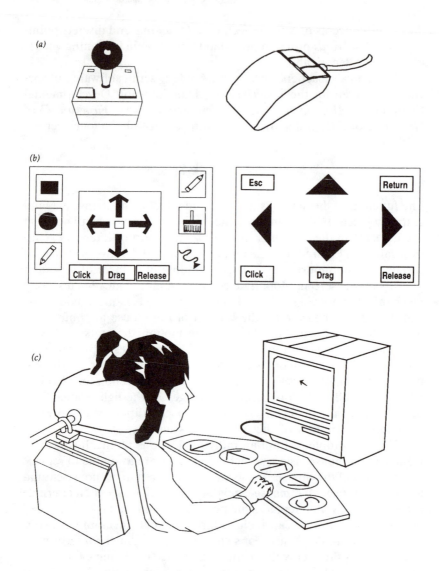

Figure 5–6

(a) Typical joystick and mouse peripherals. (b) Alternative keyboards with custom overlays can be used to emulate mouse or joystick input. (c) Some alternative keyboards use switches to emulate mouse input. The switches are used for cursor control. Five input switches are used to produce up, down, left, and right cursor movement and mouse button action.

tion are duplicated by changes in the position of an object on the computer monitor. Joystick control is often used with computer games, drawing programs, and educational software.

A wide variety of modified joystick systems are available for users who are physically disabled. These systems provide users with access to entertainment systems, microcomputers, and communication aids. For example, KY Enterprise's *Mouth Operated Joystick* provides access to the popular Nintendo video game systems. McIntyre Computer Systems Division's *MacIntyre* provides a software and hardware solution for access to Apple Macintosh microcomputers. Prentke Romich's *JS-4 Joystick* provides access to communication aids. Lovejoy Electronics' *Lite Touch* uses a light-activated joystick emulator for Apple II series, Commodore, and IBM PC systems.

Table 5–5 lists general guidelines to use when considering the use of mouse or joystick systems.

Brian: Mousing Around with Exploratory Play

Brian is a 5-year-old child who had a head injury that caused bleeding in the left pyramidal tract of his brain, resulting in right-side spastic hemiplegia. Brian has increased muscle tone in his arm so that muscles are stiff and movements are difficult. He has visual motor problems that affect his ability to integrate visual-motor tasks. He has normal intelligence. In classroom situations, Brian ambulates with the

Table 5–5. Design considerations for mouse and joystick systems.

1. What cognitive, sensory, motor, and related factors have an impact on the client's use of the mouse or joystick?

2. Does the client have the visual-spatial skills for mouse or joystick control?

3. Does the client have the motor control and functional range of movement for accessing a mouse or joystick?

4. If the mouse cannot be used, does the mouse or joystick application software have equivalent keyboard characters for operation? Can these equivalent keystrokes be used with a more accommodating alternative access method?

5. Can a mouse or joystick emulator be used with the computer? Can the computer accommodate the expansion interface? What cables are necessary for connection?

6. Does the emulation technique provide equivalent mouse or joystick funtions?

7. Can mouse or joystick macros be used to make access to menus and commands more efficient?

8. Can the mouse or joystick emulator slow down high-speed arcade-type software?

9. Can the mouse or joystick emulator adjust the speed and rate of mouse or joystick cursor movements? Can the emulator adjust button selection rates?

use of a wheelchair. Special education teachers wanted to get Brian more involved in cooperative play activities with other students. The class had been using several new exploratory play programs on the classroom computer. Brian expressed great interest in using these software programs. However, the software was designed for "mouse-only" operation, and Brian's motor impairments restricted his ability to use the mouse.

The school district's technologist had used an expanded keyboard and a keyboard emulator successfully with Brian and other students earlier in the school year. It was recommended that Don Johnston Developmental Equipment's *Adaptive Firmware Card G32e* and Unicorn Engineering's *Unicorn Expanded Keyboard Model II* be used as a mouse emulator. Because Brian's classroom teachers had little experience in creating setups for the Unicorn keyboard and Adaptive Firmware Card (AFC), the technologist suggested the use of preprogrammed AFC utility software, called setup disks. These disks provide access to commercial software programs through a collection of custom-designed overlays that provide immediate access to the AFC and Unicorn keyboard. Unicorn Engineering's *Mousing Around* AFC setup disk was used as the mouse emulation program. The mouse emulating software came with a number of colorful overlays that controlled cursor movements. The teachers selected the appropriate overlay for use with the mouse-driven software. In selecting the *Unicorn Keyboard* overlays, much consideration was given to Brian's motor and language processing skills. His skill levels determined the number and types of symbols to put on the overlay and how to arrange the symbols. With training, Brian was able to work with his classmates while exploring Lawrence Productions' *McGee* and Broderbund's *Playroom*.

Speech Recognition

The ultimate goal of speech recognition is to provide computers with the ability to process and understand continuous human speech. The promise of this technology is tempered by problems associated with variabilities in speech, complexities of semantics, and limitations of existing technology. The current generation of speech recognition systems process discretely spoken utterances or words if they are separated by a silent pause. The user has to speak slowly and clearly, over pronouncing each word. Nevertheless, microcomputer speech recognition systems can offer disabled individuals flexible access options for information input.

Microcomputer-based **speech recognition** is based on the concept of speech template matching. The process begins with the identification and listing of keyboard commands and alphanumeric keys necessary to run the user's application software. The user then **trains** the computer to understand his or her voice. This is accomplished by repeating a particular utterance or word several times. Each utterance is sampled and analyzed by the computer, the electronic patterns produced are then combined to create a single target template for that utterance. The **template** conveys information about the variability of electronic patterns across training utterances. Creation of a 100-word vocabulary file can take up to several hours to complete. After training, templates are matched to the user's list of keyboard commands and alphanumeric keys and saved to disk in a file called a **vocabulary**.

To use speech recognition, the user utters a word to be recognized, the pattern of that word is then compared to each target template in the RAM resident vocabulary file. The comparison method the computer uses to recognize each word is based on a set of "minimum match rules." These rules are user selectable so that each template can be personalized. For example, users often are provided with the ability to change word reject thresholds, adjust word separability differences, microphone gain, word gain, word boundary, and filter recognition levels. Assuming that minimum match rules are satisfied, the computer recognizes the utterance with the target template it most closely matches. The size of the typical vocabulary file can range from 50 to 1,000 words. The size of the active file usually depends on the amount of available RAM space.

The recognition accuracy of this approach can vary from 60 to 90 percent for typical application vocabularies. This technology does not always work for some individuals. For example, people with dysarthria have difficulty with the coordination of the muscles of respiration, phonation, articulation, and resonation, leading to slurred and imprecise speech. As a result, the individual's utterances or words may not match previously stored templates.

Examples of speech recognition systems include Voice Connection's *Introvice I* and *II* (Apple II series) and *Introvice V, VI, Micro Introvicer* (IBM PCs, PS/2, and MS-DOS compatibles); Kurzweil Applied Intelligence's *Kurzweil Voice System* (IBM PCs); NEC America's *SAR-100 Voice Plus* (IBM PCs); Covox, Inc.'s *Voice Master* (Apple II series, Atari, and Commodore); and TASH's *Voice-Key* (IBM PCs).

Another discrete utterance speech recognition system available to disabled users is Dragon System's *DragonDictate*. Unlike other speech recognition units, which require preliminary training, *DragonDictate* incorporates phonetic models built for 25,000 words, so the user does not have to train new words. The speech recognition process is flexible enough to account for slight differences in individual pronunciations, so multiple users can access the system. In addition, the system interactively learns a user's vocabulary and speaking style. *DragonDictate* uses natural language recognition, so the user speaks normally. The system also is capable of learning an additional 5,000 user-specific words. *DragonDictate* is available for IBM PC and compatible microcomputers configured with a 80386 CPU. Articulate Systems, Inc., has licensed Dragon System's speech technology to provide speech recognition for the Macintosh computer (Articulate System's *Voice Navigator II*).

Speech recogniton systems are connected to the microcomputer via an interface card, software, and headset or stand-alone microphone. The recognition software operates in the background as a TSR program. Most speech recognition systems operate transparently with applications software. However, specific software compatibility questions should be investigated prior to acquiring a speech recognition system. Most systems will allow the user to define additional computer commands and add them to specific vocabulary sets. Computer memory limits the size of the active vocabulary set available to the user at any time. To make vocabulary sets more functional and run faster, users often organize vocabularies according to specific applications.

Table 5–6 lists adaptive access guidelines to use when considering the use of speech recognition systems.

Table 5–6. Design considerations for speech recognition systems.

1. What cognitive, sensory, motor, and related factors have an impact on the client's use of the speech recognition system?

2. Does the client's voice articulation, pitch, or loudness change regularly? Does the client's articulation, pitch, or loudness fatigue easily?

3. What application software will be used with the speech recognition system?

4. How large a vocabulary file is needed? How large a vocabulary file will the speech recognition system accommodate? Can the computer's RAM and disk storage systems accommodate the vocabulary files?

5. Can the user define specific vocabulary files for specific applications?

6. Does the speech recognition software include predefined templates for application software?

7. How easy is it to train, edit, and add words to the vocabulary?

8. How many keyboard commands can be stored for one template or word?

9. Will the user change locations when using the speech system?

10. Can the user's computer accommodate the speech recognition system's interface card and cable system?

11. Is the speech recognition system compatible with all existing computer hardware and software systems?

Kerry: Opening Doors with Words

Kerry is a 26-year-old office worker who suffered a C-7 spinal cord injury in an automobile accident. The accident left Kerry a quadriplegic in a power wheelchair. Kerry had no residual cognitive deficits secondary to the accident. While extensive rehabilitation efforts were underway for Kerry, her therapists and family were raising questions regarding her ability to return to work and live independently. The occupational therapist referred her to the center's rehabilitation technology department for services.

Kerry, despite her long-term disability, was determined to be self-sufficient. With the help of her job counselor, she pursued a wide range of job options, including her former office position. Kerry's employer had always thought of her as a very qualified, dependable, and industrious employee. However, her manager had concerns about her ability to compete in the office workplace. After several meetings with therapists, technologists, counselors, and Kerry's former employer, the decision was made to adapt Kerry's office work station.

Kerry had no functional use of her upper extremities, but she managed very well with verbal communication. The major demands of the technology solution required the following: (1) the approach had to offer speed, accuracy, and manageability; (2) the access method had to work with the company's existing office computer work station; and (3) the access method had to be transparent to the company's existing office software systems. If these needs could be met, the company would agree to pick up the cost of the modifications for Kerry's employment.

The technology solution incorporated Dragon Systems' *DragonDictate* speech recognition system. The speech board and software were compatible with the company's Compaq *386 Deskpro* systems. Because Kerry was responsible for accounting functions, it was vital that the speech system be compatible with the company's *Lotus 1-2-3* spreadsheet and *WordPerfect* word processing systems. The technology team added 8 MB of extended memory to the company's computer to accommodate all the application software. The *DragonDictate* system allowed Kerry to set up and use all of the Compaq *Deskpro's* editing and control commands with both *Lotus 1-2-3* and *Word Perfect*. To speed up tedious computer operations, "voice macros" were added to Kerry's *DragonDictate* vocabulary. **Macros** allow the user to group computer commands together as a unit and execute them with one or two keystrokes. In office field tests, Kerry and her speech recognition system were able to achieve nearly 39 words per minute on word processing tasks. The system also allowed her to create extensive accounting applications for the company.

Switch Access Systems

Single-, dual-, and multiple-switch access methods incorporate a series of hardware devices designed to be used in place of standard keyboards. Switches provide individuals with severe motor control problems with the ability to operate microcomputers, communication devices, adaptive toys, home appliances and related environmental control systems. The operation of a switch is straightforward. **Switches** either open or close an electronic circuit, controlling the flow of electricity to an electronic device, much like a light switch in the home turns the lights on (closed circuit) or off (open circuit).

In accessing computers, switches are often interfaced with the "game I/O" connector. This connector is normally used for joysticks and game paddles. However, switch interfaces can be designed to allow switch access to microcomputers (see Figure 5–7). Apple II series computers, for example, use internal and external game I/O connections that provide an easy means for connecting switches. To function, the switch's **plug** must be connected to a switch interface, which in turn connects to the computer's game I/O socket or port. The computer reads a low signal when the switch is off and a high signal when the switch is on. To use this access method, software programs must include software drivers that look for switches connected to the computer's game I/O. Don Johnston Developmental Equipment and Laureate Learning Systems publish a wide variety of games, early vocabulary, and language development software that is compatible with game I/O switch access. For a detailed explanation of adaptive switches, readers are referred to Chapter 6.

Because many switches are similar in operation, they may be used across a wide variety of electronic devices. Users should note, however, that switches are manufactured with dissimilar sizes of miniature plug connectors (see Figure 5–7). The switch interface, toy, or related electronic device must include the same size **jack** to accommodate a switch plug. Typical sizes include ⅛-inch, ¼-inch, and ½-inch diameter plugs and jack mounts. To alleviate size incompatibilities, plug adapters are available to allow the user to convert plugs to fit different sized jacks. A number of vendors offer switch interfaces for game I/O access: AbleNet's *Computer Switch Interface* (Apple II series); Don Johnston Developmental Equipment's *Switch Interface* (Apple II series); Dunamis, Inc.'s *Switch Interface Box* (Apple II series); and TASH's *Switch Adaptor* (Apple II series). These switch interfaces are connected to the computer's game I/O port. The switch interface has jacks which are accessible for switches. Game I/O interfaces can only be used with software compatible with game I/O switch access.

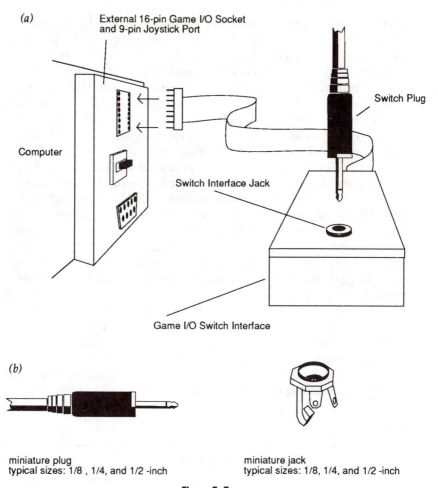

(a)

External 16-pin Game I/O Socket
and 9-pin Joystick Port

Switch Plug

Computer

Switch Interface Jack

Game I/O Switch Interface

(b)

miniature plug
typical sizes: 1/8 , 1/4, and 1/2 -inch

miniature jack
typical sizes: 1/8, 1/4, and 1/2 -inch

Figure 5–7
(a) A game I/O switch interface which connects to the game port of a microcomputer. (b) Typical miniature switch plugs and jacks.

In addition to game I/O switch access, computers also can accommodate switches with the use of keyboard emulators. Using this approach, switches can operate standard hardware and software transparently. Because switch users are employing an indirect access method, the keyboard emulator incorporates an intermediate selection scheme for sending characters to the computer. The two most common categories of indirect selection schemes are encoded and scanning methods.

Morse code is a very popular switch encoding scheme for use with computers. **Morse code** uses one or two switches to send sequences of signals to the keyboard emulator. These signals are the intermediate step in the process. The signals are called **dit** (short signal [.]) and **dah** (long signal [—]) codes. The keyboard emulator then translates the sequence of dits and dahs into keyboard characters that the computer understands. There are a number of variations on the Morse code system (Friedlander & Rahimi, 1979; Washington Research Foundation, 1983). Table 5–7 lists common Morse code equivalents for letter, number, and punctuation keys. The codes for computer function keys vary dramatically across keyboard emulator systems.

Several switch options are available to Morse code users. Single-switch **plain Morse code** requires the user to open and close one switch for short and long durations to send dits and dahs. In single-switch **tone Morse code** the user presses the switch in coordination with audible high- and low-pitched tones to send dits and dahs. Two-switch **automatic Morse code** has two switches for dits and dahs, so users alternate between switches to send the appropriate sequence of dits and dahs. In general, disabled individuals must have good motor control to correctly time signals when using plain Morse code with one switch. Because tone Morse code provides a clear auditory distinction between dits and dahs, users are better able to synchronize and confirm switch closures. Automatic Morse code puts no timing demands on the user; but users must be able to activate two switches.

Scanning is another indirect approach for using switches with computers. **Scanning** uses one or more switches to select items from an

Table 5–7. Morse code input.

Letters and Numbers

A	.—	H	...	O	———	V	...—	0	—————	7	——...
B	—...	I	..	P	.—..	W	.——	1	.————	8	———..
C	—.—.	J	.———	Q	——.—	X	—..—	2	..———	9	————.
D	—..	K	—.—	R	.—.	Y	—.——	3	...——		
E	.	L	.—..	S	...	Z	——..	4	....—		
F	..—.	M	——	T	—			5	.....		
G	——.	N	—.	U	..—			6	—....		

Punctuation Marks and Symbols

[.]	.—.—.—	[(]	....	[>]	....——	[!]	..—.
["]	—...—	[)]	......—	[?]	..——..	[@]	.———..
[$]	—...—.	[,]	——..——	[:]	—..—..	[']	...—..
[+]	..—..	[;]	——..—.	[*]	.———.	[/]	—..—.
[—]	.—.——	[<]	....—.	[%]	.——.—.	[#]	.—..—.
Space	..——						

array. An **array** is a sequence of characters, numbers, or symbols. The array is the intermediate step in entering information into the computer. Each selection in the array represents a keyboard character that can be sent to the microcomputer. There are a number of variations on how scanning arrays are presented to the user (see Figure 5-8). For example, scanning arrays may utilize graphic images, characters or symbols, or even auditory synthesized speech commands. When selecting scanning arrays, clinicians should consider how the client's cognitive, sensory, and motor skills may affect scanning array design.

Before users can interact with scanning arrays, they must first select a scanning method. Many scanning methods are available for operating microcomputers. The most conventional methods include automatic linear scanning, step linear scanning, inverse scanning, and frequency-of-use scanning. Each of these methods may operate using two mutations: one-item-at-a-time or group-item scanning. For example, one-item-at-a-time scanning moves the cursor from item to item. Users wait until the cursor reaches the desired item and then press the switch. This scanning variation is a very time-consuming process. To expedite matters, users may consider using group-item scanning. In this variation the cursor moves from group to group in an array, users wait until the cursor reaches the group containing the desired item and press the switch. The cursor then begins to move from item to item within the group; users wait until the desired item is reached and press the switch.

Automatic linear scanning is the simplest and most common scanning method. To use this method, the user presses the switch to bring up the array. A cursor then starts moving across the array of selections using either one-item-at-a-time or group-item scanning. The user waits until the cursor is on the desired item and then presses the switch.

Step linear scanning is a manual method of moving the cursor across the screen and selecting items. A user presses a switch to bring up the array. The user then presses and releases the switch each time to move the cursor across the array. This process repeats until the cursor is on the desired item. Clearly, users are required to make many more switch closures using this method. Group-item scanning combined with step linear scanning can reduce the motor demands on the user.

Inverse scanning is the opposite of automatic linear scanning. Users are required to hold the switch closed to start the cursor moving. The user continues to press and hold the switch until the cursor reaches the desired item. Only then does the user release the switch. Again, group-item scanning can speed the selection process.

Frequency-of-use scanning is a dynamic approach to scanning. This method uses statistics and frequency counts to determine which items in the array are used most often by the client. Special software

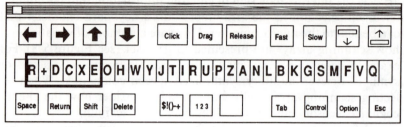

(a)

_R_ < #.+ A B C D E\ F G H I J =K L M N O P Q R S T U V W X Y Z . ^ *
_R < A . 0123 4567 89.+ *-/=

QEC>^V.,?!; "#$%&' ()*+-@/:<=> [\]^` AODT

(b)

SPACE RETURN UP   DOWN   LEFT   RIGHT
ESC   DELETE

(c)

Go to DOS	Esc	! / ,	@ / 2	# / 3	$ / 4	% / 5	^ / 6	& / 7	* / 8	(/ 9	) / 0	{ / [	} /]	abbreviation
Array Up	Tab	- / ,	< / ,	> / .	P	Y	F	G	C	R	L	? / /	+ / =	absolutely
Array Down	Ctrl	A	O	E	U	I	D	H	T	N	S	=		accessories
Word Prediction	Shift	: / ;	Q	J	K	X	B	M	W	V	Z	~ / `	| / \	accommodate
ADD word/ Abbrev	caps lock	Alt	@		K		Backspace	PgDn	PgUP				amazing
DEL Word/ Abbrev	F1	F2	F3	F4	F5	F6	F7	F8	F9	F10	F11	F12		

(d)

Figure 5–8

Scanning methods use arrays to represent keyboard characters, numbers, and symbols. (a) Graphic scanning arrays can use icons, pictures, letters, and words to represent keyboard and mouse commands. (b) Textual arrays use letter groups to represent keyboard commands. (c) Scanning arrays also can use single words to simplify keyboard input. (d) Scanning arrays also can be configured as full keyboard layouts with frequency-of-use, word-prediction, and word-abbreviation schemes.

then dynamically changes the order of items from the most to the least frequently used. The idea behind this approach is to reduce scanning time by avoiding irrelevant items and grouping commonly used items together in the array.

A client's cognitive, sensory, and motor profile will affect his or her ability to interact with scanning arrays and scanning methods. Table 5–8 lists design considerations as options for augmenting scanning arrays and scanning methods. Most keyboard emulators will allow clinicians to use these and other methods to individualize the scanning process.

Yvonne: Switching from Motor Training to Pre-Scanning Skills

Yvonne is a 4-year-old child with multiple cognitive, speech, and motor handicaps. She has been diagnosed with severe spastic quadriplegia, a form of cerebral palsy, and severe mental retardation. Speech

Table 5–8. Design considerations for switch access.

1. What cognitive, sensory, motor, and related factors have an impact on the client's use of the switch access method? Can the client use any other direct selection method? Can the client use multiple switch inputs?

2. Will the client use the game I/O switch input? Is the application software compatible with the game I/O switch input?

3. Does the switch system require a keyboard emulator? Can the computer accommodate the expansion interface? What cables are necessary for connection? Is switch encoding or switch scanning more appropriate for the user?

4. Can the user understand and efficiently operate an encoding switch system? Can the client use two-switch Morse code? Is plain or tone Morse code more appropriate for the user?

5. Can the client understand and efficiently operate a switch scanning process? What sensory modalities are most appropriate when determining the array format? How easy is it to train the client to use the scanning array?

6. Can the client understand and use multiple screen arrays? Can the client understand and use interbranching arrays?

7. Are the size, spacing, organization, and feedback of the array appropriate for the client?

8. What type of scanning method is most effective with the client — automatic linear scanning, step linear scanning, inverse scanning, or frequency-of-use scanning? Can the client use group-item scanning with the major scanning method?

9. Can the keyboard emulator change the scanning method? Can the emulator adjust the rate, location, and format of the scanning array?

10. Can macros, abbreviation-expansion, or word-prediction software reduce the number of switch selections required by the user?

and psychological testing identified language skills at an 18-month level and reasoning abilities at the 2-year-old level. Early intervention programs concentrated on developing Yvonne's early communication and motor skills through the use of switches. Therapists used switch-activated toys and cassette players to indicate choices, encourage head control, coordinate arm movements, and develop motor control. She communicated using an eyegaze E-Tran system with eight pictures presented at a time. In order to move to a more complex augmentative communication system she would need to learn scanning skills. Yvonne's speech-language pathologist and teachers decided to pursue computer-based activities for developing pre-augmentative communication switch scanning skills. It was felt that computer-based aids could help Yvonne to interact more effectively with those around her and might provide significant educational or vocational benefits for her long-term treatment. The goal of the technology intervention was to develop Yvonne's ability to control simple switch-input software as a precursor to more advanced scanning methods.

It was decided to continue using her low-profile, large single switch with a homemade game I/O switch interface (see Figure 4–6) and an Apple *IIe* computer. Because of Yvonne's severe motor impairment, previous switch training had concentrated on developing motor skills that were consistently accurate. The computer-based switch activity was a continuation of this training, but also directed attention to the application software. Programs from Laureate Learning System's *Creature Chorus* and *Creature Antics,* Exceptional Children's Software's *Rabbit Scan,* and Don Johnston Developmental Equipment's *Join the Circus* were used for teaching various switch skills. The games introduced the following skills: (1) pressing and releasing a switch on command; (2) making multiple switch closures; (3) holding a switch closed for a specific time duration; and (4) waiting for the software to scan through choices to get to the target item.

Mark: Encoding with Augmentative and Written Communication

Mark is an 18-year-old who was involved in a diving accident that resulted in a C-3 spinal cord injury. He is totally dependent on others in self-care. Mark operates a specially adapted electric wheelchair with a portable ventilation system. He controls the wheelchair with a "sip-and-puff" switch. Rehabilitation following Mark's accident has involved an interdisciplinary team of experienced professionals. In addition to psychosocial interventions and caregiver training, the team included provisions for the design of specialized technology equipment to enhance Mark's independence and quality of life.

The technology team was looking for techniques that would support planned vocational programming, promote the resumption of meaningful life roles, and facilitate opportunities for community reintegration. Although Mark could communicate orally, his speech was slow, difficult to understand, and fatiguing for him to produce. Over time he was unable to sustain adequate breath support for speech. Speech recommendations included the need for a backup speech communication capability as Mark fatigued. In addition, vocational programming strongly supported a written communication requirement.

Mark's needs were addressed with the use of a laptop computer. A Toshiba MS-DOS laptop computer provided the foundation for the portable system. Mark's dependency on others for self-care needs necessitated the use of a hard disk system. Access to the computer was accomplished using Mark's dual-action sip-and-puff switch and a supporting keyboard emulator. The sip-and-puff switch is really two switches in one. A sip sends one signal, and a puff a second signal, giving Mark the ability to use automatic Morse code as a computer input method. Words+ Inc.'s *Morse Code WSKE II* program provided keyboard emulation, word prediction, and abbreviation expansion capabilities for use with Mark's word processing software. In addition, *Morse Code WSKE II* provided software-based, text-to-speech synthesis for generating speech output while concurrently running other application software. The software-based speech synthesis provided the laptop with true portability.

Adaptive Output Systems

This section will provide the reader with information on the wide assortment of computer output methods available to disabled users. Standard computer output systems are ineffective or unaccessible to disabled users. Therefore adaptive output systems are needed to augment a user's sensory deficits. These aids include screen magnification systems, braille devices, and speech synthesis techniques.

Screen Magnification

Computer accommodations for users who are visually impaired often involve adaptations to the computer monitor. **Screen magnification** involves the enlargement of the monitor's character display capability. Depending on the system, characters can be enlarged 2 to 15 times the normal size. Screen magnification devices are available to users as hardware only, software only, and as combination systems.

The simplest solution for enlarging the screen display involves the use of powerful **fresnel lens**, which more than double the size of images on any standard computer monitor. These hardware devices come with adjustable and removable frames that attach to the computer screen. In addition, these devices often have built-in glare protection to minimize visual fatigue associated with glare on the monitor. A fresnel lens solution will work with virtually all computer systems and requires no special hardware or software adaptations to the computer system. Lastly, these systems are capable of enlarging both text and graphic screens. AbleTech Connection's *Compu-Lenz* is an example of a fresnel lens system (Apple II series, Macintosh, IBM, Tandy, Commodore, and MS-DOS compatibles).

The next type of screen magnification modification involves the use of software-based screen enlargement systems. These systems are very portable and are designed to work with standard computer monitors. The concept behind this approach is to use TSR memory resident software that is capable of on-demand text enlargement. However, compatibility among these programs with standard application software varies dramatically. Many IBM and compatible computers offer various text and graphics display modes (see Chapter 2) which may not work with these software-based systems. For example, some screen enlargement software can be used only with "nongraphic" MS-DOS application programs. The programs generally are designed for text-based word processing applications. Clients interested in using more sophisticated applications involving windows, graphics, menu bars, or video games may have difficulty using these magnification systems. However, some new generation screen enlargement systems are entering the market that accommodate Color Graphics Adapter (CGA), Enhanced Graphics Adapter (EGA), and Video Graphics Adapter (VGA) display modes. Finally, software-based approaches are slower, but less expensive and easier to upgrade than hardware and software combination approaches.

Software-based screen enlargement programs provide users who are visually impaired with a wide variety of features. **Zooming** features allow users to magnify the entire screen, single lines, or a portion of the screen. **Magnification size** features allow clients to adjust the enlargement of character sizes. **Tracking** features provide manual and automatic methods for the user to control horizontal and vertical screen movement, plus continuous screen scanning. Examples of software-based screen enlargement software include: AI Squared's *Zoomtext* (IBM PCs and MS-DOS compatibles); Arts Computer Products' *PC Lens* (IBM PCs, MS-DOS compatibles, Tandy); Berkeley System's *inLarger* (Macintosh); Optelec's *LPDOS* (IBM PCs and MS-DOS compatibles); Microsystems Software's *MAGic* and *MAGic Deluxe* (IBM PCs and MS-DOS compatibles).

Combination hardware and software screen magnification systems may involve the use of large-screen monitors with graphics adaptor boards or closed-circuit cameras with special large-screen monitors. Large-screen monitor solutions vary. Some vendors use multiple monitor systems that provide a monochrome monitor for text display and a graphics monitor for the magnification process. Others use one graphics monitor that switches back and forth from regular to enlarged screen displays. Finally, video camera systems use proprietary closed-circuit televisions (CCTV) in conjunction with a video camera to allow regular and enlarged material to appear on the monitor in separate screen windows. These enlargement devices generally are more expensive than either magnification lens or software-based techniques. However, they usually are faster and provide improved hardware and software compatibility. Examples of hardware-based systems include Telesensory Systems' *Vista* and *Vista-Vert Plus* (IBM PCs); Optelec's *20/20+ High Resolution Monitor*; VTEK's *DP-10* large-print monitor (Apple II series), *DP-11 Plus,* and *DP-11 PLus MCA* large-print monitors (IBM PCs, PS/2).

Braille Access Systems

For individuals with very limited or no usable vision, computer options include braille input and output devices. **Braille** is a system of writing for the blind that uses characters made of raised dot patterns. Each character can be represented by six or eight dot patterns, depending on the braille system used. Braille input systems include special braille-style keyboards, terminals, or standard keyboards. Figure 5–9 provides a list of six-dot braille characters and their American Standard Code for Information Interchange (ASCII) computer equivalents.

Three kinds of braille are available on personal computers: Grade 1, Grade 2, and computer braille. Grade 1 and Grade 2 braille systems were in use long before the introduction of microcomputers in the consumer market. Grade 1 braille operates using a one-to-one letter correspondence to English. For example, the word "dog" is spelled out as "d o g" using three braille cells. A **braille cell** is a group of six dots that when raised in combinations forms patterns to represent letters (see Figure 5–9). Because the six-dot cell system cannot represent all upper- and lowercase letters, numbers, and punctuation symbols, Grade 1 braille incorporates special symbols to indicate numbers and capitalization. In practical computer applications, Grade 1 braille is not the preferred form of braille for an experienced braille reader. The heavy paper used to retain cell impressions is cumbersome and heavy for long documents. In addition, a braille page contains a maximum of

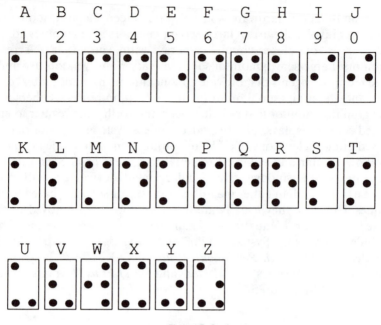

Figure 5-9
Six-dot braille coding.

1,080 cells or about 27 lines of 40 cells, greatly reducing the amount of information that can be presented on a single page.

Most users prefer Grade 2 braille, a shorthand version of braille in which contractions are used to build words. For example, the word "education" is formed from the letters "e d u c a" and the contraction "tion." Grade 2 braille has the advantage of reducing the size of the printed document and allowing the user to read braille faster.

Computer braille is an addition to both Grade 1 and Grade 2 braille. This braille system adds the special keyboard characters that are unique to microcomputer systems. Computer braille uses braille cells to represent computer control codes. For example, a braille user would represent the Return key with two cells which represent the computer code "control M."

Microcomputer braille input and output requires a software and hardware combination that translates English characters and computer commands into braille and back again. With braille input, the keyboard sends braille to software which converts it into computer ASCII codes. The output process involves converting computer ASCII codes into a braille format that a braille printer or screen reading device can understand. Flexible braille conversions should include keyboard alphanumerics, computer commands, and screen display attributes.

American Printing House for the Blind's *APH Pocket Braille* is a portable, rechargeable braille device for the input, storage, and editing of braille. The system can output files to printers, braille embossers, and personal computers. Telesensory System's *Braille Interface Terminal* allows input and screen review with IBM PCs or MS-DOS compatibles.

Telesensory's *BrailleMate* is a portable hand-held braille keyboard with a built-in speech synthesizer. The system can organize, store, and retrieve information. Users can enter text as Grade 1 or Grade 2 braille. The system can automatically convert Grade 2 braille to standard text for speech and print output.

A number of manufacturers produce rechargeable battery-operated laptop systems for braille input, speech output, and transparent operation with application software. Syntha-Voice Computers, Inc.'s *Nomad* is an IBM PC laptop with braille or Qwerty keyboard input, braille translation software, screen reading software, and speech output. Telesensory Systems' *VersaBraille II+* is a dedicated braille input-output device. It includes word processing, braille translation software, and keyboard emulation for IBM PCs.

A number of braille printers, or "embossers," are available for producing output for blind users. A few examples include American Thermoform Corporation's *Braille 400 S* (Apple II series, IBM PCs, Tandy); Enabling Technologies Company's *Marathon Braille* (Apple II series, Macintosh, IBM PCs, and Tandy); and Telesensory Systems' *VersaPoint-40 Braille Embosser* (Apple II series, Macintosh, IBM PCs, Tandy, Commodore, Atari).

Generally low-cost braille printers average 20 to 40 characters per second (cps). For higher speeds, the price increases dramatically. Braille **cells**, the six- or eight-dot matrix over which a character is produced, can vary from printer to printer, and some braille output may feel different to the user. Finally, braille printers may require additional software and interface hardware to communicate properly with microcomputers.

Adaptive Speech Output

Software programs that read the computer screen and output the information through a speech synthesizer are called **screen reading** programs. These TSR programs provide access to word processing, spreadsheet, database and other application software. Screen reading software is often used in conjunction with screen magnification systems for users who are visually impaired or blind.

Some important features of screen reading software include the ability to speak keyboard characters, capitalization, punctuation, screen colors, and formatting codes. The ability to speak and spell individual words, entire lines, paragraphs, and multiple pages is also important. The flexibility to read and speak the application program's menus, prompts, and status is also critical to screen reading programs. Finally, the ability to disengage from application software and use speech with the computer's operating system can also be advantageous to users who are visually impaired.

Computer Conversation's *Verbal Operating System* software and a speech synthesizer can provide IBM PCs and PS/2, MS-DOS compatibles, and Tandy computers with the ability to read and speak application software and the disk operating system. Artic Technologies' *Artic Vision* and *Artic Business Vision* with its required speech synthesizer also can process screen and keyboard output into speech. The program can follow the screen cursor, speaking material automatically, or change to user-definable reading windows. Artic Technologies' program series supports IBM PC computer systems. Berkeley System's *outSpoken* is a Macintosh screen reading program that can read graphic elements off the computer monitor. The program is capable of reading letters, words, lines, menus, icons, windows, and other graphic elements. No additional speech synthesizer is necessary; *outSpoken* uses software-based speech synthesis. American Printing House for the Blind's *Talking Utilities for DOS 3.3* and *ProDOS* provides speech output for disk operating functions and ASCII text files on Apple II series microcomputers. Telesensory sells *Vert Plus, Personal Vert, Soft Vert* and *Screen Reader* systems provide screen reading capabilities using synthesized speech.

Another application of microcomputer-based speech output is in the role of an augmentative communication aid. These systems produce speech synthesis through software and hardware techniques. Software-based approaches generally use two variations of text-to-speech synthesis. These include phoneme- and diphone-based voice synthesis. **Phoneme-based** speech systems use the smallest elements of speech (phonemes) to model and reproduce speech by electronically combining phonemes to produce words. The intelligibility ratings for an unfamiliar listener can vary from 30 to 70 percent. **Diphone-based** speech uses the last half of a phoneme and the first half of the next phoneme combined. This approach provides greater information about speech. As a result, the intelligibility of diphone-based speech is greater than phoneme-based approaches. Software-based speech synthesis does not require additional hardware and or an external power supply. As a result, software-based systems are highly portable. First Byte's *SmoothTalker 2.0* (phoneme-based) and *SmoothTalker 3.0* (diphone-based) are software-based speech systems. They are available for use with Apple II series, Macintosh, Atari, Commodore, IBM, and Tandy systems.

Hardware-based systems incorporate the same text-to-speech technologies as software-based approaches. The intelligibility of these systems is equivalent to software-based systems. However, hardware-based speech systems can add additional capabilities to improve intelligibility. For example, some systems record digital diphone sounds to produce even greater intelligibility. The results are speech synthesizers that sound like human speech. In addition, pronunciation and intonation can be controlled and users can choose male or female voices. The disadvantages of hardware-based approaches are the additional hardware components that increase the weight and complexity of the computer system, and often demand an AC power source. As a result, some hardware-based speech systems are not truly portable communication systems. Digital Equipment's *MultiVoice DECtalk* (Apple, Acorn, Macintosh, IBM, Atari, Commodore, Tandy) and Adaptive Communication System's *RealVoice PC* (IBM PCs and MS-DOS compatibles) are two examples of hardware-based speech solutions.

A number of augmentative communication programs are available to run software- and hardware-based speech synthesis on microcomputers. In fact, these programs often give users the flexibility to choose from a wide variety of speech synthesis systems. A few examples of speech software include: Words+, Inc.'s *Equalizer II, E-Z Talker, Talking Board,* and *Talking Screen* (IBM and MS-DOS compatibles); World Communication's *Help U Type and Speak, Help U Key and Speak,* and *Help U Keyboard and Speak* (IBM PCs and PS/2); Microsystems Software's *HandiCHAT* (IBM PCs and PS/2); and Dunamis, Inc.'s *SimpleCom I & II* (Apple II series).

Customizing User Interfacing

The last section of this chapter will provide the reader with methods for simplifying the user interface. The methods presented are illustrative of the wide array of techniques often used to lessen the complexities associated with the integration and daily use of assorted hardware and software systems.

The special adaptations made to microcomputers play a significant role in providing access to disabled users. Well-designed technology solutions are made as transparent to the user as possible. By insulating users from irrelevant technical complexities, assistive technology can help users perform complex tasks in the simplest, most familiar, and most meaningful way possible. Careful adaptation of the user's interface can greatly improve the success of technology implementations.

Customized adaptations to an input device involve designing a completely new arrangement. Clinicians should consider layout alternatives that facilitate easy operation. Planning should include identification of and familiarization with the software the individual will use. Clinicians then should make lists of all keys and key combinations necessary to run the software. This also provides a method for isolating and eliminating relevant keyboard commands. Decreasing the number of keys can reduce visual scanning demands on some users. In addition, by identifying frequently used key combinations, technologists can help reduce selection demands on the user by utilizing macros. **Macros** store multiple key sequences so that users can repeatedly execute the sequence with just a few keystrokes.

The arrangement of keyboard characters also can increase user proficiency. An analysis of the frequency of key use can help determine where to locate frequently used keys. In addition, nonreading users may find color-coded keys, simplified mnemonics, or different tactile designs helpful. Auditory learners and users who are visually impaired or blind may find speech feedback very important.

Redefinition involves the rearrangement of the standard input device's letters, numbers, or computer keys. For example, changing the standard keyboard layout to an alphabetical or statistical format could be beneficial to some users. Similarly, macros can be implemented with redefinition software and/or hardware.

Alternative keyboards and keyboard emulators usually provide users with options for adjusting the **rate of acceptance**, the time necessary for the keyboard to respond to a key press; **auto-repeat defeat** functions that enable or disable the duplication of keys when continuously pressed; and **sticky key** or **one-finger access** functions that provide key latching, which eliminates the need for single-finger operators to hold two or more keys down at the same time. Clinicians can save these individualized parameters to disk as setup files. **Setup files** allow the user or caregiver to quickly load adaptive settings into the computer from a menu of choices. This eliminates the need for continual reprogramming and allows individuals who are unfamiliar with the system to operate the adaptive equipment.

When a technology solution requires running multiple TSR programs and application software, the clinician should consider automatic loading of the programs by adding them to the computer's boot operations. For example, Apple Macintosh computers use "INIT" files which are small programs that load into RAM memory every time you start up the computer. IBM and MS-DOS compatible microcomputers use the "autoexec.bat" file to load executable programs automatically.

For novice or part-time MS-DOS users, entering commands and running DOS batch files requires correct spelling and syntax for file names and path statements. This process can be tedious and confusing for users with many files on large hard drive systems. A number of DOS-menuing software packages are available to help technologists design and build friendly menus. These packages allow users to build multiscreen menu systems to start software programs, run DOS commands and DOS files, and move between screens through menu linking. Progressive Computer Services' *EZ-Menu* and Fifth Generations Systems' *Direct Access* provide individual users with the ability to automatically build hierarchical menus with no programming experience. These and other menu building programs run on low-end PCs with as little as 256K RAM and a single 360K floppy disk drive.

SUMMARY

Assistive technology solutions require clear identification and understanding of patient needs. The design of technology solutions is based on the individual client's cognitive, sensory, and motor profile. After the patient's technology needs are defined, technologists can explore a variety of computer access methods, including alternative keyboards, touch windows, voice recognition, and switch systems. Adaptive computer solutions also can be augmented with a variety of adaptive output systems such as screen magnification, speech output, and braille. Because technology systems are not always intuitive and simple to operate, the technologist also must carefully plan and design the user's interface. Effective interface design helps to integrate computer components so users can operate and use the system more effectively.

REFERENCES

Batshaw, M. L., & Perrett, Y. M. (1987). *Children with handicaps* (2nd ed.). Baltimore: Paul H. Brookes.

Cress, C., & French, G. (1991). Age-related differences in interface control in normally developing children. In *Proceedings of the RESNA 14th Annual Conference* (pp. 257–259). Kansas City, MO: RESNA.

Church, G., & Bender, M. (1989). *Teaching with computers: A curriculum for special educators.* Boston: College-Hill Press.

Friedlander, C. B., & Rahimi, M. A. (1979). EMG activated spatial Morse code general purpose communication device. *IEEE Engineering in Medicine and Biology, 15,* 298–299.

Joyce, B., & Showers, B. (1980). Improving inservice training: The messages of research. *Educational Leadership, 37,* 379–385.

Karat, J., McDonald, J. E., & Anderson, M. (1985). A comparison of selection techniques: Touch panel, mouse, and keyboard. In B. Shackel (Ed.), *Human-*

computer interaction — INTERACT '84. North Holland: Elsevier Science Publishers.

Mandal, A. C. (1982). The correct height of school furniture. *Human Factors, 24,* 257–269.

Meadow, K. P. (1980). *Deafness and child development.* Berkeley: University of California Press.

Warburg, M., Frederickson, P., & Rattleff, J. (1979). Blindness among 7700 mentally retarded children in Denmark. *Clinical Developmental Medicine, 73,* 56–67.

Washington Research Foundation. (1983). *Morse code teaching instructions.* [Available from author, Suite 222, U District Building, 1107 N. E. 45th, Seattle, WA 98105.]

6

Adaptive Toys and Environmental Controls

■ Sharon Glennen, PhD ■
■ Gregory Church, MS, MAS ■

Assistive technology allows individuals with handicaps to obtain control over the environment. This empowerment is important in the areas of communication, mobility, and education. It is equally important in the areas of play, leisure, and daily living activities. For the young child, empowerment through play allows a chance to develop new skills in fun nonthreatening situations before using them in day-to-day interactions. For the older child, the ability to participate in games or to control leisure activities provides an opportunity to interact with peers on an equal status. For an adult, the ability to control the environment is necessary to promote independence at home and work.

In addition to viewing play and leisure skills as methods of developing empowerment, it is also important to develop these skills because of their intrinsic value. The ability to play is an important part of childhood. A child who cannot participate in play activities is missing an opportunity to experience normal development through play (Musselwhite, 1986). Many adults with disabilities have large quantities of unstructured time in their days (Bender, Brannan, & Verhoven, 1984).

The development of leisure skills will help both children and adults manage such time by teaching them how to independently participate in enjoyable activities. This chapter will review assistive technology for adaptive play and leisure activities, and assistive technology for environmental control.

ADAPTIVE PLAY TECHNOLOGY

Stages of Play Development

When considering adaptive play technology for a child or adult it is important to determine the individual's level of play development. Toys that are appropriate for individuals at some stages of play are inwappropriate for other stages. Children with severe physical disabilities need adapted toys appropriate for each stage to develop skills at each play level. Musselwhite (1986) lists six stages of adaptive play based on the works of Wehman (1979). These six stages are: (1) exploratory, (2) independent, (3) parallel, (4) associative, (5) cooperative, and (6) symbolic.

Exploratory play is the first stage of play development. Most play at this level consists of sensory and causative explorations with toys. Children at this stage of play development enjoy grasping and squeezing toys, mouthing toys, and batting and dropping them. The child may repeat actions over and over to test all possible outcomes with a toy. Although play at this stage is purposeful, objects and toys are not used for their appropriate functions. For example, a child at this stage might mouth a block, drop a block, or bat it off a wheelchair tray. Adapted play at this stage might consist of batting at objects suspended from toy bars or grabbing objects using assists such as hand splints or special velcro hand mitts. These techniques are described later in this chapter.

Independent play is the second stage of play development. Children at this stage realize that objects have functions. They are able to play appropriately with simple objects but tend to play by themselves. Children at this stage enjoy repetitive play such as stacking blocks, filling and dumping boxes, spinning tops, and turning pages of books. Adapted play might consist of activating simple switch toys, or simple cause-and-effect software using the computer.

During **parallel play** the child continues to play independently but will make sure that he or she is near another child. Two children might build separate stacks of blocks near each other, or might push separate cars along the floor. The fourth stage, **associative play**, is similar to parallel play except that the children will briefly make eye contact or physical contact with one another. Two children might color near each other and periodically look at each other and giggle. **Cooperative play** occurs when the child seeks turn-taking interactions during play activities. Playing catch, taking turns stacking blocks, and looking at a book with an adult are examples of cooperative play. Across these last three stages, adaptive play should consist of activities that gradually require peer participation. For example, at the parallel play stage, two children might initially play near each other with separate switch toys. At the associative stage, they might play with toys that move, such as remote control cars, and send them toward each other. At the cooperative stage, the children would share a switch toy and take turns activating it.

The final stage of play development is **symbolic play**. Children who are capable of symbolic play are able to use objects for make-believe functions and can participate in pretend play. Examples of symbolic play include playing house, puppet play, dress-up, and pretend cooking. Adaptive play might consist of attaching puppets to wrist bracelets, using velcro play mitts to assist with holding dolls, or using sophisticated computer games such as William K. Bradford Publisher's *Explore-a-Story* to enact fantasy games.

Play as Therapy

Facilitating the development of play skills can be an important method of developing skills in other areas. Play activities can be used to motivate a child to attempt new and challenging skills (Musselwhite, 1986). A child who is frustrated attempting to make certain motor movements in therapy may try harder when given the opportunity to use the same motor movements in play. Play activities also can enhance opportunities for generalizing learned skills to other environments and activities. Participating in play motivates the child as well as adults and peers in the child's environment. This motivation ensures that others are likely to help the child practice play skills in new situations. Finally, play is a fun method of giving a child the opportunity to practice learned skills over and over again (Manolson, 1984).

Play and leisure skills can be used to promote development in many areas. Gross motor and mobility skills can be developed easily through play. The ambulatory child can develop gross motor skills by participating in playground activities such as tag and ball play. Play can also be used to motivate a child to participate in range of motion or positioning activities. Individuals with physical disabilities spend large portions of their days standing, lying on their sides, or in other positions. The ability to participate in play in these various positions will make these times more enjoyable. An individual confined to a wheelchair can learn mobility skills through play. Races and obstacle courses can be used to teach speed and control for moving a wheelchair. Children also can participate in treasure hunts in which prizes are hidden in different rooms that must be maneuvered into. By gradually increasing the obstacles that must be maneuvered around, an individual can learn visual motor planning skills with a wheelchair.

Fine motor skills can be significantly enhanced through play activities. Many toys are small and require good reaching, grasping, and releasing skills to manipulate. Moving small objects from one location to another, or one hand to another, also requires the development of visual motor coordination and motor planning.

Self-help and vocational skills also can be taught through play activities. Feeding, dressing, cooking, and hygiene skills can be taught through pretend play with dolls. Play also is important in the development of vocational skills. Play gives children an opportunity to act out future vocations, such as being a mommy, daddy, storekeeper, or teacher. Older individuals can use role-play interactions to practice job skills such as greeting customers, making change, or typing memos. The opportunity to participate in vocation-oriented play is important in establishing job skills in individuals with disabilities.

Play also can be used to develop cognitive skills. At early levels, play is an important method of teaching object permanence, cause-effect, and means-end schemes. A child can learn to hit a switch to see what will happen on a computer screen. At higher levels, play is used to explore relationships between objects and the environment. A child might squish various objects into Play-doh to see what shapes are made in the indentations, or might play a computer game such as Broderbund's *The Playroom* which allows some exploratory play.

Social and communication skills also can be developed through play. Play is ideally suited for the development of turn taking and cooperation. These social skills are developed in the planning stages of play when individuals are deciding what to do with their leisure time and during participation in actual play. Computer games with more than one player give individuals with physical disabilities an opportunity to participate in the turn-taking process. Both receptive and expressive communication skills are enhanced through learning to follow and give directions in play.

Strategies for Adapting Play Materials

Many individuals with physical, cognitive, or sensory disabilities are not able to play with commercially available play materials. Toys and games must be adapted to allow independent play. Williams, Briggs, and Williams (1979) have developed several strategies used to adapt play materials for individuals with handicaps. The first strategy is to stabilize materials. Individuals with physical disabilities often need toys affixed to a stable surface so they will not move. A wheelchair tray can be lined with strips of dual-lock plastic velcro, and various toys can have velcro attached to their bases. The toys then can be affixed to the wheelchair tray and held in a stable position to allow the child an opportunity for play. This can be done with a playhouse, toy dishes, and plastic baby dolls.

The second strategy is to enlarge materials to enhance visual perception and to decrease the need for fine motor coordination. An expanded computer keyboard such as Unicorn Engineering's *Unicorn Board* can be used to operate computer games instead of a standard keyboard. A child can be given a large plate switch to operate a switch toy instead of a small button switch. Similarly, the next strategy is to prosthetize. Parts are added to toys to make them more accessible and easier to manipulate. Handles can be attached to puzzle pieces, puppets are attached to wristbands, and items such as brushes, magic markers, and spoons are given large foam handles to make them easier to hold.

Another strategy is to make play materials more familiar and concrete. Some toys are highly abstract and do not resemble the real objects they represent. For example, Fisher-Price people are more abstract than most baby dolls. Playing a board game with three dimensional pieces is more familiar than playing the same game on the computer. By using play materials that are concrete and familiar, the individual who is disabled will be better able to relate play skills to everyday activities.

The next group of strategies involves removing extraneous cues and stimuli and enhancing important stimuli. Removing extraneous stimuli allows the individual to focus more easily on important factors of a toy or game. Puzzles that have solid color backgrounds are easier to learn than puzzles in which the background is a multicolored picture. Similarly, some computer games have extremely busy backgrounds which make it difficult to focus on important stimuli on the screen. When necessary, cues can be added to help an individual focus on important stimuli. Textured cloth can be attached to switches to make them more attractive to touch. Similarly, plastic mirrors or colored pictures can be attached to switches to make them more visually attractive. Cardboard covers that hide all but the most important stimuli can be added to computer screens, computer keyboards, and communication boards. Computer keys can be color-coded by adding minidot stickers to important game keys such as Return, Space Bar, and Escape.

Finally, play materials should be adapted to make them safe and durable. Sharp edges should be sanded to make them smooth. For some children, toys need to be protected from saliva by covering them with nontoxic sealants, clear plastic laminate, or clear contact paper. Any part that can easily be loosened by an individual should be removed or fastened in a more permanent manner. Computers can be adapted by covering the keyboard completely with a plastic cover, adding moisture guards to the keyboard, or removing the keyboard and accessing programs through alternate switches.

In addition to the strategies just listed, Musselwhite (1986) suggests that all play materials should be accessible. Individuals should be able to physically select and choose their own toys and games. For children in wheelchairs, toys can be attached to the wall at an appropriate height with dual-lock velcro strips, or placed in a toy net or on shelves which are hung at chair height. Children who lack arm or hand control to retrieve their own toys should be able to choose play activities by grossly pointing toward a desired toy. Toys should be arranged so that they are easy to point to, or simple communication boards can be developed so that the child can choose play activities by pointing to a picture of the activity or toy.

Individuals with computer skills who are physically disabled should have access to games on a computer hard disk. The hard disk allows them to independently choose between games without waiting for others to switch floppy disks for them. If a hard disk is not available, the user should be able to request software by pointing to individual disks or pictures of computer games on a communication board. If the user has some manual dexterity, adding tabbed handles to the outer edge of floppy disks, and providing a disk guide can facilitate independent computer use.

Toy, Game, and Appliance Adaptation Ideas

Switch Toys and Appliances

Using switches to activate toys allows individuals who are physically disabled to play with most battery-powered, remote-control, or electric toys and appliances. **Switch toys** are an ideal way to teach cause-effect skills and control of physical movements to a child who is physically disabled. Young children often learn to control motor movements by accidentally hitting a switch. The movement is positively reinforced by activating a toy, which encourages the child to attempt the movement again. When developing switch toys, the switch being used, the connecting cable, and the toy or appliance it controls need to be considered.

A wide variety of adaptive switches are available either commercially or through homemade plans. Virtually any body part that has controlled motor movements can be used to activate an adaptive switch. This includes the head, arms, hands, fingers, legs, knees, and feet, as well as eye blinks, brow movements, breath control, and muscle movements that are not observable to the naked eye. Each individual must be evaluated to determine which body movements and which switches provide the most control. In general, individuals with spastic motor movements require durable switches that can withstand sudden rough movement and some range of motion to activate the switch. Zygo's *Tread Switch,* Prentke Romich's *Wobble Switch,* and large push switches such as Able Net's *Big Red Switch,* often are appropriate for this population (see Figure 6–1). Individuals who have hypotonic motor disorders need switches that are sensitive to light, minimal movements. Zygo's *Leaf Switch, Lever Switch* and Kaynor Toys for Special Children's *Large Plate Switch* are appropriate. In addition several touch-sensitive switches are available that operate with computer chip surfaces that register the slightest pressure on the switch. TASH's *Plate Switch* is a flat surface switch that comes in four different colors. Touching any part of the colored surface activates the switch (see Figure 6–1).

Individuals who have spinal cord damage or other motor disorders resulting in paralysis require switches that measure almost imperceptable motor movements (see Figure 6–2). Words Plus makes an *Infrared Switch* that sends an infrared light beam from the switch to a surface which then reflects back the light. Any "break" in the light beam changes the reflecting surface and activates the switch. This switch can be operated by eye blinks, minimal hand and finger movements, or other body movements that can break the light beam. *Sip-and Puff-Switches* often are used for individuals with cervical spinal cord injuries. These switches operate on breath control. Finally Prentke Romich's *P-Switch* consists of a small piezoelectric sensor which is strapped onto any body surface such as the forehead, cheek, forearm, or thigh. Any muscle tensing is picked up by the sensor and relayed to the switch.

Most switches have only one possible electronic connection. Touching the switch activates the connection which in turn activates the device the switch is connected to. Some switches, called dual switches, have the capability to perform more than one task. Prentke Romich's *Rocking Lever Switch* can turn a device on when pushed on one side, and turn the device off when pushed on the other (see Figure 6–1). *Sip-and-Puff Switches* can turn on devices with an intake breath, and turn them off with an outward puff of air. Dual switches also can be used for Morse code operation. One switch operation acts as the "dit" and the other as the "dah."

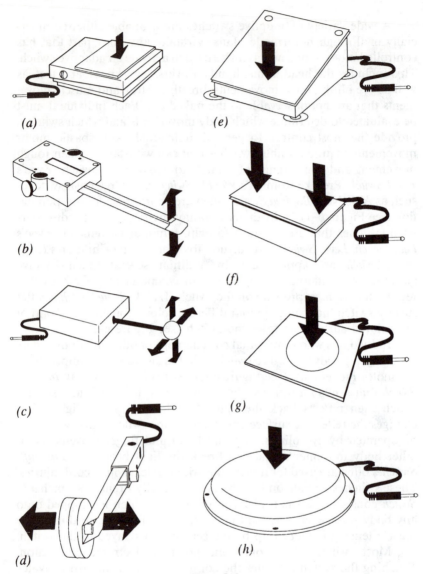

Figure 6-1

Adaptive switches. (a) Zygo *Tread Switch:* requires downward pressure on the plate surface and gives audible feedback. (b) Zygo *Leaf Switch:* bending the wire in the plastic casing to the right or left activates the switch. (c) Prentke Romich *Wobble Switch:* moving the ball minimally in any direction activates the switch, which gives audible click feedback. (d) Zygo *Lever Switch:* requires minimal downward pressure on the padded foam surface. (e) Toys for Special Children *5 × 8 Plate Switch:* minimally pressing on the surface activates the switch. (f) Prentke Romich *Rocking Lever Switch:* pressing downward on the right or left side activates selections on the device. (g) TASH *Plate Membrane Switch:* minimal pressure in the circled area activates the switch. (h) Able Net *Big Red Switch:* downward pressure on the large circular surface activates the switch.

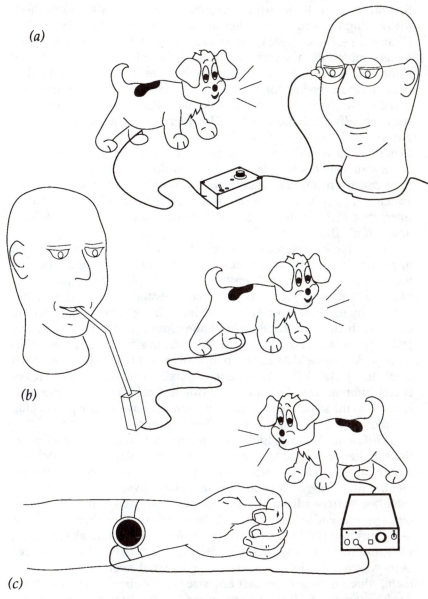

Figure 6–2

Switches for individuals with paralysis. (a) Words+ *Infrared Switch:* eyeblinks activate the switch which is connected to a toy via a control interface. (b) *Sip-and-Puff Switch:* air inhalation or exhalation through the pneumatic tube activates sensors in the control interface which is connected to a toy. (c) Prentke Romich's *P-Switch:* a piezoelectric sensor is strapped to the skin; minimal muscle tension sends signals to the control interface which is connected to a toy.

Several "how to" books which describe plans, materials, and methods for making homemade switches are available (Burkhart, 1980, 1982; Charlebois-Marois, 1985). Most switches can be made using store-bought materials, a soldering gun, and tin snips. Radio Shack and similar electronics stores sell most of the wire, jacks, plugs, and electrical tape necessary for making homemade switches. Homemade switches can be inexpensive to make but often are not as durable as commercially available switches. However, some unusual switches are not available commercially. These include Burkhart's (1980) puzzle switch which is activated when a puzzle piece is put in place and a coffee-can switch which is a pressure-sensitive switch in which children can drop objects. Once a certain weight level is achieved, the switch will activate a toy. The coffee-can switch can be used to promote interactive play similar to children's games such as "Pick Up Sticks" and "Don't Break the Ice."

Adaptive switches can be attached to a variety of battery-operated or electronic toys and appliances. The cables necessary for connecting the switch to the toy will vary. The cable's plugs must match the switches' and toy's receptors. Most commercially available switches have ⅛-inch, ¼-inch, or ½-inch female phone jacks. They require cables with similarly sized male phone plugs (see Figure 6–3). Phone jacks that range in size from 1/32 to 1/16 inches in size are called subminiature jacks. Those that range in size from ⅛ to ¼ inches are called miniature jacks. Adaptors are commercially available to convert between different sizes. In homemade switches, cables often are internally wired to the switch with a soldering gun but have a male phone plug attached to the end of the cable (see Figure 6–3).

Different toys and appliances require different cable configurations. Battery-operated toys that have not been adapted for switch use require a metal switch interruptor inserted into the battery compartment. These interruptors are commercially available as either **toy cables** or **battery adaptors.** These cables have standard male phone plugs on one end and copper toy interruptors on the other (see Figure 6–3). Burkhart (1980) gives instructions for making homemade cables with aluminum interruptors. The interruptor consists of two flat pieces of metal separated by a nonconducting material, such as cardboard or foam, which is usually circular and sized to the circumference of standard batteries. The interruptor is placed in the battery compartment between the battery and one of the metal battery contacts (see Figure 6–3). When the toy is turned on, it will not operate until the switch is activated. The advantage of this method is that any commercially available battery-operated toy can be adapted using these techniques. One disadvantage is having to insert the switch interruptor into the battery compartment. Some toys have an extremely tight fit between the bat-

Adaptive Switch and Toy Configurations

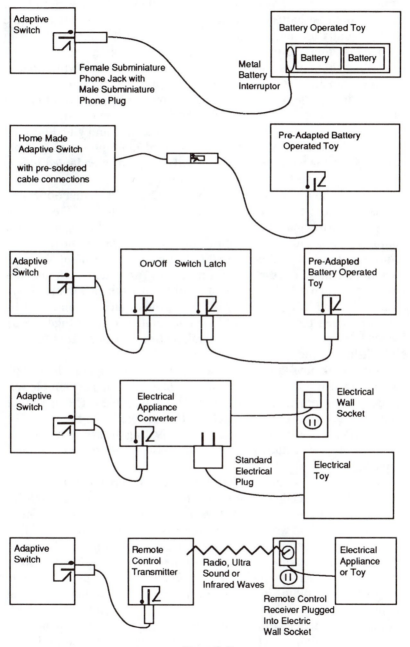

Figure 6–3
Adaptive switch and toy configurations.

tery and the metal contacts, which makes it difficult to insert the interruptor. The authors have broken many cable wires by trying to force interruptors into battery compartments that were too small. Separate cables usually are needed for each toy because it is inconvenient to keep reinserting the interruptor over and over again.

Many companies manufacture battery-operated and wind-up toys that have already been adapted for switch use. Kaynor's Toys for Special Children, Able Net, and Burkhart's Toys for Special Children sell these toys at reasonable prices. Preadapted toys come with either ¼-inch or ½-inch female phone jacks already drilled and glued into the toy (see Figure 6–3). An appropriately sized male phone plug cable connects the toy with the switch. An advantage of preadapted toys is the ease of connecting cables to the toy.

One problem in using adaptive switches with battery-operated toys is that the switch must be pressed continually to keep the toy running. This movement is the opposite of skills needed to operate most communication aids and computer games. Most communication aids require that the switch be pressed and immediately released. A **switch latch interface** will circumvent this problem. The switch latch operates like an on-off switch. One press of a switch turns the toy on, a second press is needed to turn the toy off. The switch latch is connected by cables between the switch and battery-operated toy (see Figure 6–3). Switch latches are available commercially from Kaynor's Toys for Special Children, and Able Net.

Electronic toys and appliances also can be operated through switches by using special **electronic control units**, which are simple versions of environmental control units (see Figure 6–3). The appliance plugs into the control unit, which is then plugged into the wall. The switch also plugs into the control unit. Activating the switch causes the toy or appliance to turn on. Able Net sells a control unit for electronic toys.

Electronic toys and appliances also can be operated through remote control. Special control units are plugged into wall receptacles (see Figure 6–3). Appliances or toys are then plugged into the control unit. The individual who is handicapped is given a remote control that can turn the control units on and off. Remote control signals can be sent using ultrasound, radio, or infrared signals. Adaptive Communication Systems manufactures the *ToyPac,* which operates remote control toys via radio signals. The *Toypac* can be adapted for several methods of access, including direct selection, single and double switch scanning, directed scanning, and joystick use. More information on remote control units will be given in the Environmental Controls section of this chapter.

Adapting Toys for Communication

Play activities provide an ideal means of introducing the communication skills of making choices and turn taking. Communication-oriented play can be facilitated by use of both low- and high-technology equipment and games designed to facilitate decision making and interaction. One of the easiest ways to introduce communication into play activities is to give an individual the opportunity to choose play activities. Play activity choice boards are one method of providing this communication skill. Objects or pictures representing play activities are arranged on a communication board. The individual then can choose play activities by pointing to the appropriate symbol (see Figure 6–4). Individuals who cannot use simple, direct selection communication boards can use an **Eye Gaze Object Box**, which is a clear plexiglass box with small toys arranged inside (see Figure 6–4). For individuals who need to use scanning methods of access, choice boards that attach to a single switch are available commercially (see Figure 6–4).

Another version of choice boards is the use of play vests (Goosens & Crain, 1986). Play vests are made of heavy-duty material such as ripstop nylon or denim and have velcro strips sewn across the front. A variation is to have clear plastic pockets sewn into the front of the vest (see Figure 6–4). Small objects can be attached to the vest with velcro or pinned to the vest. Similarly, pictures representing play activities can be attached to the vest with velcro or pins or placed into clear plastic pockets. The vest is worn by a trainer who sits in front of the child. The child can request play activities by pointing to pictures or objects arranged on the vest.

Choice boards and play vests can be used to give an individual choices between play activities. Once a play activity is chosen, topic-oriented communication boards are needed to give the individual a method of participating in turn-taking exchanges within the play activity. Goosens and Crain (1986) recommend that an individual be given access to simple topic-oriented communication boards during routine play activities. The boards are developed with pictures depicting typical subjects, objects, actions, and descriptions needed for communication within the activity. For example, one topic board might be developed for playing with dolls, another for cooking activities, and another for blowing bubbles. Topic-oriented boards should be located near the play area so that an individual learns to automatically retrieve the communication board along with the toy. Communication symbols can be attached to a toy by arranging symbols on a flat toy surface and covering the surface with clear contact paper. This idea works well for Fisher-Price buildings, child-sized play kitchens, and some game

Play Activity Choice Boards

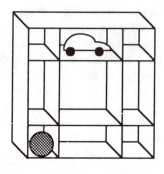

Plexiglass Eye Gaze Object Box

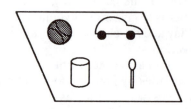

Object Choice Board

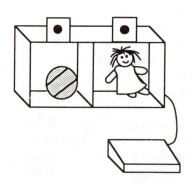

Scanning Choice Board with Switch

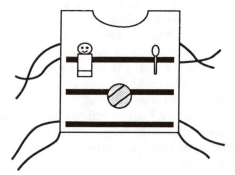

Play Vest with Objects

Figure 6–4
Play activity choice boards.

boards. Toys with small parts can be stored in plastic containers with the container lid used to construct a topic-oriented communication board. Other toys can be stored in tote bags with a communication board slipped into a plastic pocket sewn onto the outside of the bag.

Loop tapes can be used as a communication tool in play activities (Goosens & Crain, 1986). Loop tapes are cassette tapes similar to those used by phone answering machines. The cassette recorder has to be adapted for single switch use or have a remote control input jack. Cassette recorders that have already been adapted can be purchased, or a metal battery interruptor cable can be placed into the battery compartment of a standard cassette recorder (see Figure 6–3). A message is then recorded on the loop tape. By pressing the switch the message can be played over and over again. An individual can use messages such as "more tickles please," "turn the page," or "throw the ball" to initiate play activities. By using more than one switch-activated loop tape system, the individual can make choices between play activities.

Many adaptive play activities can be used to foster interactive turn taking. One method is to place a small rolling object, such as a ball, car, or block, into a cardboard tube which is held by two individuals. By taking turns lifting the tube, the toy can be rolled back and forth. Individuals who cannot lift the tube by themselves can participate in this activity by choosing which item to send down the tube and by receiving objects sent by other players.

Books can be adapted for turn-taking activities by making the pages easy to turn. Children's books with durable heavy cardboard pages work best. Clear contact paper can be used to attach 1 × 1-inch tabs to each page. The tabs should be ordered from top to bottom along the open side of the book. Some children are able to turn pages if the pages are separated for them. Sticky foam rubber or adhesive felt dots can be placed on the four page corners. These dots will separate the pages to make them easier to turn. Children can use cassette tapes in adapted single-switch recorders to read books aloud to themselves or others. Finally, augmentative communication aids can be programmed with the text of each book page. The picture symbols which will "read" the page out loud can be placed in the book on the appropriate pages. The child then presses the matching symbol on his communication aid to hear the page read. Chapter 4 gives more information on augmentative communication aids.

Finally, computer games can promote interactive turn taking. Software exists for exploratory play and game play. *Interaction Games* from Don Johnston Developmental Equipment Company is a software program specifically designed for two-person game playing using switches. *Facemaker* by Spinnaker is a computerized version of Mr. Potato Head. Two individuals can take turns selecting facial parts to develop a final funny face. MCE's *McGee* software lets children take turns letting the main character do fun activities around a cartoon house. Exploratory software such as Sunburst's *Muppets on Stage* can be used with the *Muppet Learning Keys* in group play activities. Children can take turns selecting the color and number of objects depicted on the computer screen. At higher levels individuals can work together to find Carmen in Broderbunds' *Where in the World is Carmen Sandiego?*. Chapter 5 describes methods of adapting computers.

Adapting Toys for Physical Access

There are many ways to adapt toys and games to make them physically accessible to handicapped individuals. Books and articles by Burkhart (1980, 1982), Carlson (1982), Charlebois–Marois (1985), Goosens and Crain (1986), and Musselwhite (1986) give specific suggestions, along with instructions for making each item. Many of their ideas involve adding prosthetic parts to toys to make them easier to manipulate. Small cloth toys, such as puppets, baby dolls, and stuffed animals, can have velcro wristbands sewn to them. The wristbands are then wrapped around the wrist of an individual who is handicapped making it possible to move the toy without dropping it. Similarly, gloves with velcro can be used to manipulate adapted toys. A pair of gloves can be adapted by sewing velcro to the fingertip and palm areas. Small toys can have velcro sewn or glued to their surfaces. An individual can then use the glove to pick up and move the toys. Magnets can be sewn into the fingertips of gloves to assist in picking up metal objects or pushing nonaluminum toy cars.

Play boards and toy bars can be used to stabilize toys for play. A play board is a piece of fiberboard or wood which is attached to a table surface or wheelchair tray (Carlson, 1982). The play board has long slots cut into it, with toys such as play cars or people attached by nuts and bolts through the slots (see Figure 6–5). Other toys, such as a play bed, are simply bolted into place on the surface of the play board. The child can easily push toys in their slots without knocking them off the edge of a wheelchair. A toy bar is a wood or plastic piping frame that is attached to a wheelchair tray or table surface (see Figure 6–5). Toys are attached to the toy bar by string or by plastic chain links. The toy bar prevents the toys from falling out of reach. For young children who like batting at toys, the toy bar is made tall so the toys will hang in the air. Older children who want to manipulate the toys need shorter toy bars with longer strings so they can move the toys to various locations on their wheelchair trays. A toy or pencil edge can be made to rim the surface of a wheelchair tray. The toy edge prevents objects from accidentally falling off the edge of the tray. Toy edges can range in height from ¼-inch to 3 inches. The size of the edge depends on the size of the objects typically played with, the age of the individual, and the physical skills of the individual.

ENVIRONMENTAL CONTROLS

Assistive technology devices can give disabled users control over many elements in their environment. Adaptive toys allow young children to

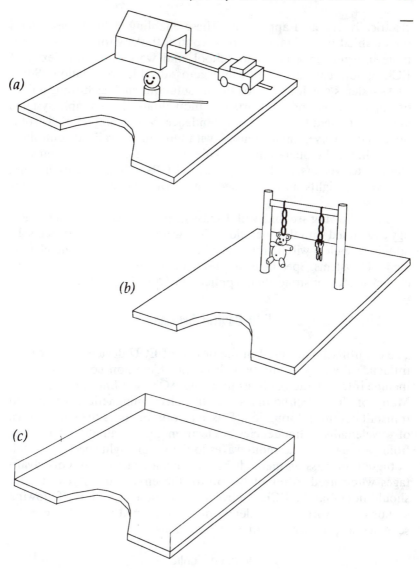

Figure 6–5
Toy stabilization methods. (a) Play board built into a wheelchair tray. (b) Toy bar attached to a wheelchair tray. (c) Wheelchair tray with a pencil or toy edge.

participate in critical areas of play, leisure, and daily living activities. A further refinement in the continuum of technology solutions for achieving control over the environment are environmental control systems.

Environmental Control Units (ECUs) are hardware and software systems that allow spontaneous and programmed control over remote, electrically operated appliances. These enabling technologies extend the disabled individual's ability to control the environment and promote independence at home, school, and work. The complexity of ECU options can vary significantly across disabled populations. Some ECU systems are designed for simple solutions such as turning a light or appliance on and off. For some individuals, these simple systems are not sufficient to provide independence. More complex ECU solutions may involve "smart houses" with built-in centralized controllers that manage the operation of a wide variety of electrical systems including, televisions, kitchen appliances, VCRs, stereo systems, heating and cooling, lights, automatic beds and doors, telephones, and burglar alarm systems.

The following sections will discuss general concepts and terminology associated with the operation of environmental control systems. In addition, readers will be introduced to a variety of simple and elaborate ECU systems. Specific examples of commercial systems will be included to demonstrate their application with disabled users.

ECU Control Schemes

The control schemes used in the design of ECU devices significantly influence their applicability with clients. Common control schemes include infrared, radio, ultrasound, and AC power line carrier signals. Many of these technologies use the electromagnetic spectrum to transmit control information. This spectrum includes the entire range of wavelengths of frequencies of electromagnetic radiation extending from gamma rays and radio waves to the visible light spectrum. Each of these transmission methods has distinct advantages and disadvantages when used to remotely control the environment. The reader should note that the ECU control schemes described in the following sections can work independently or be combined with other control schemes to produce hybrid ECU solutions.

Infrared Control

Infrared (IR) control methods are commonly used in consumer TV, stereo, and VCR home electronic units. The technology is based on digital Infrared Pulse-Code Modulation. The control process begins with the emission of digital signals which represent control codes or commands that operate the remote device. The digital signal is then converted into infrared pulses that are transmitted remotely to the electronic unit. Because infrared signals extend beyond the visible light spectrum of the human eye, users cannot see these signals in operation.

The two major components of infrared controls are the transmitter and receiver subsystems (see Figure 6–6). The transmitter is responsible for generating digital commands, converting the commands into infrared pulses, and transmitting them to the remotely operated device. The receiver subsystem is responsible for detecting the infrared pulses, converting them back into digital signals, and routing them to appropriate electronics which execute the control commands.

Infrared technology has a number of advantages for remote control. First, infrared is a very flexible method for coding control commands. Any digital signal can be easily converted into complementary infrared pulses. In addition, infrared is not affected by the technical limitations associated with bandwidth, which is the range of frequencies available for signaling. This gives the user a wide spectrum of sig-

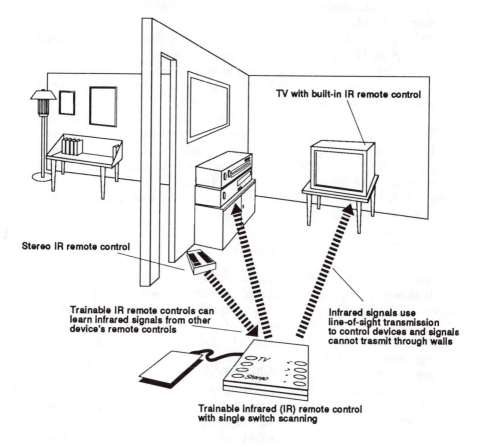

TV with built-in IR remote control

Stereo IR remote control

Trainable IR remote controls can learn infrared signals from other device's remote controls

Infrared signals use line-of-sight transmission to control devices and signals cannot trasmit through walls

Trainable infrared (IR) remote control with single switch scanning

Figure 6–6
Environmental control unit with infrared (IR) control scheme.

nal options for remotely operating electronic devices. Lastly, the microelectronic circuitry associated with this technology encourages the design of highly portable ECU solutions.

A disadvantage of infrared is the need for "line-of-sight" operation. Basically, the user must have no obstacles or objects between the transmitter and receiver. Some environmental impediments might include room layout, walls, furniture, or the client's location. Another disadvantage of infrared relates to one of the strengths of this technology. The flexibility of digital coding schemes often results in incompatibilities across different remote control systems. As a result, individuals often are required to use separate remote controls for the TV, stereo, and VCR. New "trainable" remote controls are now entering the market. These units have the ability to watch and learn the infrared pulses of different systems so that a single trainable transmitter can control a wide number of infrared devices.

Technical Aids and Systems for the Handicapped Inc. (TASH) markets an IR environmental control system for the disabled called *Relax*. The *Relax* system is an infrared transmitter that can be operated with adaptive switches. This ECU is a trainable transmitter capable of learning, storing, and transmitting 50 different control codes, allowing clients to control TV, VCR, and any other appliance that uses IR control schemes. The system can control up to six different appliances. The client can access *Relax* using a single switch or an expanded keypad with 15 keys (2.75 inches in size). An indicator light and a scan array are used for making function selections. The *Relax* system can use TASH's *2 IR* infrared receiver or the X-10 remote control system, which is discussed later in this chapter.

Radio Control

Radio control methods are commonly used in consumer toys, automatic door openers, and other miscellaneous home electronic equipment. This technology uses radio frequencies (RF) to transmit control codes to appliances. The spectrum of radio waves is designated in different frequencies called bands. These radio bands allocate specific segments of the radio spectrum for specific uses. The measure of frequency or bandwidth is called Hertz (Hz).

A wide range of radio bands in the electromagnetic spectrum is used for various telecommunication uses. For example, Medium-Frequency (MF) radio operates in a band from 300 kHz to 3 MHz. This band is used mainly for AM radio broadcasting. The Very High Frequency (VHF) radio band, operating from 30 to 300 MHz, is used for FM radio, television, car phones, and personal paging systems. The demand for mobile radio is increasing rapidly, which means that this part of the radio spectrum is becoming overcrowded and there is an ever-growing shortage of these frequencies. The Ultra High Frequency (UHF) radio band operates from 300 to 3000 MHz, nearly ten times the capacity of VHF band. This band has been allocated for television, mobile radios, radar, and navigational devices.

Environmental control systems using RF transmission must operate within a specific radio band to broadcast control codes to operate a remote device. The most common radio band used with ECUs is the UHF band. Radio control systems use a transmitter that beams radio waves to a receiver. The receiver then sends control signals to the electronic device (see Figure 6–7).

Radio's through-the-air broadcasting method makes for wireless, flexible environmental control systems. Because radio signals can be transmitted through walls, users are not limited to the "line-of-sight" operation associated with IR control units. This allows radio control systems to transmit and control a wide range of appliances around the home from one central location. In addition, this control method can be used in remote locations without running unwieldy wires and purchasing expensive cabling. The compact design of RF systems and the simplicity of the transmission mechanism makes for highly mobile ECU solutions.

Radio control techniques do have some limitations related to the transmission of the control signal. The major limitation of radio-controlled ECUs is the limited distance control signals can travel. Most RF environmental control systems function only within a specific operational radius. This radius usually extends from 50 to 200 feet, depending on the transmitter. When the control unit leaves its control radius, receivers lose the transmitter's control signal. Because of overcrowding on certain radio bands, control transmissions also are subject to interference. Inadvertent radio signals also may be detected by RF receivers, resulting in false or inappropriate device operation.

Radio frequency transmitters are often used with AC power line control methods. The most commonly used AC power line system is called X-10, after the manufacturer, X-10 (USA), Inc. X-10 technology is used by many different companies in the manufacture of ECU devices. This technology is discussed in detail later in the chapter.

Prentke Romich Company's *Scanning X-10 Powerhouse* environmental control unit is a wireless radio-controlled ECU. The system can operate up to 16 appliances and/or lights inside or outside. The user has access to this environmental control by using either a single or dual switch or using the input controller for Invacare Corporation's *Arrow* powered wheelchair. The *Scanning X-10 Powerhouse* ECU is made up of a portable, battery-operated visual display transmitter and a receiver subsystem. The display transmitter provides visual and audi-

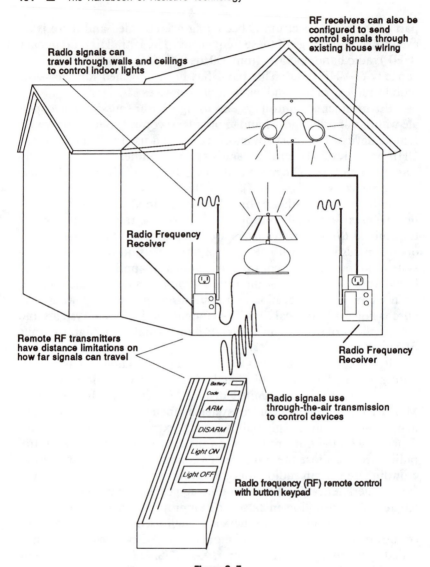

RF receivers can also be configured to send control signals through existing house wiring

Radio signals can travel through walls and ceilings to control indoor lights

Radio Frequency Receiver

Remote RF transmitters have distance limitations on how far signals can travel

Radio Frequency Receiver

Battery
Code
ARM
DISARM
Light ON
Light OFF

Radio signals use through-the-air transmission to control devices

Radio frequency (RF) remote control with button keypad

Figure 6–7
Environmental control unit with radio frequency (RF) control scheme.

tory feedback as the user scans the appliance list. The user of an *Arrow* powered wheelchair activates a switch to select between wheelchair functions and ECU mode. The receiver subsystem consists of an *X-10* wireless transceiver and the appropriate number of *X-10 Powerhouse* appliance modules. The transceiver sends control signals to appliance modules over the dwelling's electrical wiring. X-10 (USA) Inc. sells the same system without the adaptive switch scanning in a system called the *Wireless Remote Control System RC5000.*

Finally, X-10 (USA) Inc. also markets a radio-controlled unit that extends the range of existing infrared (IR) remote controls. *Powermid* consists of a radio frequency (RF) transmitter and transceiver. The user points an IR remote control at the *Powermid* RF transmitter which then converts the infrared signals into radio waves and sends them to a second *Powermid* transceiver located in another room. The transceiver then converts the radio signals back to identical infrared signals and sends them to the user's stereo, TV, VCR, CD player, cable box, or any other IR-controlled appliance. This system can eliminate line-of-sight problems associated with IR environmental control units.

Ultrasound Control

Ultrasound control schemes are based on the use of very high frequency sound waves. The sound wave vibrations are of the same physical nature as sound but use frequencies above the range of human hearing. Consequently, ultrasound signals are not audible to people. The control process begins with the emission of an ultrasound signal representing a control command. Because ultrasound is non-directional, sound waves emitted from the transmitter will bounce around the room's walls until the receiver can detect the sound wave. The receiver then converts the sound wave into control commands that activate the appliance (see Figure 6–8).

A major advantage of ultrasound is that it does not require line-of-sight operation. The user's ultrasound transmitter can be located anywhere in a room and still send signals to the receiver. Because ultrasound signals cannot go through room walls, accidental triggering of receivers in other rooms is eliminated. An added advantage of ultrasound control systems are their wireless setup and operation. The user's home requires no additional cabling or wiring. Lastly, ultrasound transmitters generally are small and conducive to portable ECU solutions.

A limitation of ultrasound is that the system can operate only appliances located in the room with the transmitter. A user cannot transmit ultrasound signals to appliances in other rooms without first entering the room with the transmitter.

Technical Aids and Systems for the Handicapped, Inc. (TASH) markets a variety of ultrasound environmental control systems. These systems, which include *Ultra 4S, Ultra 4L, Ultra 4J, Ultra 2P,* and *Ultra 2T,* consist of color-coded transmitters and receivers. Up to four distinct color-coded ultrasonic signals can be sent to receivers of the same color code. A 1.5 volt AA-size alkaline battery powers each transmitter for up to 1 year. The *Ultra 4S* is a hand-held transmitter ($4 \times 2.5 \times 1$

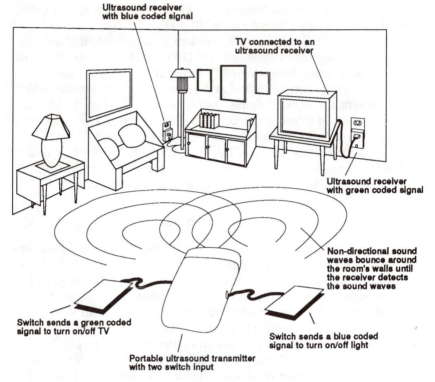

Ultrasound receiver with blue coded signal

TV connected to an ultrasound receiver

Ultrasound receiver with green coded signal

Non-directional sound waves bounce around the room's walls until the receiver detects the sound waves

Switch sends a green coded signal to turn on/off TV

Switch sends a blue coded signal to turn on/off light

Portable ultrasound transmitter with two switch input

Figure 6–8
Environmental control unit with ultrasound control scheme.

inches) with four small buttons with color codes. This transmitter is intended for use by individuals with very good hand and finger control. The *Ultra 4L* is designed to mount on the user's wheelchair. It has four color-coded buttons recessed on a small keyboard (5 × 8.25 × 1.5 inches). Each button is 1 inch in diameter and is designed for individuals with limited hand and finger dexterity. The *Ultra 4J* uses a joystick with four directional switches. The system is designed to mount on the user's wheelchair or table top. The *Ultra 2P* is a pneumatic transmitter operated by puffing and sipping on the mouthpiece. This transmitter can only send two, color-coded ultrasonic signals. The *Ultra 2T* transmitter is operated with any two single or one dual switch and can send two ultrasonic signals. Both the *Ultra 2P* and *Ultra 2T* transmitters have dimensions of 4 × x 2.5 ×1 inches and can be mounted on a wheelchair or table. All of the these ultrasound transmitters must be used with appropriately colored *Ultra 4 power modules.* The modules are plugged into 115V AC home outlets. Appliances are then plugged into the power modules.

AC Power Line Control

AC power line carrier signals are another popular method for controlling the environment. This control method gives the user control of lights and appliances from anywhere in the home or apartment using the building's existing electrical power lines. The system consists of three major components: a command control center, a base receiver, and appliance modules.

The command control center is responsible for sending digital signals over the existing power lines of the user's residence. The control center acts as the transmitter and can be configured as either a remote or plug-in unit. A remote control center usually sends command signals to a base receiver via radio or infrared control (see Figure 6–9). The base receiver then transmits control codes to appliance modules. A plug-in control center typically transmits signals directly to appliances via the home's AC power line. There are also methods that allow the client to interface a control center to a personal computer. In this configuration the computer is used to program all home control information into the command control center. The control center then can be detached from the computer and operate in remote or plug-in configurations.

The second element of AC power line control is the base receiver. This subsystem acquires remote signals from the command center. The base receiver plugs into a dwelling's AC power receptacle. The base receiver can be configured to accept signals from infrared (IR) or radio frequency (RF) sources. The unit then sends control signals to appliance modules. These modules come in a wide variety of configurations. For example, they can be configured as seperate modules that plug into standard AC electrical outlets around the home. The module allows the user to turn on and off any appliance that is plugged into it. Modules also may be configured as wall switches (see Figure 6–9). In this configuration, a module replaces the standard wall switch, enabling the user to turn lights on and off from anywhere in the house, including inside and outside locations. A third option, the wall receptacle module, replaces the standard AC power wall outlet (see Figure 6–9). The module looks just like a regular wall outlet but can control any appliance plugged into the receptacle. The replacement process involves minor rewiring of the module into the wall receptacle.

Power line control methods are very flexible. The user can configure simple or sophisticated ECU solutions. Because the system uses the home's existing wiring, users are not required to perform complex setup or rewiring. The command control center allows users to operate lights and appliances from a single remote control. Portable control centers that incorporate RF signals provide users with the ability to control lights and appliances inside and outside of the home. The

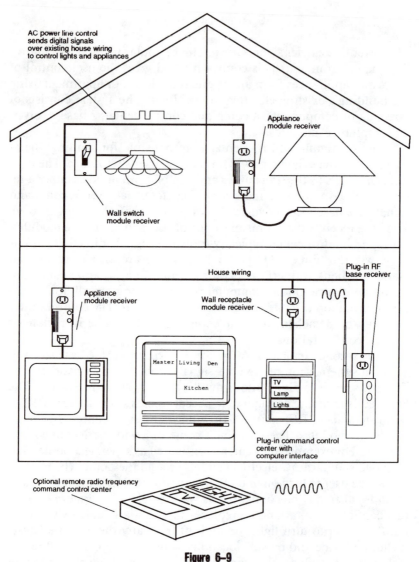

AC power line control
sends digital signals
over existing house wiring
to control lights and appliances

Appliance
module receiver

Wall switch
module receiver

House wiring

Plug-in RF
base receiver

Appliance
module receiver

Wall receptacle
module receiver

Master | Living | Den

Kitchen

TV
Lamp
Lights

Plug-in command control
center with
computer interface

Optional remote radio frequency
command control center

Figure 6-9
Environmental control unit with AC power line control scheme.

radio waves allow the remote signal to travel through walls and ceilings directly to the receiver module.

Although no wiring is necessary for using power line control methods, careful planning and arrangement of ECUs in the client's environment is necessary. Careful planning determines the type and location of the command control center and provides data on the number of device control options required by the user. In addition, the command control center will require some programming. This usually involves setting up unit and house codes to group lights and appliances appropriately for the client.

AC power line control systems are referred to as "X-10" units, named after the developer and manufacturer, X-10 (USA) Inc. A wide variety of X-10 modules and controllers are used by other companies in the manufacture of consumer home automation and security systems. The major systems are differentiated by how the user activates the control center, how the control center transmits signals to control modules, and how many devices can be managed by the control center. In general, most ECU systems that use X-10 technology for control require a transmitter, a base receiver, and appliance modules.

DU-IT Control Systems Group's *Deuce* is a multipurpose environmental control unit. It consists of a master unit that measures 8 × 14 × 4.75 inches. The master unit is designed for use on a work station or table. It can transmit control signals to four internal 110V AC outlets for appliance control and four internal ECU switch closures for electronic devices utilizing switch-based control methods. *Deuce* also can control any standard or speaker phone using either pulse or tone dialing. The system's telephone control functions include pick-up, number dialing, and hang up tasks and memory storage of 18 telephone numbers. To transmit AC power line control signals, an X-10 command control center must be plugged into the *Deuce* master unit. This configuration allows the user to operate up to 16 different appliances. The *Deuce* unit transmits control commands to the X-10 command control center which then sends control commands to individual appliance modules plugged in all around the user's home. The *Deuce* control unit provides the user with several input options including direct selection, dual switch input, and IR remote control.

An X-10 system can be controlled from wheelchairs using DU-IT Control Systems Group's *Mecca*. This control system provides the same functionality of the *Deuce* unit but is integrated into the user's powered wheelchair. The system uses radio control to transmit X-10 control commands to the telephone, lights, and appliances.

Prentke Romich Company's *Control 1* is another multipurpose environmental control unit. It consists of a master control unit that measures 11 × 17 × 3.75 inches and is designed for use on a work station, desk, or table. The master control unit is designed for computer use but can be used independently. The *Control 1* has eight receptacles for the control of a TV, intercom system, call bell, electric bed, or other electronic devices. The unit also can answer phones, dial numbers, and store up to ten phone numbers. The control unit is compatible with both pulse and tone dialing. The system's X-10 control options require the use of separate X-10 appliance modules. Users have a variety of options for accessing *Control 1*. First, users can purchase Prentke Romich's *Control 1 Input Display* (CID). The *CID* can be connected to the *Control 1* via a cable or operated as a remote unit using radio signals. *CID* uses a dual-switch system for scanning and Morse code input. The *Control 1* also can be operated from a microcomputer or communication aid such as Prentke Romich's *Light Talker* or *Touch Talker*. A special adapter cable is required for use with a communicator as on any other device with an RS 232C interface.

X-10 (USA) Inc.'s *Home Control Interface* is an X-10 environmental control system that gives users the freedom to program their environments using a microcomputer. The *Home Control Interface* connects to the computer's serial port using the supplied cable. In addition, the system includes menu-driven software and the X-10 command control center required to transmit control functions to lights and appliances. Users purchase appliance modules separately as needed. The *Home Control Interface* can control up to 256 differently coded X-10 light and appliance modules. The control unit can be programmed for up to 128 separately timed events involving the control of several appliance modules. This includes the ability to program timed events for different rooms on different days. The *Home Control Interface* system is available for IBM PCs, IBM compatibles, Apple Macintosh, Apple *IIe* and *IIc,* and Commodore *64* and *128* microcomputer systems.

The Heath Company's *Mini* and *Maxi Command Centers* and *X-10 control modules,* KY Enterprises' *EZRA,* Stanley's *LightMaker Home Controls,* Radio Shack's *Plug 'n Power System,* X-10 (USA) Inc.'s *X-10 Powerhouse,* Sears' *Home Control System*, Ultratec, Inc's *Super Signal System* are other examples of command control centers, base receivers, and appliance modules for X-10 use.

Finally, TASH's *Kincontrol* is a scanning ECU that allows control of up to 10 different functions. The *Kincontrol* can be operated with any single or double switch, an *Ultra 4* transmitter with an *Ultra 2R* receiver, the *Relax* trainable infrared transmitter and 2IR receiver, or X-10 controllers. The *Kincontrol* features adjustable settings for scanning modes, scan speed, and channel selection.

Miscellaneous Control Schemes

Selection of an ECU should be based on the user's control needs and the specific appliance functions needing control. A number of single-function environmental control units that allow users to control a single device with one or two switches are available. For example, a user may wish to turn a fan on or off after a specific period of time. The solution could involve the use of a single-function ECU. TASH's *Power Minder* is a self-contained power cord with a built-in timer and power interrupt switch for small appliances that plugs into any standard 110V AC power outlet. A momentary contact on the connected switch turns the power on and the timer turns the fan off after a 15-minute interval.

In another example, a user may desire to turn a microcomputer, monitor, and printer on and off with single switch input. In this control application the computer system's power cables are grouped into one multioutlet power bar or power strip. The power strip is then attached to the wall outlet. TASH's *Ultra Power Bar* allows users to operate the unit by any switch plugged into the jack on the power bar. In addition, the power bar can be operated by an ultrasound transmitter. Either access method gives the user the ability to turn on the computer system components at the same time.

A more intricate single-control application is the operation of a television. A user may wish to control the television's power, volume, and channel functions. TASH's *Unicontrol TV Converter* provides a single-control solution for operating the TV. The system consists of a TV converter and switch-operated remote control that replace the television's standard infrared remote control and receiver. The TV converter acts as the receiver and the remote control operates as the transmitter. A single or dual switch can then be connected to jacks on the remote control unit. The remote control, with or without the switches connected, can then be used to control the TV. One switch may be used to turn the TV on and off while the other operates channel and volume functions.

Guidelines for Selecting ECUs

The multiplicity of control schemes available to individuals who are disabled provides for great flexibility in design and implemention of environmental control systems. When service providers consider plans for the selection of ECUs, it is helpful to identify the key factors that will influence the successful implementation of the control system.

Assessing the needs of the user is an important part of any environmental control prescription. This can be accomplished through client-family interviews, formal testing, or related protocols. The purpose of the evaluation is to give the team an understanding of the user's control needs and how these control needs relate to the individual's functional environment. It is helpful to begin the assessment process by developing a physical layout of the client's environment. This usually involves mapping out various rooms of the client's residence, locating electric wall receptacles, and identifying any unique room features that may affect remote operation. This diagram provides the technology team with a method to illustrate important design variables in the user's environment.

The team then can generate a list of lights and appliances in each room that the user wishes to operate. The device list then can be applied to the user's dwelling diagram to detail frequently used rooms and the locations of important lights and appliances. Careful attention should be given to how the user operates and utilizes lights and appliances. For example, can the client operate appliances as a group or will each appliance require single-switch operation? Information regarding the frequency of appliance use gives the technology team information on how the user interacts daily in his or her environment. These data provide meaningful information on where the client might wish to control frequently used electronic devices. It also provides information on ways to optimize the location and control of individual appliances.

The transmission of control signals to appliances can be accomplished using infrared, radio, ultrasound, and AC power line carrier signals. The location of appliances plays an important role in the selection of these control schemes. Information about specific room arrangements in the client's environment details the location of electric wall receptacles, unique room features that may affect ECU operation, and the location of appliances the user wishes to control. These data provide the team with estimates on how many devices the ECU needs to control. Further, knowledge regarding the specific operation of appliances gives the technology team insight into what appliance functions need to be controlled by the ECU. The information on the location of appliances throughout the user's environment also helps the team determine whether the user will need direct- or remote-control options.

The user's cognitive abilities play a large role in the selection and design of ECU systems. The user's cognitive abilities certainly will influence the complexity of environmental control systems. For example, a user with severe mental retardation may only be capable of using a control system that turns a radio on and off. More intricate ECU applications, such as the control of television channels and volume control, usually demand higher levels of cognitive functioning. The user's association skills are key factors in the successful use of environmental controls. The user of the ECU must instinctively identify and remember the relationship between what he or she does and what follows. The correspondence between a user's skills, the interface, and the user's control needs are critical to the ECU design process.

An individual's motor abilities also have a significant impact on the selection and use of ECUs. Motor deficits that result in limited range of movement, reduced tactile sensation, weak or low force movement, or misdirected movement are a few examples of motor factors that affect ECU access. Many consumer products use hand-held remote controls to operate the main unit. Unfortunately, most commercial remote control transmitters are not accessible to individuals who are disabled and use a single switch or require larger keypads. Selection criteria for transmitters should include an analysis of the unit's input facilities. Can the user control the ECU through a variety of input options? Input options include direct selection on a keyboard, single- and multiple-switch scanning, and switch encoding schemes. To augment the user's motor abilities, ECU designs should accommodate alternative input devices such as alternate keyboards, joysticks, light pointers, single or multiple switches, communication aids, or computers. Similarly, consideration should be given to the flexibility of the input method and its selection process. Input considerations might include the need for single- or multiple-switch access. The flexibility of the scanning interface also is important. Consideration should also be given to systems that allow customization of the scanning array, including optional array symbol sets, alternate scanning methods, and adjustments for scanning speed. Attention to input and selection issues like these is important for accommodating the needs of individuals who are disabled.

Attention also should be given to the user's mobility requirements. The location of the user when operating appliances plays an important role in the selection of control schemes. For example, if the user is confined to a bed, the ECU transmission method requires control from a central location. From this single location, the user may need to control devices in the immediate room and throughout the house. This application requires the transmitter to communicate with many receivers throughout the dwelling. Alternatively, if the user can ambulate freely throughout the environment with a wheelchair or walker, a portable transmitter design may be more appropriate. The portable transmitter configuration may require consideration of ECU access methods. For example, the technology team may contemplate user access through the wheelchair joystick control or as a totally separate control system mounted on the wheelchair or walker. ECU control considerations might entail designing a system that uses the wheelchair's input controller. In this implementation, electronics compatibility, power requirements, and interfacing would be considerations. Similarly, the user's ability to independently select between wheelchair drive functions and the environmental control mode might be an issue.

Sensory impairments also are important factors in the selection of ECU systems. The technology team should evaluate the appropriateness of the ECU's control interface. For example, ECU lights, blink rates, auditory feedback, or activity of the visual field could produce startle responses in users. This can interfere with the control process. Careful attention also should be given to how the ECU communicates various modes of operation to the user, system errors, presenting and selecting desired choices, and adjusting or changing environmental control functions. The need for assistive output is a key factor for users who have sensory impairments. For instance, speech synthesis can provide voice prompting to announce and confirm control functions for users who are visually impaired. Computer-based ECUs might employ monitors or screens with large text menus so that clients with low vision can more easily view listings of controllable lights and appliances.

SUMMARY

Environmental control systems can offer users who are disabled increased independence so they can interact more fully in recreational activities, work, and home control activities. The critical element in the success of environmental control technology is the technology team. When planning to make control technology more effective for users, team members must be knowledgeable about the function and capabilities of the technology being prescribed. Members of the technology team must use this knowledge to integrate control systems with the control needs of clients. Hence, the technology implementation process should consider the wide variety of control schemes available to users who are disabled. In addition, a number of human and hardware factors influence the effectiveness of ECU control schemes. Technologists should identify critical factors and determine what effects they may have on the user's control needs. Identifying and planning for these factors can greatly aid technologists in making and designing effective environmental control systems.

REFERENCES

Bender, M., Brannan, S. A., & Verhoven, P. J. (1984). *Leisure education for the handicapped: Curriculum goals, activities, and resources.* San Diego, CA: College Hill-Press.

Burkhart, L. (1980). *Homemade battery powered toys and educational devices for severely handicapped children.* College Park, MD: Author.

Burkhart, L. (1982). *More homemade battery devices for severely handicapped children with suggested activities.* College Park, MD: Author.

Carlson, F. (1982). *Prattle and play.* Omaha, NE: Meyer Children's Rehabilitation Center, Media Resource Center.

Charlebois–Marois, C. (1985). *Everybody's technology: A sharing of ideas in augmentative communication.* Montreal, Canada: Charlecoms.

Goosens, C., & Crain, S. (1986). *Augmentative communication intervention resource.* Wauconda, IL: Don Johnston Developmental Equipment.

Manolson, A. (1984). *It takes two to talk: A Hanen early language parent guide book.* Toronto, Canada: Hanen Early Language Resource Center.

Musselwhite, C. (1986). *Adaptive play for special needs children.* San Diego, CA: College-Hill Press.

Wehman, P. (1979). Toy play. In P. Wehman (Ed.,) *Recreation programming for developmentally disabled persons.* Baltimore, MD: University Park Press.

Williams, B., Briggs, N., & Williams, R. (1979). Selecting, adapting, and understanding toys and recreation materials. In P. Wehman (Ed.), *Recreation programming for developmentally disabled persons.* Baltimore, MD: University Park Press.

7

Integrating Assistive Technology in the Classroom and Community

■ Joan Carney, MA ■
■ Cynthia Dix, MS ■

For many individuals with multiple handicaps, accessibility to assistive technology is comparable to barrier-free architecture in promoting independence. Utilizing electronic and computer assisted technology to address disability-related needs allows many functions to be performed without the aid of other persons, thus reinforcing the individual's view of him- or herself as competent (Burkhead, Sampson, & McMahon 1986). In addition, for children with multiple handicaps, assistive devices can aid parents and clinicians in better assessing psycholinguistic abilities and thereby in optimizing the child's potential.

Although prescribing assistive technology for youngsters with multiple handicaps can be quite complicated, even the most careful matching of devices with a student's needs will be lost if the client is not shown how to integrate these prosthetics into his or her life. Those responsible for implementing integration of the technology must be identified, receive training, and develop a plan for fostering acceptance of the assistive devices. This chapter will discuss these issues, as well as outline sample integration plans for students with varied needs.

THE INTEGRATION TEAM

Just as earlier authors have proposed an interdisciplinary model for evaluation of the student and prescription of assistive devices, individuals responsible for integration strategies must also work as a team to produce optimal results. Utilizing the interdisciplinary team model fosters the "whole child" approach of considering intellectual, physical, sensory, and psychosocial factors.

A growing number of students are employing assistive technology in educational settings. Due to varying practices of local school systems regarding educational placement, students who are handicapped may be centralized in one location or assigned to a neighborhood school. Such local practices have an impact on the availability of staff members with experience in assistive technology and may influence the composition of the integration team for each student. For example, a center-based program for students with multiple handicaps is more likely to have staff members who have experience in planning and implementing the use of assistive technology; whereas staff at a neighborhood school may need the assistance of outside resources to participate on the integration team.

The most obvious, but frequently overlooked, member of the integration team is the student. Successful use of assistive devices can be expected only if both the student's needs and desires are addressed. Family and community caregivers are equally important and need to be encouraged to actively participate as members of the integration team. Although the use of technology may begin in the classroom, each team's long-term goal should be to strive for integration not only in the school but, also in the home and the community. This generalization of use from one environment to another can only be achieved if caregivers actively participate in the process.

Classroom staff also are essential members of the integration team. The primary teacher and support staff are asked to carry out the integration plan, but are not always included in its development. This can set the plan on a course for failure. Classroom staff will have ownership of the components of the plan only if they are allowed to develop them to suit not only a particular student but all who share the educational environment.

Staff experienced in the field of assistive technology also must be included on the integration team to provide consultation and training. Optimally, the local educational agency will have a team of professionals from various disciplines ready to serve in such a capacity. Disciplines represented may include speech-language pathology, occupational therapy, physical therapy, psychology, special education, vision services, and rehabilitation engineering. In many school systems such a team is not in place. Other sources of professional assistance include agencies that have prescribed the equipment, selected clinicians in the school system who have had previous experience integrating the use of assistive devices, or school-based therapists who are willing to approach this endeavor with careful consideration and enthusiam. Prudent selection of the integration team lays the groundwork for success in the incorporation of assistive technology in the classroom and the community.

In the interdisciplinary model, the roles of the various members will become more and less prominent as the plan progresses. This concept of a "fluid team" allows a more natural approach. One team member, however, should be identified as the case manager whose role is to provide coordination and continuity.

Staff Preparation

Assistive technology has the potential to expand educational opportunities for students with disabilities; however, the manner in which technology is integrated into the classroom setting is dependent, in part, on the amount and type of preparation school staff receive prior to its introduction into the classroom. Ideally, school staff who work with children undergoing evaluation for technology are included on the team of professionals selecting equipment and developing strategies for its integration in the classroom. In some cases, a student is evaluated by an outside agency with very little input from school staff. When the technology arrives, however, school staff frequently are asked to provide the student with training in its use and to integrate the equipment in their existing educational programs. Training for school staff is therefore crucial to the student's successful use of assistive technology.

Two models of staff preparation appear to exist across educational settings. These are (1) group training and (2) individual training. The first model provides staff with general information related to assistive technology. This information may or may not be specific to immediate needs of the student population. Courses offered at the college or university level, conferences and workshops offered by local, state, and national organizations, and training seminars offered by vendors to familiarize individuals with specific equipment may be included in this model. School staff members choose to participate in these activities to broaden their knowledge base in assistive technology. Thus, when their students begin using technology, they already possess information that will assist them in participation on the technology integration team. In some cases, such staff members may take on the role of technology expert. This model of staff preparation is a "hit or miss" proposition, and even the most motivated staff members may find it difficult to locate courses that provide training in integration of assistive technology in the educational setting. In a survey of 50 school districts, Mokros and Russell (1986) found that only two thirds of the special education teachers who utilized computer technology in their classrooms had received some training in the use of technology. The others were self-taught. The reported focus of most of the training they had received was on computer programming (BASIC and LOGO). Others reported having been provided with "computer literacy" courses and instruction in operating computer hardware. None reported receiving training in incorporating either the devices or available software into their curriculum. What they had learned in training sessions was only vaguely related to what they were doing with their students.

Introduction to the use of assistive technology for individuals who are handicapped should begin at the university level. This topic could be included in a teaching methods course syllabus, a series of classes on the needs of students who are physically handicapped, or in a course that specifically addresses computer-assisted instruction and technology for environmental control and augmentative communication. Teacher preparation courses and inservice training sessions designed for teachers working in the field should cover accessibility, a review of the available hardware and software, and actual experience with a variety of devices, as well as some focus on the integration of technology into school and community use. Optimally, such training would be a long-term endeavor, allowing the introduction of new devices as they become available, in addition to providing enough time and ongoing support for professionals to practice integration techniques. The increased use of assistive devices in all educational environments would seem to warrant such ongoing training within educational agencies.

Inservice programs for school staff offer an excellent opportunity for individuals who use similar curricula to learn the basics of assistive technology and then brainstorm methods for integration. School staff members who are responsible for designing and presenting inservice training on assistive technology will meet with the highest degree of participation if they begin by conducting a needs assessment of school staff. In most cases, school staff will present a range of expertise, and the skills that individual staff members need to develop are determined largely by the technology needs of the students they serve. The following topics were identified by a needs assessment conducted in the Howard County, Maryland Public School System (1990):

1. Overview of augmentative communication
2. Low-tech augmentative communication aids and techniques

3. Make-and-take session for low-tech augmentative communication aids
4. Overview of high-tech augmentative communication aids
5. Vocabulary selection for augmentative communication aids
6. Interaction strategies
7. Introduction to computer-assisted instruction
8. Adapted peripherals and computer adaptations for students with physical disabilities
9. Software selection and integration utilizing software activity kits
10. Word processing for students with disabilities
11. Technology applications for young children

Evaluation forms completed by participants in the inservice programs listed above revealed some general trends regarding the preferred format of these inservice programs. Most participants desired practical "how to" information and wanted a minimum of theory. "Hands-on" time with the technology equipment was also highly valued by the participants. Videotaped segments that illustrated techniques and student performance were reported to be of value as was detailed literature that provided participants with information for reference and minimized the need for taking extensive notes. Participants also greatly enjoyed door prizes. These items were usually materials which staff members frequently used to make classroom materials, such as colored markers, velcro, or glue sticks, but could also be blank computer disks or materials donated by a vendor. One of the most highly rated training modules was the "Make and Take" session. During this presentation participants had the opportunity to create materials, such as topic communication displays or overlays, with guidance from others with more experience. Participants shared materials they had created and made copies of materials that others presented. A camera was available to take photographs of communication displays for students who needed photographic symbol representations.

Although group inservice staff development and training has many benefits, it does not replace the need for the second model of staff preparation. This model involves individualized training for school staff in the use of the specific technology equipment selected for a particular student. This training addresses operational procedures for the various devices, the selection of vocabulary or programming of software, if applicable, troubleshooting techniques, and the selection of target activities, as well as strategies for integration. The integration team must seek such training from any available resource. These may include identified team members, clinicians from an independent agency who have prescribed the devices, local college or university faculty, or the equipment vendors.

Some local education agencies across the United States are identifying staff members to attend training given by outside organizations and agencies. Their role is then to train other school staff members. Several features of this "training of trainers" model make it an attractive option for school systems. First, the cost and number of professional days required for a few staff members to receive training outside of the school system is less than would be required to provide such training for all school staff members. Second, once these trainers have received instruction related to specific assistive technology equipment, their expertise may then be applied to other students who will be using similar equipment. Last, and perhaps most important, the individuals from the educational setting who are trained are an ongoing resource to all staff members in the school system. It is crucial, however, that technology resource staff members have continuing opportunities to update their skills by attending conferences and workshops. Frequent new developments in assistive technology demand that technology resource staff members remain up-to-date to provide the best service to staff and students.

Individualized training for staff members should emphasize a "hands-on" approach. Using this method, the individual providing the training typically takes on the role of a facilitator or coach. The trainer may provide brief information about the equipment, demonstrate its use, and then verbally guide the trainee through hands-on practice. As a last step, the user should attempt to complete a specific operation using written directions only, with the trainer available to assist if difficulties are encountered. By this time, the trainee should have developed a high degree of independence and should be able to complete the same tasks independently.

Many school staff and family members find that manuals prepared by manufacturers of assistive technology equipment are not "user-friendly." Trainers often find that they must develop simplified, step-by-step "how to" guides which provide individuals new to the equipment only with the specific information required to operate, care, and/or program the equipment relative to the specific student's needs. Use of these abbreviated "how to" guides can decrease the amount of training time required to assist school staff in developing basic competencies for the operation of assistive technology equipment.

Following instruction in the mechanics of operating assistive technology equipment, individualized training in the use of specific strategies and integration techniques is necessary. This involves a three-step process. The first step includes a discussion of the student's needs and the identification of strategies and techniques that have been found useful for students with similar needs. This phase usually is best accomplished at a staffing or conference. Next, the trainer models the use of the identified strategies in the educational setting during a selected activity. This coaching model has been utilized successfully to assist school personnel in developing competency in the use of strategies and integration techniques. Last, following demonstration by the trainer, the staff member employs the targeted skills while the trainer observes and provides feedback.

In some cases, the student and his or her family are the integration team members who receive the training in the use of the prescribed assistive technology. Having received this training from an outside agency, they then have the responsibility of training school staff members who may have been unable to attend the training due to the distance involved, inability to procure leave from their school duties, or other logistical problems. A helpful practice in this case is to arrange for the training sessions to be tape recorded or videotaped so that lessons may be reviewed at a later date by school staff members and also can serve as a reference to the student and family members.

Peer Preparation

The frequently overlooked partners in technology integration in the educational setting are classmates. New technology in the classroom, such as a voice output communication aid or a power wheelchair, is usually of interest to all students, even if it is intended for use by one individual. Normal curiosity does not need to be discouraged; it is an excellent investment of time and planning to satisfy this curiosity. A classroom activity that addresses both awareness of the special needs of classmates who have disabilities and introduces the technology to them is one way of accomplishing this goal. The student for whom the device was prescribed may assist the teacher or other staff member in demonstrating the equipment. This presentation may take place during a sharing time or other regularly scheduled classroom activity.

The initial goal of the peer preparation activity is to establish the purpose of the equipment. Because many popular toys utilize computer technology, speech synthesizers, and powered mobility, it is important for classmates and peers to understand the more essential purposes of the assistive technology.

Another goal of the introductory activity for peers is to establish the rules governing use of the equipment. Students who use the technology equipment, their families, and school staff should discuss, in advance of this activity, whether they will implement a "hands-off" policy for other classmates or permit peers to try the device. Unfortunately, a hands-off policy makes use of the device more enticing and may, in some cases, increase the likelihood that other students will attempt to use it without supervision. If at all possible, classmates should be allowed to try the equipment during this introductory activity.

A third goal for the introductory activity is to establish the skills of the student who will be using the technology. For example, in the case of a student who will be using a voice output communication aid, introduction of the device represents a change in their potential for participation in communication. Awareness of this potential change sets the stage for future emphasis on strategies to be used by communication partners to enhance communication. Preschool and early elementary classroom activities such as "Simon Says" have been successful in establishing communication aid users as active communicators in the eyes of their classmates. In addition, it encourages the students using the communication aids to adjust their own self-concepts.

Students who utilize communication aids very often have definite ideas about what they would like their classmates to know about their devices. Planning sessions to select and program appropriate messages in the communication device are very helpful and serve to enhance the concept of ownership for the student who will be using the device. Students utilizing other assistive technology equipment also should be encouraged to plan their presentations to the class and take the role of presenter during the activity. The teacher may then become the facilitator by introducing new topics and asking pertinent questions.

The final goal for a peer preparation activity is to provide classmates with information about how they can help the student who will be using the technology. In many cases, peers are willing to help individuals with handicaps but often tend to anticipate their needs and discourage the independence of those using assistive technology. Classmates usually need reminders to ask whether assistance is required or desired before providing it.

Discussion during an introductory activity may provide an arena for students who have unanswered questions regarding the disabilities classmates present. In most cases, students who have had the opportunity to obtain information about persons with disabilities in an open, nonthreatening discussion are more likely to treat their classmates with respect and equality.

PHYSICAL ENVIRONMENT

Issues of handicapped accessibility and architectural barriers have become prominent in many aspects of the construction and renovation of public structures. The school building and instructional space available to a student with physical handicaps who is fitted with assistive devices must be carefully considered. For example, power mobility often requires special arrangements due to the dimensions of the wheelchair or scooter and can require transportation adaptations for safety and to allow for the nature of the power source. These fundamental considerations should be resolved prior to their introduction into the educational environment. Although a student previously may have utilized power mobility, the addition of an augmentative communication device and its mounting mechanism may alter accessibility to the school or classroom because of the added physical dimensions.

For the student with handicaps, classroom layout needs to be assessed for safety and ease of accessibility to educational materials. In general, wide spaces between desks and direct aisles are preferred. The tendency of some teachers to group desks in clusters around the room may be problematic when including a student with assisted mobility. Students with physical handicaps should have easy access to the teacher and their peers to facilitate socialization and requests for assistance.

Church and Bender (1989) offer several suggestions on appropriate lighting of the classroom space to reduce glare on the viewing surfaces of some adaptive devices. Ideally, the classroom should not have windows to reduce the glare from direct sunlight. When this is unavoidable, anti-reflective screen covers should be considered. Because most classrooms are equipped with overhead lighting, placement of the youngster who must view the screen of an assistive device needs to be adjusted around that light source. Lighting levels may need to be reduced when employing the screened application; but other activities, such as reading printed material, may require increased levels of lighting.

Noise level should always be considered in an instructional environment. The introduction of a new assistive device can change the noise level in different ways. Power mobility produces little noise and is not often operated once instruction is in progress. Voice-output augmentative communication devices vary in the quality and intelligibility of synthesized speech. Devices should be prescribed with this in mind. Volume levels need to be adjusted for the user and for his or her communication partners. Some teachers will find that once a voice output device has been introduced, a once quiet youngster becomes quite talkative. This needs to be managed just as unacceptable amounts of discussion would be with other class members. Appropriate conversation should always be encouraged.

Computers used for instructional purposes generally produce only a low-level hum. On the other hand, some software is specifically chosen for students with handicaps because it provides auditory feedback for reinforcement. When a student is using software with auditory feedback, specific arrangements need to be made to reduce the competing noise so that instruction may proceed elsewhere in the classroom.

Utilization of a computer for written communication and word processing involves the use of a printer. Depending on the location and type of printer, as well as the frequency of its use, the noise it produces can be very intrusive (Church & Bender, 1989). Positioning of furniture and equipment in the classroom setting can assist in the reduction of computer-generated noise. Study carrels may be used at times for individualized work, but removal of the student from the classroom is discouraged. Removal sends an inherent message to users and their peers regarding their acceptance in the environment. When economically feasible, laser printers can be chosen over dot matrix or daisy wheel printers for noise reduction. Scheduling specific times for printer use or making teacher corrections directly on the computer disk are additional options.

Members of the integration team need to consider furniture requirements for the safe and effective use of assistive technology. Devices should be positioned for proper viewing, ease of access, and with consideration for physical comfort and posture. The size of a wheelchair and the incline of its seating dictate the height of the work surface and the viewing height of instructional materials. If a student is independently ambulatory but must carry an augmentative device from class to class, a reasonable work space needs to be available in each class setting.

Most importantly, a student who is just beginning use of an augmentative communication device or a computer for instruction, may experience new discomfort or fatigue as a result of improper positioning, increased noise level or suboptimal lighting. It is important that the integration team examine the physical setting for accessibility, lighting, noise level, and positioning of the student and their devices on an ongoing basis. This will increase the likelihood of successful integration of the technology.

TECHNOLOGY INTEGRATION PLAN

Integration may be defined as the act of bringing together a number of components to create a whole. As it is applied to assistive technology use in the educational setting, integration involves bringing together the identified components (hardware, software, techniques, and strategies) for each student in the context of the objectives and activities of the educational setting. Technology may be viewed as a tool to accomplish a task. Integration of the tools identified for a student does not need to be viewed as an "all or nothing" proposition. For example, it would be an overwhelming undertaking to select vocabulary and plan intervention techniques for all the activities in which the student is involved at one time. This is especially true if the student and staff require a considerable amount of training in the use of the technology to utilize the tools effectively.

An initial planning meeting with the team should include an analysis of the students' typical daily schedule and selection of target activities for technology integration. The following guidelines have proved helpful in the selection of target activities for students who employ assistive technology. The activities should:

1. Occur frequently (daily or several times per week)
2. Be motivating and enjoyable
3. Present opportunities for independence in at least one of the Following areas: verbal communication, written communication, mobility, self-care, vocational skills, or control of the environment
4. Be activities the students cannot effectively complete utilizing their nonassistive current modes or methods.

Part I of the Technology Integration Plan has been developed to provide a helpful framework to record the information that is generated by the integration team (see Figure 7-1). Team members determine the target activities for initial integration of technology by utilizing the three-point rating system indicated on the form shown in Figure 7-1. Following selection of target activities, Part II, the Action Plan, is then completed for each identified activity (see Figure 7-2). This form provides a framework for listing target skills and objectives for the selected activity, recording the specifications of suggested equipment, materials, motivators, and strategies and indicating the preparation and follow-up needed, as well as a projected date for review. Part III, the Review, is used to record all modifications to be made to the plans for selected activities following an initial attempt at integration (see Figure 7-3).

A systematic approach for expansion of activities aided by pertinent technology is crucial. Monthly reviews to identify necessary modifications to the student's current plans and to develop plans to integrate technology with additional activities are helpful; however, the frequency of these team reviews should be adjusted to reflect the pace at which the student's needs change. Technology integration is clearly not a task that can ever be checked off anyone's "to do" list. True integration is an ongoing, evolving process which requires a considerable time commitment from each team member. A typical pitfall in technology integration in the educational setting is not defining responsibility for preparation and follow-up. Use of the sample Technology Integration Plan should assist technology integration teams in clearly designating responsibilities and establishing time frames for completion of preparation activities.

Student:

Date:

Team Members:

Typical daily schedule

Directions: List all daily activities and rate each one for the listed characteristics using the following scale: 3 - high   2 - moderate   1 - low. Total the ratings for each activity and record the number in the Total column. Place a check in last column when the activity is included in the student's Technology Integration Plan.

Daily Activities	Current Mode(s) of _____	Motivation	Opportunities for Independence	Present mode(s) Ineffective	Total	Included in Plan
Other routine events (at least once per week)						

Figure 7-1

Technology Integration Plan Part I. Preparation Sheet.

218

Student's Name: Date:
Team Members:

Target activity:

Target skills (objectives):

Suggested equipment:

Target vocabulary to be represented by ____ Photos ____ Symbols ____ Words/Sentences
Suggested materials/motivators:

Preparation needed	Person(s) responsible	Target date

Suggested strategies:

Anticipated date of review:

Figure 7-2
Technology Integration Plan. Part II. Action Plan.

219

Target activity:
Team Members revising Plan:

Date of initial Action Plan

Date of review	Modifications	Person responsible	Initiation date	Review date

Figure 7–3
Technology Integration Plan. Part III. Review.

Examples of Technology Integration Plans

The Technology Integration Plan will include different information depending on the needs and abilities of the students. To illustrate some possible uses of this format, two sample Technology Integration Plans will be presented. The two students discussed in this section could be of any chronological age. The examples are intended to represent composites of students with distinctly different needs for assistive technology rather than individual case studies. Although some students initially may present needs that are similar to Student A and transition to needs represented by Student B , all students do not necessarily follow this sequence of skills.

Student A: Sarah

Sarah is a student with physical disabilities and severe speech impairment. She receives the majority of her instruction in a special education setting with an emphasis on development of functional skills. Written communication is not currently included in her individualized education program. She was evaluated by an Assistive Technology Team and a voice-output augmentative communication aid accessed via a lightpointer was prescribed. It was also determined that she could access a plate switch with her right hand when it was placed to the right of midline on her lap tray. She had received initial training in the use of the lightpointer and was able to target four light-activated switches. Some of Sarah's educational goals that could be achieved through the use of assistive technology are:

1. Initiation of interactions with others
2. Communication of choices, wants, and needs
3. Expansion of expressive language skills
4. Control of the environment for exploration and play or recreation

Sarah's Technology Integration Plan, Part I, was completed by her classroom teacher, instructional assistant, speech-language pathologist, occupational therapist, physical therapist, and parents. Typical daily activities were listed for school and home. Play and recreation was selected as an initial target activity at school. At home, play and recreation time after dinner was selected. The activities selected for home and school represented very similar technology needs. Sarah's family chose to participate in the plan developed for school use before beginning implementation at home (See Figure 7–4).

Part II, the Action Plan for play time, was developed by the Integration Team to incorporate all of the educational goals listed above.

Student: Sarah   Date: 12-10-91
Team Members: Sarah, Sarah's mother, classroom teacher, instructional assistant, speech language pathologist, occupational therapist, physical therapist

Typical daily schedule

Directions: List all daily activities and rate each one for the listed characteristics using the following scale: 3 - high 2 - moderate 1 - low. Total the ratings for each activity and record the number in the Total column. Place a check in last column when the activity is included in the student's Technology Integration Plan.

Daily Activities	Current Mode(s) of Communication	Motivation	Opportunities for Independence	Present mode(s) Ineffective	Total	Included in Plan
Arrival	facial expression/vocalization	3	3	1	7	
Opening	eye gaze	3	2	2	7	
Seat Work	eye gaze	2	2	3	7	
Playtime/Speech	vocalizations/eye gaze	3	3	3	9	✓
Snack	vocalizations/eye gaze	3	3	1	7	
O.T.	facial expression	2	2	2	6	
Small Groups	vocalization/eye gaze	2	3	2	7	
P.T.	facial expression	1	2	2	5	
Outside Play	facial expression/vocalization	2	3	3	8	
Story Time	eye gaze	3	1	2	6	
Dismissal	facial expression/vocalizations	1	2	2	5	
Other routine events (at least once per week) Computer	facial expression/vocalization	3	3	3	9	add

Figure 7–4

Part I. Preparation sheet for Student A (Sarah).

The team identified several components for typical play time routines which could be addressed employing the following assistive technology equipment: several of Sarah's favorite toys adapted for switch input, pictures of the toys, a plate switch for Sarah to activate with her right hand, four light-activated switches, and the prescribed voice-output communication aid. With information from Sarah's family, it was determined that the best motivators would be those with visual and auditory feedback.

Prior to implementation of the Action Plan, the team identified that the following preparation was necessary: vocabulary for the play routines needed to be selected and programmed in the communication aid, appropriate picture symbols needed to be chosen, the light-activated switches needed to be mounted on Sarah's tray, and her communication device needed to be mounted on her wheelchair. The team members assigned responsibilities and chose a target date to begin this activity (see Figure 7–5).

The team identified strategies to facilitate Sarah's independent use of the assistive technology. The first activity would involve Sarah's use of a lightpointer to select a message on her communication aid that would summon a classroom member; she would then indicate to the individual what toy she wanted to play with. That toy would be operated with a plate switch attached to the right side of her tray and a picture of the toy would be placed on the switch. Messages available to Sarah on her communication device would be changed so that Sarah could comment on the activity, ask another student if she or he wanted a turn, ask for help, or request a different toy. Vocabulary was selected to provide a variety of communicative intents and opportunities for Sarah to interact with adults and peers and was based on a script of the activity which was prepared by her classroom teacher after observation of Sarah's usual play with the toy. The linguistic complexity of the messages was adjusted to reflect Sarah's receptive language skills. This activity was designed to allow maximum independence for Sarah during play and to place her in an active, rather than passive, communicative role.

Initially, it was anticipated that Sarah might need some facilitation to utilize the assistive technology selected for her. The strategy that the Integration Team selected to achieve this goal was to arrange for an instructional assistant to act as a facilitator for Sarah during this activity. The assistant would provide prompts for Sarah to summon another classroom member and to communicate her choice of a toy. As Sarah's response time was slow, use of ample wait time to allow Sarah to initiate was recognized as an important strategy. Another identified strategy was the use of prompts in a hierarchy progressing from verbal, to gestural, to physical assistance. Information from *Partners in Augmen-*

Student's Name: Sarah   Date: 1-10-91

Team Members: Sarah, classroom teacher, instructional assistant, speech language pathologist, occupational therapist, physical therapist

Target activity: Playtime / Speech

Target skills (objectives): During playtime Sarah will: (1.) initiate interactions with teachers or peers 1 time per 15 minutes, (2.) communicate choice of activity once daily, (3.) utilize more than one type of communicative attempt, and (4.) engage in the operation of switch activated toys.

Suggested equipment: switch activated toys, pictures, plate switch, light activated switches, communication aid with multiple switch input capability

Target vocabulary to be represented by ___ Photos ✓ Symbols ___ Words/Sentences ___
Suggested materials/motivators: and pictures

Preparation needed	Person(s) responsible	Target date
vocabulary selection	classroom teacher	1-14-91
vocabulary programming	speech language pathologist	1-20-91
selection of pictures	instructional assistant	1-14-91
mounting of switches	O.T. and P.T.	1-20-91
mounting of device	assistive technology team	1-21-91

Suggested strategies: wait time, use of prompt hierarchy, aided language stimulation
Anticipated date of review: 2-10-91

Figure 7-5

Part II. Action Plan for Student A (Sarah).

224

tative Communication Training (Culp & Carlisle, 1988) was identified as a helpful resource for facilitation techniques. It was also determined that all classroom staff would utilize "aided language stimulation," as described by Goosens' and Crain (1988). Using this strategy, staff members would point to pictures representing their messages as they interacted with Sarah, thus providing excellent modeling of picture-based communication techniques.

Follow-up goals identified by the team included monitoring of Sarah's continued interest in the selected toys and development of scripts for additional toys as needed. Materials available from Burkhart (1980, 1982) and Levin and Scherfenberg (1986, 1987) were identified as resources. The classroom teacher and instructional assistant would learn to program the communication aid so that they could quickly change or add new messages as Sarah's interests changed. An anticipated review date for this target activity was set by the team (see Figure 7–5).

When the Action Plan was reevaluated, Part III, Review, was completed. At this time the team decided that an additional activity option would be added to Sarah's play time. It was observed that she frequently watched other students using the computer during play time and enjoyed using a variety of single-switch software. The team gathered information regarding early educational software suitable for Sarah and determined that it was of two basic types: (1) cause and effect and (2) content (labeling, concepts). Attractive qualities were color, movement, and sound. The Integration Team determined that Sarah displayed competency in many of the component skills for computer use as identified by Behrmann, Jones, and Wilds (1989):

1. Consistent volitional motor response
2. Visual tracking, discrimination, and figure-ground
3. Mastery of cause and effect
4. Object permanence
5. Sustained attention
6. Imitation
7. Desire
8. Receptive ability to follow simple commands (oral or gestural)

The Technology Team utilized the following teaching hierarchy to identify the entry level skills for Sarah's computer use and to develop a long-term plan for her use of computer-assisted instruction:

1. Cause and effect — touch for feedback
2. Selection of an item for reinforcement — student selects any item without need for a single correct response
3. Symbolic play — selection and manipulation of items for play scenarios

Target activity: _Playtime_   Date of initial Action Plan: 1-10-91
Team Members revising Plan: Sarah, Sarah's mother, classroom teacher, instructional assistant, speech language pathologist, occupational and physical therapists

Date of review	Modifications	Person responsible	Initiation date	Review date
2-10-91	Develop scripts for additional toys	speech language pathologist and classroom teacher	2-17-91	3-17-91
2-10-91	Add computer assisted instruction time as new target activity:			
	add pictures and program communication aid	speech language pathologist	2-17-91	3-17-91
	select single switch software	classroom teacher	2-17-91	3-17-91
	provide switch interface	assistive technology team	2-17-91	3-17-91

Figure 7-6

Part III. Review for Student A (Sarah).

4. Socialization — turn taking or parallel play
5. Selective discrimination — student selects appropriate response

Sarah was currently demonstrating use of switch-activated toys, therefore, she would be expected to generalize to the use of software providing cause-and-effect and selection of items for reinforcement. Her target skills for computer use were identified as symbolic play, socialization, and selective discrimination. The equipment needed for this activity included the Apple II computer available in the classroom, a switch interface, the same plate switch used to activate the adapted toys, and appropriate software. Materials available in Trieschmann and Lerner (1990) were identified as resources. The preparation that would be needed included the computer as a choice during play time, development of a script for the communication aid related to computer use, programming the communication aid, selection of appropriate picture symbols, and selection of appropriate software. Strategies utilized during this activity were similar to those previously identified; however, additional modeling was necessary when a new software program was introduced. A few other students in Sarah's classroom who were familiar with the software were enlisted as peer tutors. This arrangement provided numerous opportunities for communication and allowed the adult facilitator to fade direct intervention in this activity.

The Integration Team continued to use this format in making modifications and additions to Sarah's Technology Integration Plan at each review date (see Figure 7–6).

Student B: Paul

Paul is an elementary student with physical disabilities and severe speech impairment. He previously was in a special education program for students with physical disabilities, but is now ready for mainstreaming for all of his academic instruction with support from an individual aid and the special education teacher, as needed. Paul successfully used a voice-output augmentative communication aid via scanning with preprogrammed words and phrases, but needed a method to construct novel messages. He has had experience with computer-assisted instruction, but only limited exposure to word processing software programs. Paul's technology needs also included ongoing access to assistive devices for written communication and access to environmental controls for increased independence in the educational setting.

When Paul was evaluated by an Assistive Technology Team, a voice-output communication aid with text-to-speech and message storage capabilities was prescribed for verbal communication. Paul's written communication needs were addressed with a laptop computer accessed via his communication device. Paul had already demonstrated successful use of a joystick for independent power mobility. This selection technique was also chosen for the communication aid. Setup of the communication device featured a 128-location display with a Qwerty keyboard arrangement. A page turner was prescribed for classroom use as well as remote controlled switches to adapt selected devices in art and music classes at a later date. Some of Paul's educational goals that could be enhanced through the use of assistive technology included:

1. Expansion of expressive language to include novel messages
2. Development of written communication skills to complete class assignments and homework
3. Increased physical independence in the classroom setting

The Technology Integration Plan was developed by team members beginning with Part I, the Preparation Sheet. Paul's previous special education teacher and his regular education teacher played important roles in completing this section of the Integration Plan. A specific social studies unit was identified as the target activity. Not only was this a highly rated activity, it was also judged to be one that incorporated the objectives identified for Paul (See Figure 7–7).

Part II, the Action Plan for social studies, was developed to include specific objectives for a planned social studies group activity, necessary equipment, and suggested strategies. Team members assigned responsibilities for preparation tasks and set dates for initiation and review (see Figure 7–8)

At the review meeting of Paul's Technology Integration Plan, modifications to enhance his rate of production of written work were identified. At this time, Action Plans for additional activities were also developed to expand the integration of assistive technology in the educational setting (see Figure 7–9). In discussing Paul's need for environmental controls, it was felt that the page turner could be easily integrated in Paul's primary classroom, especially with the assistance of his individual aid. Future team plans included the development of an additional Technology Integration Plan targeting increased physical independence in art and music classes using environmental controls. A smaller task force would be assigned the task of adapting such devices as a slide projector, a camera, a tape recorder, and an electronic keyboard toward that objective.

PLANNING FOR THE UNEXPECTED

Even a plan that has been carefully developed and implemented has the potential for problems. Anticipating common problems and plan-

Student: Paul
Date: 1-10-91
Team Members: Paul, Paul's father, best friend Tom, classroom teacher, special education teacher, speech language pathologist, occupational therapist, physical therapist, computer coordinator, individual aid

<u>Typical daily schedule</u>

Directions: List all daily activities and rate each one for the listed characteristics using the following scale: 3 - high 2 - moderate 1 - low. Total the ratings for each activity and record the number in the Total column. Place a check in last column when the activity is included in the student's Technology Integration Plan.

Daily Activities	Current Mode(s) of verbal + written communication	Motivation	Opportunities for Independence	Present mode(s) Ineffective	Total	Included in Plan
Language Arts	Throughout his school day Paul utilizes a combination of: facial expression, communication aid, vocalization, and yes no head nods for verbal communication	1	3	3	7	
Mathematics		3	1	2	6	
Social Studies		3	3	3	9	✓
Music/Art		3	2	3	8	add
Lunch		3	3	2	8	
Science		1	2	3	6	
Adapted Physical Education	He relies on his individual aid for written communication	2	2	2	6	
Therapy (SLP, OT, PT)		1	2	2	5	
Other routine events Media Center (at least once per week)	"	3	1	2	6	

Figure 7-7

Part I. Preparation Sheet for Student B (Paul).

Student's Name: Paul   Date: 1-30-91

Team Members: Paul, Paul's father, best friend Tom, classroom teacher, special education teacher, speech language pathologist, occupational therapist, physical therapist, computer coordinator, individual aid

Target activity:

Social Studies Group Project

Target skills (objectives): Within the 4 week group project time Paul will: (1) contribute 3 ideas using his voice output communication aid, (2) complete a written outline of topic ideas, (3) write a paragraph related to his assigned topic, and (4) participate verbally in the group presentation.

Suggested equipment: voice output communication aid with text-to-speech and message capabilities, laptop computer, word processing software, printer

Target vocabulary to be represented by ___ Photos ✓ Symbols ✓ Words/Sentences

Suggested materials/motivators:

Preparation needed	Person(s) responsible	Target date
vocabulary selection and programming of communication aid	speech language pathologist	2-15-91
train Paul in word processing	computer coordinator and individual aid	2-15-91
train peers	speech language pathologist	2-15-91
environmental assessment	occupational and physical therapists	2-15-91

Suggested strategies: (1) Provide Paul with a programmed message that he is formulating a novel message, (2) teach outlining and composition via teacher/student collaborative method, (3) use role play to prepare verbal presentation

Anticipated date of review: 3-15-91

Figure 7-8

Part II. Action Plan for Student B (Paul).

Target activity: Academic Classes   Date of initial Action Plan: 1-30-91
Team Members revising Plan: whole team as designated on initial action plan

Date of review	Modifications	Person responsible	Initiation date	Review date
3-15-91	Provide Paul with a means to increase his rate of production of written work (i.e. software with prediction, abbrieviation and expansion capabilities)	computer coordinator and special education teacher	3-30-91	4-30-91
3-15-91	Introduce Page turner in primary classroom.	classroom teacher and individual aid	3-30-91	4-30-91
4-30-91	Develop a Technology Integration Plan for increased independence in Art and Music via environmental controls.	technology integration team	5-15-91	6-15-91

Figure 7-9
Part III. Review for Student B (Paul).

ning for their resolution can assist the student in remaining functional in the educational environment during any "down time" with their assistive technology.

Hardware Glitches

Before a student receives any assistive device, the team should identify a resource for resolving hardware breakdowns, mishaps, or malfunctions. This might be a representative of the vendor, a member of the integration team, or a local rehabilitation engineer. A preliminary contact will confirm the resource person's availability for assistance and a projected time frame for repairs. Anticipating that hardware problems may arise and considering how long a student might be without equipment allows the team to arrange alternative systems for such an event.

Software Crashes

Software problems should also be anticipated. Some programs are available for review on a trial basis from the distributor to assess applicability to an individual student's needs. This hands-on trial is encouraged before ordering. Once software programs are purchased, appropriate members of the integration team should become familiar with their use. Back-up disks, if not provided, should be made or otherwise obtained. Storage of the back-up disks needs to be considered in the early stages of the plan; copies of programs important to communication or vocational pursuits need to be readily available when problems occur.

FINDING VERSATILE SOFTWARE

Several publications offer software descriptions and reviews for consideration in selecting programs for educational and clinical use. A wide selection of software is available for the able-bodied user. Use of general software for students with handicaps must be considered in light of each student's specific strengths and needs. Although many software features, such as authoring capabilities, variable entry levels, variable instructional levels, and printouts of student records, would benefit all students, particular features must be considered when selecting software for students who present specific physical and sensory deficits. Eiser (1986) offers several considerations for "retooling" software (see Figure 7–10).

One area to consider is the student's response rate. Programs that offer control over speed of presentation, use of a single key to continue,

	NONSPEAKING	LIMITED ACCESS METHODS	VISUAL DEFICITS	HEARING IMPAIRED	ATTENTION DEFICITS	UNMOTIVATED	SLOW RESPONSE TIME	IMPULSIVE RESPONDING	MEMORY DEFICITS
AUDITORY FEEDBACK	✔		✔		✔	✔			✔
ADJUSTABLE VOLUME	✔		✔	✔					
LARGE SCREEN PRINT			✔						
SIMPLE GRAPHICS			✔		✔				
ADJUSTABLE PRESENTATION SPEED		✔	✔	✔	✔	✔		✔	✔
ADJUSTABLE RESPONSE TIME		✔	✔		✔	✔	✔	✔	✔
IMMEDIATE FEEDBACK	✔				✔	✔	✔	✔	✔
TRACKING OF RESPONSES						✔			✔
STORAGE OF PARTIAL DATA						✔			✔
REPETITION PROVIDED	✔			✔	✔		✔	✔	✔
VARIABLE INSTRUCTION LEVELS						✔			
VARIABLE ENTRY LEVELS						✔			
REDUCED KEY RESPONSES		✔					✔		
ATTRACTIVE GRAPHICS				✔		✔			
IMPORTANT DATA HIGHLIGHTED			✔		✔			✔	✔

Figure 7–10
Software selection criteria for individuals with assistive technology needs.

and storage capacity for the option of completion at a later date may be appropriate. Students with visual perception or discrimination deficits may require programs that have clear, simple, or reduced amounts of graphics. Software programs with the option of offering large print or accompanying auditory feedback also should be sought. A student's attentional difficulties may necessitate a search for software programs that highlight essential information, provide sound or color cues, or allow for the storage of partial data to be used for future reference.

Motivational problems may exist from the outset or develop later for any number of reasons. Software that optimizes participation under these conditions would possess optional feedback frequency (immediate reinforcement if desired), record-keeping options to chart and track progress, offer tasks for the development of executive functions (reasoning, strategy) rather than drill and practice, or reflect age-appropriate interests at varied ability levels.

A student's preferred learning style may suggest software programs that provide auditory feedback, display a simple visual layout with the option of reducing the amount of print presented to the student, or allow for teacher control of the content and vocabulary. Difficulties in encoding, or physical limitations that inhibit efficient direct selection via the keyboard, can be modified with software that allows for one key or limited key responses. Programs that predict vocabulary from initial characters or whose designs are well-suited to alternative keyboard use should also be considered. Software that addresses memory deficits should provide review and repetition, allow for immediate feedback, or provide cues (auditory or visual) for memory aids. The capacity to store data and organize it logically for future reference is also desirable to assist in compensation for memory problems (see Figure 7-10).

USER REJECTION

Matching technology to the student and inclusion of the student in all aspects of the Technology Integration Plan does not always prevent user rejection. Many of these children and adolescents have adjusted to their previous means of functional communication or mobility, and although seemingly improved, the new alternative causes anxiety. Attitudes of communication partners toward synthesized speech can be openly rejecting, or avoidance of the student can send a more subtle message. Approaches for better acceptance might include introducing the student with a new augmentative device to a peer mentor who has had success in similar circumstances. It would not be unreasonable to find that the introduction of a new technology draws additional attention to students' disabilities and thus heightens the anger and frustration they feel because they are not able-bodied. These students may be open to sorting out their feelings through counseling or discussion.

Any time a student rejects a device, even after gradual integration and preplanning, the team needs to regroup to problem solve. A careful and considered look at each part of the process may reveal the difficulty. If it is stigmatism in the community, small positive experiences may build confidence. If the problem exists in the complexity of the system, the team may wish to try a less-sophisticated device and upgrade later. Comfort in positioning for system use and sensory needs should be reconsidered because it may not be obvious to the student why he or she is experiencing discomfort. When all else fails, the team may conclude that assistive technology is not the answer for this student at the time.

DENYING ACCESS

Students who utilize assistive technology are not commonplace and persons who come into contact with them must often alter their thinking. First and foremost, these devices are meant to promote independent functioning to the degree possible. Once the device has been integrated, refusing the student access, even for part of the day, is discouraged. It is not uncommon to hear that a teacher has removed a communication device because a student has become too talkative or because verbal responses were not required at a particular time. Most school policies would not allow such physical restraint of a speaking individual. Similarly, power mobility has been excluded from some school environments because it requires additional student supervision or gives the youngster the independence to leave an undesired, but compulsory, situation. In general, these prosthetic devices need to be considered a part of the student's personality. Unless safety is an issue, behavioral problems that result from their use should be handled the same as they would be with any other class member.

COMMUNITY

The educational setting is a microenvironment for each student. Successful implementation of assistive technology in this setting is often viewed as a primary goal by families and school staff; however, the educational setting represents only part of a child's life. Educational goals are meant to prepare students for life in general and thus teach many social and community living skills. Generalization of such learning is especially difficult for many students with multiple handicaps. The technology integration team should also address ways to integrate assistive technology into the home and community. Following completion of Part I, Preparation of the Technology Integration Plan (see Figure 7-1), it may be clear that some students experience most of their communication needs with unfamiliar communication partners in the community. This occurs because numerous opportunities exist for interaction, and the students present communication modes, such as gestures, sign language, or partially intelligible speech are not understood by community members. It is also true that students who utilize power mobility typically experience the greatest need for independent mobility in the community. Thus, integration of technology in the community setting may begin as soon as the technology is delivered, or may be included in the student's Technology Integration Plan later, after some success with integration in the educational setting has been experienced.

The Community Integration Team

The make-up of this technology integration team varies greatly. Depending on the curriculum followed in the student's educational setting, school staff may be involved with community training; however, in many cases, the family or community caregivers are the team members who actually implement the plan. Ideally, school staff and family members will meet to develop ideas for community integration. Other community members, such as a play group leader or recreation center employee, also may be recruited to participate. When appropriate, the student should be included on the team. Primary therapists should remain involved to adjust the student's strategies and techniques for variables that arise in the community. Individuals who will provide technical support for the family members must also be identified. Ideally, this support will be ongoing so that family members may learn the basic care and operation of the devices and have assistance in troubleshooting when the unexpected occurs.

Preparing The Community

Within the immediate neighborhood or community, prominent participants in usual routines should be informed ahead of time about the youngster's means of interaction. This should start out small, perhaps in one setting such as the post office or small grocery store. Sharing information ahead of time allows community members to communicate more effectively with the individual who is handicapped and to promote the most independence possible. In each case, the community member needs to be provided with expectations. This information does not need to be delivered in a formal conference. A special message which explains the purpose of the equipment and requests the individual's cooperation in taking part in communication assisted by a speech synthesizer might be programmed into voice-output communication aids for unfamiliar communication partners. Another option would be to display a printed message with similar information in a prominent place on the child's device or wheelchair. The student may direct the attention of community members to the message when appropriate. The parent may model appropriate interaction with his or her child in view of the community member or "coach" them through the process the first few times. Community members usually will follow the parent's lead.

Some community activities lend themselves to the integration of individuals with disabilities better than others. Many leaders of community activity groups, play groups, scouts, and church congregations have had some experience or training in working with individuals with handicaps and are willing to make accommodations and adaptations if provided assistance. An excellent starting point is an initial meeting with these activity leaders. This gives the parent and student an opportunity to share information about what the student can do independently and to identify those aspects of the activities in which he will require some assistance. For example, a student who utilizes power mobility might be able to participate independently in a game of jump rope by turning the rope and taking a turn going under the rope rather than jumping. The same youngster could actively participate in a swimming activity, but would need assistance to get in and out the pool. All environments are not conducive to electronic equipment; a decision is sometimes made to utilize a low-technology approach. This is especially true in the case of communication aids when the activities involve fingerpainting, swimming, or other similar activities. The emphasis should be on achieving the highest level of participation with the fewest accommodations. This is especially important if the accommodations require considerable setup or staff time; in the community, staffing ratios usually do not allow the dedication of a staff member's time to one child.

Environmental Considerations

Considerable efforts have been made by lobbyists and families of the disabled to provide free access to the community. Recent changes in the codes for public building construction now require some arrangements for handicapped accessibility in most areas, but not without great effort on the part of the individual with disabilities. In reality, individuals with physical disabilities are virtually banned from many establishments. Therefore, to provide successful community integration of assistive technology, the integration team needs to assess each environment prior to planning a student's visit. Attention must be paid to the width of doors and aisles for wheelchairs and any additional mounting devices. Many buildings are not accessible from the front door but provide a side or rear entrance that is ramped or at grade for deliveries. Even many accessible entrances have manually opened doors. Buildings with electronic doors may be more desirable for the youngster in question. Cashiers and merchandise need to be within reach or a clerk needs to be available for assistance. Handicapped-equipped bathrooms are becoming less of an oddity in public buildings, although their availability cannot be taken for granted.

Noise levels should be considered if there are hearing deficits or if a voice-output communication device is to be utilized. Lighting needs must be met for students with devices requiring the viewing of a screen or students with visual deficits. Areas that are highly stimulating due to their level of activity or amount of visual stimuli should also be examined as to their potential effect on the client.

Planning For Success

Successful integration of assistive technology in the community may be measured by the degree to which the student is able to participate in typical activities engaged in by peers. The key to successful integration is planning and back-up planning. As in the school setting, integration of assistive technology should not be viewed as an "all or nothing" proposition. The task is more achievable if a technology integration plan identifies the skills the student will be targeting, lists the preparation and equipment needed, includes a systematic method for evaluating the effectiveness of the plan, and lists modifications and additions in the use of assistive technology. Asking too much of the student, too soon could lead to anxiety and frustration, and therefore avoidance of further interaction with the equipment or the community activity.

Vocabulary selection for students who use a voice output communication aid in targeted community activities sometimes presents a great challenge for the integration team. It is necessary for the individuals who assist the student to have detailed information regarding the activity. Similarly, when planning independence in power mobility, each environment needs to be explored for accessibility and terrain. Information for these situations may best be obtained by "shadowing" the student during the activity and then developing a script and adapting for any communication barriers. Because many community activities occur less frequently than daily routines, it is sometimes helpful to role play the interactions to allow students to develop some confidence prior to the activity; however, life is not a dress rehearsal. Sometimes, it works out best for students and their technology team members to prepare for the activity and then jump in. Flexibility is important because technology is notorious for failing when it is needed the most. The back-up plan can make the difference between no participation in the activity and partial participation.

Lack of Community Acceptance

Lack of recognition of individuals with handicaps as "whole persons" is long-standing. Historically, we are in a better position than we were several decades ago in awareness, if not acceptance. Research has shown that not only stated opinion, but rather unstated attitudes and behaviors provide the critical measure of acceptance (Blackstone, 1989). Typically, rejection of handicapped persons can be diminished with information and positive experiences. As discussed by Blackstone (1989), such positive exposure yields varied acceptance for advanced technology use in assistive devices. For example, those with little experience with nonspeaking individuals tend to have positive reactions to electronic aids, whereas some more familiar communication partners prefer the interactive nature of a nonelectronic communication board. Similar attitudes have been expressed toward power mobility and its actual reduction of time spent with able-bodied peers, because they are no longer required for mobility. Parents and professionals need to consider both the promotion of independence and the alteration of interaction with peers and caregivers in their quest to improve each person's quality of life.

Promoting acceptance is a continuing goal in each step of the integration process. Ongoing school and community training of peers and caregivers, mentor and buddy programs for students, and societal exposure through literature and films all promote acceptance of persons with disabilities.

REFERENCES

Behrmann, M., Jones, J., & Wilds, M. (1989). Technology intervention for very young children with disabilities. *Infants and Young Children, 1*, 66–77.

Blackstone, S. W. (1989). For consumers: Societal rehabilitation. *Augmentative Communication News, 2*, 1–3.

Burkhart, L. (1980). *Homemade battery powered toys and education devices for severely handicapped children.* College Park, MD: Author.

Burkhart, L. (1982). *More homemade battery devices for severely handicapped children and suggested activities.* College Park, MD: Author.

Burkhead, E. J., Sampson, J. P., & McMahon, B. T. (1986). The liberation of disabled persons in a technological society: Access to computer technology. *Rehabilitation Literature, 47*, 167–168.

Church, G., & Bender, M. (1989). *Teaching with computers: A curriculum for special educators.* Boston, MA: College-Hill Press.

Culp, D. M., & Carlisle, M. (1988). *PACT: Partners in Augmentative Communication Training.* Tuscon, AZ: Communication Skill Builders.

Eiser, L. (1986). "Regular" software for special ed kids? *Classroom Computer Learning, 7* (2), 26–30.

Goossens', C., Crain, S., & Elder, P. (1988). *Engineering the preschool classroom environment for interactive symbolic communication.* Paper presented at the International Society for Augmentative and Alternative Communication Biennial Conference, Anaheim, CA.

Howard County Public School System (1990). *Guidelines for the augmentative communication and technology team.* Ellicott City, MD: Howard County Public Schools.

Levin, J. & Scherfenberg, L., (1986). *Breaking barriers.* Minneapolis, MN: Ablenet.

Levin, J., & Scherfenberg, L. (1987). *Selection and use of simple technology in home, school, work, and community settings.* Minneapolis, MN: Ablenet.

Mokros, J. R., & Russell, S. J., (1986). Learner-centered software: A survey of microcomputer use with special needs students. *Journal of Learning Disabilities, 19,* 185–190.

Trieschmann, M., & Lerner, J. (1990). *Using the computer to teach children with special needs.* Evanston, IL: National Lekotek Center.

8

Assistive Technology Product Directory

■ Sharon Glennen, PhD ■

One of the difficulties encountered in providing assistive technology services is researching the thousands of hardware and software products available for individuals with disabilities. With increasingly rapid changes in the computer industry, new technologies are created faster than professionals can keep track of them. This directory is an attempt to list frequently used hardware and software products that are mentioned throughout the text. It is by no means a comprehensive listing of all products available on the market. Other sources of assistive technology hardware and software products can be obtained from the resources listed in Chapter 9.

HOW TO USE THIS CHAPTER

The hardware and software products listed in this chapter are organized in alphabetical order by their primary function. Each product listing indicates the product name, manufacturer, and description Products such as keyguards that are made by several manufacturers are listed by the generic name. The products are arranged into the following categories.

1. *Adaptive Switches and Play.* This section lists single switches, joysticks, and hardware devices that assist in connecting switches to simple battery-operated devices.
2. *Augmentative Communication.* This section lists dedicated augmentative communication systems. Augmentative communication systems that consist of software written for nondedicated computers are listed in the Software section of this chapter.
3. *Braille Input–Output Devices.* This section lists hardware that provides individuals who are visually impaired with access to computers through braille technologies.
4. *Computer Access Devices.* These devices include alternate keyboards, add-on internal computer cards, speech recognition systems, and other peripherals that provide adapted access to computers.
5. *Computer Output Devices.* This section lists technologies available for adapted computer monitor output and adapted printer output.
6. *Environmental Controls.* Assistive technologies that control electronic appliances or operate integrated systems consisting of many home and computer devices are listed in this section.
7. *Power Mobility.* The four basic power mobility systems are described in this section of the chapter.
8. *Synthesized Speech.* This section lists synthesized speech technology that can be purchased separately and added to augmentative communication aids or computer systems.
9. *Software.* The final section is also the largest section. Software programs written specifically for users of assistive technology or adapted input computer devices are listed in alphabetical order in this section.

Once the reader has identified assistive technology hardware or software products that meet their specific needs, the reader should refer to Chapter 9 for specific vendor address and phone information.

ADAPTIVE SWITCHES AND PLAY

This section describes adaptive switches that can be used for activating toys, computers, augmentative communication aids, power mobility systems, and environmental controls. Joysticks and variations of joysticks are also listed. Finally, this section contains information about assistive technology to assist with battery-operated toy play activities.

Device/Manufacturer(s)	Description

Asaflex Switch

Asahel Engineering

This switch detects slight movements such as eyeblinks, muscle tightening, and soft sounds. Two sensors are attached to the body to record these movements.

Battery Adaptor

AbleNet
Don Johnston
  Developmental Equipment
Zygo Corporation
Toys for Special Children

A cable that connects switches to battery-operated devices such as toys or tape recorders.

Battery Device Timer

AbleNet

A timer that extends the operation of switch toys from 3 to 30 seconds for those who are unable to maintain switch closure.

Big Red Switch

AbleNet

This switch is 5 inches in diameter and requires minimal pressure to activate.

Computer-Activated Environmental Control Unit

Toys for Special Children

This device connects to the game port of any Apple II series computer. A switch-operated device is attached. Activating any computer key turns on the device.

Computer Keyboard Switch

Toys for Special Children

This is a large switch that operates through touch pressure. The switch looks like a computer keyboard.

Delay Timer

Arroyo & Associates
Technology for Language and
  Learning

This device prevents switch users from making double hits with a switch. The timer can be adjusted to create an interval during which additional switch activations are ignored. The timers can be used with adapted toys and some computers.

Device/Manufacturer(s)	Description

Ellipse Switch

Don Johnston
 Developmental Equipment

The Ellipse series of switches consist of almost flat, low-profile circular switches that operate with downward pressure on the switch surface. The switch gives an audible click when pressed successfully. The Ellipse comes in three sizes.

Flat Aid Cushion Switch

Arroyo & Associates

This switch operates with light pressure that triggers a puff of air to activate the switch.

Flexi-Form Board

Adaptive Communication
 Systems

This is a form board puzzle that can be used to activate switch toys. When an individual places a shape into the proper location, the switch toy is activated.

Infrared Switch

Words+ Incorporated

This switch produces an infrared light beam. When the beam is interrupted by body movement or eye blinks, the switch is activated.

Joystick

Apple Computer
Computability
Don Johnston
 Developmental Equipment
Prentke Romich
TASH

A joystick is an alternate input device for computers, augmentative communication systems, environmental controls, and wheelchairs. Joysticks can be proportional (the movements of the joystick translate into graded movements of the device) or binary (the joystick's movements translate into on-off directional movements). Proportional joysticks typically are used for wheelchair steering. Binary joysticks are used for computers, environmental controls, and augmentative communication systems.

Leaf Switch

Zygo

This is a sensitive switch which consists of a wire encased in a plastic sleeve. Bending the wire activates the switch. It comes in long and short versions.

Lever Switch

Zygo

The lever switch is a spring-loaded, snap-action switch that requires minimal movement to activate. The switch consists of a long "lever" with a padded surface at the end. Pushing the padded surface activates the switch.

Device/Manufacturer(s)	Description

Light Pointer

Adaptive Communication Systems

This light pointer is battery operated and produces a bright red light that can be seen easily even in bright rooms. It can be used separately to point to simple communication boards or objects or to access the Eval Pac.

Mercury Tilt Switch

Luminaud

This switch is filled with mercury, which responds to changes in gravity as the switch is moved. The individual tilts the switch to activate the device.

Mouth-Operated Joystick

KY Enterprises
Custom Computer Solutions

This company manufactures a series of mouth-operated joysticks that can operate Atari and Commodore computers and Nintendo video games. The joystick has a puff switch to initiate action and game selections. The joystick is operated by user chin movement.

P-Switch

Prentke Romich

This electronic switch senses slight muscle movements through a piezoelectric sensor. The sensitivity of the small coin-sized sensor can be adjusted. It can be taped or held by velcro bands on any part of a user's body.

Pillow Switch

TASH

This switch is a small soft "pillow" that activates devices when squeezed.

Plate Switch

Adaptive Communication Systems
TASH

A thin membrane switch that is activated by light pressure.

Plate Switch

Toys for Special Children

This switch comes in several different sizes. Pushing the "plate" surface downward activates the switch.

Puff–Sip Switch

DU-IT
Zygo

This switch operates using respiratory exhalation (puff) and inhalation (sip).

Device/Manufacturer(s)	Description

Rocking Lever Switch

Don Johnston
  Developmental Equipment
Prentke Romich

The rocking lever switch consists of a metal plate attached to a switch base. Rocking the plate by pressing it activates the switch. Some rocking lever switches have dual left-right rocking capabilities that can turn devices on and off.

Series Adaptor

Ablenet

The Series Adaptor interfaces between a battery-operated toy and two switches. The user must press both switches to activate the toy. This promotes bilateral hand use.

String Switch

Ablenet

A slight pull on a string attached to the microswitch base activates this switch.

Switch Latch Interface

Ablenet
Toys for Special Children

This interface connects a switch and a battery-operated device. Pressing the switch once turns a device on. A second press turns the device off.

Switch Toys

Ablenet
Burkhart Toys
Crestwood Company
Toys for Special Children

These companies make battery-operated toys that have been preadapted for single-switch use. The toys are connected to switches using cables with subminiature phone plugs.

Tongue Switch

DU-IT

This switch is designed to be held in the mouth and operated with the tongue. It has a dual up-down movement for two switch operations.

ToyPAC

Adaptive Communication
  Systems

The ToyPAC lets a user operate remote radio-controlled toys made by Radio Shack. The ToyPAC has single-switch scanning options, joystick, and wafer board options.

Tread Switch

Zygo

This is a durable switch that is activated by pressing a rocking treadle.

Device/Manufacturer(s)	Description

Universal Input Adaptor

Toys for Special Children | Different battery-operated toys, switches, and computers require different sizes of plugs. The Universal Adaptor provides an easy way to connect different-sized plugs and connectors together.

Wafer Board

TASH | The wafer board simulates joystick operations with a series of five touch-membrane switches which control device movements.

Wobble Switch

Prentke Romich | This switch consists of a spring with a small "ball" attached to the end. Moving the ball in any direction activates the switch.

AUGMENTATIVE COMMUNICATION

Dedicated augmentative communication devices are listed in this section. The devices range from simple electronic communication aids without printed or spoken output to sophisticated high-technology systems with software acceleration techniques, digitized speech output, and built-in printers.

Device/Manufacturer(s)	Description

AIPS Wolf

Adamlab | The AIPS Wolf is a variation of the Super Wolf augmentative communication aid. This device is a low-cost system with Echo II synthesized speech output. It can be accessed by nine external switches. Each switch activates a separate spoken message. The user can program up to 90 different levels.

Canon Communicator

Canon | This augmentative communication system consists of a small alphanumeric keyboard. It produces printed output on a small strip tape printer.

Device/Manufacturer(s)	Description

DAC

Adaptive Communication
Systems

The DAC is a direct-selection augmentative communication system with up to 1 hour of digitized speech output. A total of 128 touch membrane keys can be configured into larger key groupings. This device has a letter-spelling option; however, the spelled words cannot be pronounced unless they are prestored into the system. The device also has an LCD
display.

Dial Scan

Don Johnston
   Developmental Equipment

This is a simple "clock" communicator with a rotary scanning dial. A switch is needed to activate the rotation and stopping of the dial.

DynaVox

Adaptive Communication
Systems

The Dynavox is a portable augmentative communication device with Dec Talk speech. It features a customizable dynamically changing picture symbol screen with symbols categorized into pages, or layers. It can be accessed through direct selection, single- and dual-switch, scanning, and joystick.

Equalizer

Words+ Incorporated

The Equalizer is an augmentative communication application designed to operate on IBM-compatible computers. It can be accessed through direct selection, joystick, and single-switch scanning. The software has word prediction capabilities based on the user's past word-use frequency. The prediction list changes over time. There is a music program with some preprogrammed songs.

Eval Pac

Adaptive Communication
Systems

The Eval Pac is an expanded version of the RealVoice communication system. The system consists of an Epson Hx-20 computer with add-on keyboards for direct selection with an optical light pointer, or scanning with switches, joystick, or Morse code options. The Eval Pac has human quality male or female synthesized speech, an 80-charac-

Device/Manufacturer(s)	Description

Eval Pac *(continued)*

ter LCD display screen, and a built-in printer. It can connect to most microcomputers to serve as a keyboard emulator.

Eye Typer-300

Sentient Systems Technology

The Eye Typer is an eyegaze-controlled dedicated letter spelling communication system. It can be attached to Apple or IBM computers to serve as an alternate input device.

HandiVoice 110

Phonic Ear

This device is no longer manufactured. It was one of the first dedicated augmentative communication aids with synthesized speech output.

Intro Talker

Prentke Romich

The Intro Talker is a dedicated directselection communication aid with 2 to 8 minutes of digitized speech output. The system uses a limited verson of Minspeak software.

Liberator

Prentke Romich

Liberator is a portable, dedicated augmentative communication system with DecTalk synthesized speech and a small paper printer. The system can be accessed through direct selection, Head Master, joysticks, and single switches. It has the features of picture symbol prediction, a calculator, a notebook, and a Mac scratch pad. This device uses Minspeak software and can access any computer through a keyboard emulator.

Lifestyle Personal Communicator

Cascade Medical

The Personal Communicator is a small (18 ounce) dedicated communication aid with synthesized speech output and a small LCD screen. The keyboard is designed for letter spelling. It can also be used by individuals who are hearing impaired as a TDD system.

Light Talker

Prentke Romich

The Light Talker is a portable dedicated communication aid that can be accessed via a direct optical light pointer, scanning, Morse

Device/Manufacturer(s)	Description

Light Talker *(continued)*

code, or joystick. Twenty-six different access methods are available. The system uses Minspeak software and can access any computer through a keyboard emulator. Recent models feature DecTalk digitized speech output.

Light Writer

Zygo

The Light Writer is a direct selection communication aid with a standard Qwerty keyboard. It has a bright LED print display which has two sides, one for the user and one for the listener. Synthesized speech output can be added as an option.

Macaw

Zygo

The Macaw is a small augmentative communication system with 2 minutes of digitized speech output. It can be operated in direct selection or several different scanning modes. Up to four levels of 32 symbols can be customized for the user.

Magic Wand Talking Bar Code Reader

Tiger Communication System

The Magic Wand is a voice-output communication system that uses a hand-held bar code scanner. The scanner reads bar codes corresponding to words in a communication book.

Mega Wolf

ADAMLAB

The Mega Wolf is a low-cost, direct-selection communication aid that consists of 36 membrane keys that can be arrayed in a variety of overlay configurations. The Mega Wolf can be custom programmed with over 90 different overlays and has extensive fixed vocabularies suitable for classroom activities with very young children.

PACA

Zygo

PACA, or Portable Anticipatory Communication Aid, is a dedicated augmentative communication system. PACA software is housed in a laptop computer. The system is designed

Device/Manufacturer(s)	Description

PACA *(continued)*

for single-switch row-column scanning. The software uses word prediction to present choices to the user based on frequency of use. A 24-column printer is built in, and optional synthesized speech voice output is available.

Parrot

Zygo

The Parrot is a small portable communication system with digitized speech output. Up to 16 brief messages can be recorded.

RealVoice

Adaptive Communication Systems

The RealVoice is a dedicated, portable communication aid which uses an Epson Hx-20 computer base. The system has human-voice-quality, male or female synthesized speech. An 80-character LCD display screen and built-in printer are available. The basic system is a direct-selection device. It can connect to most microcomputers to serve as a keyboard emulator.

Say It All Plus

Innocomp

This dedicated augmentative communication system has a Qwerty keyboard that converts text into speech. Up to 864 phrases or words can be stored for single-keystroke output. An LCD display gives printed output. It can be attached to a printer or computer through an RS 232 port.

Say It Simply Plus

Innocomp

This is a portable augmentative communication system that has a membrane keyboard which can be divided into a single response cell, or a 12×12 matrix. Up to 762 phrases can be stored. The synthesized speech output can be altered from low to high pitches. It can connect to printers or computers through an RS 232 port.

Scanning Intro Talker

Prentke Romich

The Scanning Intro Talker is a portable dedicated communication aid with 2 to 8 minutes

Device/Manufacturer(s)	Description

Scanning Intro Talker

(continued)

of digitized speech output. The system uses a limited version of Minspeak software.

Scan Wolf

ADAMLAB

The ScanWolf is a low-cost dedicated scanning communication aid with Echo II voice output. An array of 36 LED lights can be matrixed into a variety of overlay configurations. It can be operated in automatic- or manual-scanning modes. The device is not user-programmable. Customized vocabulary lists are sent to ADAMLAB for programming. Up to 500 words on 30 levels are available.

Scan Writer

Zygo

This device is a dedicated augmentative communication aid which can also function as an input device for Apple II series, Commodore, and IBM PC computers. The Scan Writer uses row-column letter spelling which is accessed with a switch. Synthesized speech output, and infrared remote control options are available.

Secretary

Zygo

The Secretary is a small letter-spelling, direct-selection communication system. It has printed output on a small LCD screen and paper copy. A limited number of digitized speech messages can be recorded.

Special Friend

Shea Products

Special Friend is a portable dedicated augmentative communication system with a Qwerty membrane keyboard and synthesized speech output. Phrases in categories are stored by the manufacturer. Customized phrases or words can also be stored by the user.

Steeper Communication Teaching Aid

Zygo

This device is a switch-operated scanning system in which large illuminated lights indi-

Device/Manufacturer(s)	Description

Steeper Communication Teaching Aid *(continued)*

cate the scanning sequence. Objects can be placed on the surface of the system or pictures can be mounted. It is used as a training aid with individuals who are beginning to learn the scanning process.

Super Wolf

ADAMLAB

The Super Wolf is a low-cost, direct-selection communication aid built into a Texas Instrument's Touch and Tell case. It can be programmed by the user with up to 800 words on 30 different levels. In addition, fixed vocabularies for various classroom activities are available. The Super Wolf has Echo II synthesized speech.

Switchboard Communication Training Aid

Zygo

The Switchboard is an electronic light scanning system for single-, dual-, or multiple-switch access. The device can be configured into many different scanning arrays and methods. It is used to teach scanning skills.

Talk-O

Innocomp

Talk-O offers digitized speech output in a portable augmentative communication aid. It is operated by direct selection or scanning. Up to 120 seconds of speech can be recorded.

Touch Talker

Prentke Romich

The Touch Talker is a direct-selection portable communication system that uses Minspeak software to encode words, phrases, and sentences customized for the user. Recent models feature Dec Talk digitized speech output. Printed output is available on an LCD screen.

VoCaid

Texas Instruments

This device is a low-cost communication aid with synthesized speech output. The system consists of several fixed levels of vocabulary

Device/Manufacturer(s)	Description

Vocaid *(continued)*

suitable for adults who are in acute care hospital settings who are in need of a temporary communication system.

VOIS 136

Phonic Ear

The VOIS 136 is a dedicated, portable direct-selection communication system. It has memory for over 21,000 customized entries on multiple levels. Synthesized speech output can be adjusted across ten voice characteristics.

VOIS 160

Phonic Ear

The VOIS 160 is a dedicated, portable direct-selection communication system. Up to seven levels of customized text can be accessed, giving the user 64,000 entries. Synthesized speech is available in male or female versions. A two-line LCD display shows all text entries.

VOIS Shapes

Phonic Ear

This augmentative communication system uses direct selection of 120 keys which have symbols related to sign language hand shapes, location, and movement. By sequencing the symbols together the user can access prestored words. The device has synthesized speech output and a small LCD display screen.

Whisper Wolf

ADAMLAB

The Whisper Wolf is a low-cost augmentative communication system that provides auditory scanning options. Over 90 different levels of vocabulary can be programmed into the system. There are also over 90 levels of fixed vocabulary preprogrammed by the company. While the device scans, it provides auditory information to a user through an earphone. When the user reaches the correct message, a single switch is pressed to speak the message to others.

Device/Manufacturer(s)	Description

Words+ ACES

Words+ Incorporated

The ACES (Augmentative Communication Evaluation System) is a software and hardware system for evaluating augmentative communication skills. An IBM computer is used. The system includes device emulation software that simulates many commercially available augmentative communication systems.

Zygo 100

Zygo

The Zygo 100 is a row-column scanning system that does not have spoken or printed output. It can be attached to Apple II series computers via an interface card.

Zygo Talking Notebook II

Zygo

The Talking Notebook is a portable, direct-selection communication system with synthesized speech output and a large LCD display. Notebook software includes a mini word processor, calculator, and calendar/clock.

BRAILLE INPUT–OUTPUT DEVICES

Many devices have been designed to give individuals with visual impairments access to computers using braille. The technologies listed in this section include devices such as braille keyboards, braille screen reading systems, and braille printers.

Device/Manufacturer(s)	Description

APH Pocket Braille

American Printing House for the Blind

The APH Pocket Braille is a portable computer with braille input and synthesized speech output. The system can be connected to Apple II series, Commodore, IBM, Tandy, and Texas Instruments computers through a serial port. It also can send information directly to braille embosser printers.

Device/Manufacturer(s)	Description

Brailled Keyboard Overlay

American Printing House for the Blind

This keyboard overlay has embossed braille key markings for each key. It is designed for the Apple *IIGS*.

Braille Interface Terminal

Telesensory

The BIT terminal is a 20-cell braille computer display which operates with IBM PC computers. Joystick or keyboard commands are used to move the BIT display around the computer screen.

Braille Mate

Telesensory

Braille Mate is a portable braille computer with an 8-dot braille keyboard, an 8-dot braille cell, and a built-in speech synthesizer. It can use Grade 1 or Grade 2 braille input. Grade 2 braille is printed into standard text. Braille Mate can serve as an input system for IBM PC or compatible computers.

Braille 'n Speak

Blazie Engineering

This is a portable computer system that can be used as a braille word processor. It also has talking features, a calculator, clock, calendar, computer terminal, and telephone directory. The Braille n' Speak can be connected to most computers through a serial port.

Braillex IB40 and IB80

Adhoc Reading Systems Incorporated

The Braillex is a 40- or 80-cell braille output printer system for IBM computers.

Braillo 200, Braillo 400S, and Braillo 90 Printers

American Thermofoam Corporation

These printers provide braille print for a variety of computer systems. The 200 is designed for high-speed printing with IBM computers. The 400S is a high-speed printer that also collates and can be used with IBM, Apple II series, and Tandy computers. The 90 is a small personal printer designed for use with the Apple II series of computers and IBM.

Device/Manufacturer(s)	Description

KeyBraille

Humanware

KeyBraille is used with MS-DOS series computers. It provides a 5-cell Braille display which indicates line, column, and screen attributes of the operating software.

Marathon Brailler

Enabling Technologies

This braille embosser printer can be used with Apple II series, IBM, Macintosh, Commodore, Tandy, and Texas Instruments computers.

Nomad

Syntha/Voice Computers

Nomad is a portable IBM-XT-compatible laptop computer with synthesized speech output and the option of a braille or Qwerty keyboard. It also is equipped with a cursor tracking screen reading program, and 2400-baud modem.

Notex

Adhoc Reading Systems

This is a small, portable Braille notebook computer. The system has 24-cell braille output, braille input, and word processor and calculator software.

Optacon II

Telesensory/VTEK

The Optacon II is a small portable device that provides instant braille computer output. It attaches to Apple II series, IBM, Macintosh, Commodore, and Texas Instruments computers. Optional magnifying lenses are available to enlarge print on the computer screen.

VersaPoint

Telesensory

VersaPoint is a braille embosser printer that can be used with Apple II series or Macintosh computers.

Xerox/Kurzweil Personal Reader

Xerox Imaging Systems

This device "reads" printed materials and converts them into synthetic speech. It can be used for computer data entry via an RS 232 interface and can provide Braille output.

COMPUTER ACCESS DEVICES

Individuals who are unable to use computers using standard keyboard methods can access computers using the devices listed in this section. These peripherals consist of special keyboards, add-on internal cards with RAM-resident software, speech recognition systems, and a variety of other input options.

Device/Manufacturer(s)	Description
Adaptive Firmware Card	
Don Johnston Developmental Equipment	The Adaptive Firmware Card provides alternate access methods for all Apple II series computers. It allows individuals to run any software program through a variety of input modes. These include expanded keyboards, scanning, joystick, and Morse code. The Apple *IIG32e* version includes synthesized speech features, mouse emulation, and custom macros.
AID+Me	
Computability	The AID+Me provides alternate access methods for IBM, Commodore, Apple II, and Macintosh computers. Any input device can be used, including Powerpad, Touch Window, expanded keyboards, Head Master, communication aids with serial output, and joystick.
AKI II series	
Prentke Romich	This keyboard interface provides a link between Apple II series computers and Prentke Romich augmentative communication aids. The augmentative communication aid then serves as the keyboard for the computer.
Computer Entry Terminal (CET-2)	
Prentke Romich	An alternative computer keyboard that can emulate either Apple or IBM computers. It is accessible through a variety of methods including light pointer, scanning, Morse code, and joystick. Wireless remote capability is also available.

Device/Manufacturer(s)	Description

DADA Entry

DADA

DADA Entry is an IBM-compatible keyboard emulator that operates using eight different input methods: single-switch scanning, dual-switch input, Morse code, alternative keyboards, joysticks, wafer board, and mouse. Accompanying software has word completion and abbreviation-expansion features. Speech output is available if a peripheral synthesizer is added to the system. It operates transparently to most application programs.

Disk Guide

Extensions for Independence
Prentke Romich
TASH

A disk guide attaches to the front of a disk drive to help align computer disks with the drive opening. It is available in 3.5-inch or 5.25-inch sizes for a variety of computers.

Double Switch Adaptor

Technology for Language
and Learning

This adaptor converts a single-switch jack into a two-switch jack so that more than one user can operate single-switch computer software. An Adaptive Firmware Card or Apple Computer Game I/O Switch Interface is needed.

Dragon Dictate

Dragon Systems

Dragon Dictate is a voice-operated accessing system for IBM-compatible computers. It can transparently operate any software application. The voice recognition software is designed to "learn" a user's speech patterns in a relatively short period of time. It also relies on word-prediction strategies. The recognition "dictionary" has up to 21,000 words at any one time.

Expanded Keyboard Interface

Words+ Incorporated

This interface connects to IBM computers to allow the use of a number of expanded keyboards, including the Unicorn Board, and TASH minikeyboard, with standard software. It also can be used with the Talking Board program to create augmentative communication applications. When used in con-

Device/Manufacturer(s)	Description

Expanded Keyboard Interface
(continued)

junction with the Expanded Keyboard Emulator program, it adds the features of word-prediction and abbreviation-expansion with standard software.

Expanded Keyboards

EKEG Electronics

These expanded keyboards can be connected directly to Apple II series, Macintosh, or IBM computers. The keyboard dimensions are 12×24 inches with 1½-inch keys that provide tactile and auditory feedback. Latches are provided for control, shift, and other important keys.

Expanded Keyboards for the Adaptive Firmware Card

EKEG Electronics

These keyboards were designed to operate in conjunction with the Adaptive Firmware Card. One keyboard has 48 1-inch squares; the other has 128 1-inch squares.

Eyegaze Computer System

LC Technologies

This is a computer system that is operated by eye movements. The system uses a Head Tracker, which gives it a high tolerance for head movements. The system will operate most DOS software, computer printers, telephones, and several games.

Game I/O Switch Interface for Apple II series computers

Ablenet
Arroyo & Associates
Computability
Don Johnston
  Developmental Equipment
Prentke Romich
TASH
Toys for Special Children

This adaptor connects one or two switches to any Apple II series computer through the 16-pin game port.

Free Wheel

Pointer Systems

Free Wheel is a small head-mounted optical pointer that controls cursor movement on

Device/Manufacturer(s)	Description

Free Wheel *(continued)*

Macintosh and IBM computers. The software places a keyboard image on the computer screen which is used to operate standard software. The IBM version also allows access via joystick, mouse, or single-switch options.

HandiWARE Connectors

Microsystems Software Inc.

HandiWARE interfaces an IBM PC computer with a single switch. The interface can be used to operate various Microsystems software programs.

HeadMaster

Prentke Romich

Head Master uses a headset and computer-mounted control system to simulate mouse cursor control on Macintosh, Apple *IIGS*, or IBM computers. A software program called Screen Keys places an image of a keyboard on the computer screen, which is used to operate standard software. Head Master can also be used to operate the Liberator communication aid.

Info Window Display

IBM

The Info Window Display is an IBM color monitor for PC and PS2 computers with built-in touch window capabilities.

Intro Voice I and II

Voice Connection

Intro Voice is a voice-recognition system for Apple II series computers. It has a recognition vocabulary of 80 to 160 words, which can be customized by the user. It is independent of the operating system or program language.

Intro Voice III, IV, V, and VI

Voice Connection

Intro Voice is a voice-recognition system for IBM PC or XT computers. It has a recognition vocabulary of up to 500 words, which are customized by the user. Intro Voice VI adds voice output through an on-board speech synthesizer. Micro Intro Voice can be added to IBM compatible portable computers.

Device/Manufacturer(s)	Description

Ke:nx

Don Johnston
  Developmental Equipment
TASH

Ke:nx is a keyboard emulation system for Macintosh computer systems. It can be adapted for single-switch use with scanning options, Morse code, or an alternate keyboard. Mouse emulation, customized macros, and synthesized speech output options are available.

KEII

Prentke Romich

The KEII provides keyboard emulation through Prentke Romich augmentative communication aids or any other ASCII generating device linked to IBM computers.

KeasyBoard

Parallel Systems

The KeasyBoard is a detachable computer keyboard for Apple II series computers. It operates with an optical light beam pointer. No adaptor cards are required to connect the Keasy Board.

Keyboard Covers

Toys for Special Children

A keyboard cover blocks access to some or all computer keys. Special bumpers can be attached to the underside of the keyboard cover so that pressing the cover activates selected computer keys.

Keyboard Interface for Apple II series computers

Prentke Romich

The keyboard emulator is a card that is placed inside an Apple II series computer. This card allows the connection of any external input device that sends ASCII characters. Prentke Romich augmentative communication systems can be used as keyboard emulators when connected to a computer through this interface.

Keyguard

Adaptive Communication
  Systems
Computability
Don Johnston
  Developmental Equipment

Plastic keyguards are mounted onto computer keyboards to prevent accidental key strikes. Some models come with latches to hold control or shift keys easily. Models are available for Apple II series, Macintosh, and IBM computers.

Device/Manufacturer(s)	Description

Keyguard *(continued)*

Prentke Romich
REACH
Unicorn Engineering

Keylock

Extensions for Independence
TASH

A keylock is used to temporarily hold down keys such as shift, control, or escape for individuals who cannot press two keys at once. Pressing one side of the keylock engages the key; pressing the other side disengages the key.

Keyport 60

Polytel Computer Products

This alternate keyboard has 60, ½-inch touch-membrane squares on its surface. It is designed to operate with IBM computers.

Keyport 300

Polytel Computer Products

The Keyport 300 is similar to the Keyport 60 except that it has 300, ½-inch touch-membrane squares on the keyboard surface.

King Keyboard

TASH

The King Keyboard has 1¼-inch keys which are recessed from the surface of the board. This allows users to rest on the keyboard without activating keys. The keyboard provides auditory feedback when keys are pressed. The Apple II series version connects through the Adaptive Firmware Card. The PC King is designed for IBM computers and plugs directly into the keyboard port.

Koala Pad

Koala Technologies

This small touch tablet was developed for Apple II series and IBM computers. It operates only with software written specifically for the Koala Pad.

Kurzweil Voice System and Kurzweil Voice Report

Kurzweil Applied Intelligence

The Kurzweil systems are voice-recognition input systems for IBM PC, AT, and XT computers. The Voice System recognizes up to 1,000 words, and can operate a variety of

Device/Manufacturer(s)	Description

**Kurzweil Voice System
and Kurzweil Voice Report**
(continued)

software including spreadsheets, word processing, and data bases. The Voice Report is designed as a word processor system. It recognizes up to 5,000 words and also can store macros which are triggered by a single word or phrase.

Lite Touch

Lovejoy Electronics

Lite Touch is a joystick emulator which is controlled by an optical light pointer. It can operate on Apple II series and IBM computers. Up to eight light sensors are attached to the frame of the computer screen. Pointing the optical light pointer to any of the sensors controls cursor movement in that direction.

MacIntyre

MacIntyre Inc.

This keyboard emulator for Macintosh computers provides access for single-switch users who require scanning arrays and for joystick users.

Magic Wand Keyboard

In Touch Systems

This device is a miniature alternative keyboard for IBM computers. The user touches a hand-held "wand" on the keyboard to operate it. The keyboard plugs directly into the keyboard socket of any IBM or compatible computer.

Membrane Keyboard

TASH

This keyboard measures 12 × 18 inches. Membrane keys can be activated by light touch. The keyboard connects to Apple II series computers through the Adaptive Firmware Card.

Membrane Keyboard II

Computability

This keyboard connects to Apple II series, Macintosh, or IBM computers through the Adaptive Firmware Card or PC Serial Aid. The keyboard has 128 keys and measures 13.25 × 7.25 inches.

Device/Manufacturer(s)	Description

Mini Keyboard

TASH

This small membrane keyboard connects to Apple II series computers through the Adaptive Firmware Card. The entire keyboard is 7.5 × 4.5 inches. An IBM version called the PC Mini connects directly to IBM computers.

Mini Membrane Keyboard

Computability

This membrane keyboard is only 7 × 4.5-inches large. It connects to Apple II series, IBM, and Macintosh computers through the Adaptive Firmware Card or PC Serial Aid.

Modified Power Pad for Switch Activation

Lekotek of Georgia

This is a modified Power Pad which allows the addition of up to nine switches. By pressing switches, individuals can activate Power Pad software. This system can be used with Apple II series computers.

Moisture Guard/ Keyboard Protector

Adaptive Communication
  Systems
Don Johnston
  Developmental Equipment
Hoolean
Merritt Computer Products
Prentke Romich

Clear molded plastic keyguards designed to fit over computer keyboards to prevent moisture from entering.

Mouse Emulator

TASH

This keyboard emulator for Macintosh computers with Mackeyboard software allows five different switches to control cursor movements on a display screen keyboard. A latching feature lets the user drag objects.

Multiple Switch Box

Don Johnston
  Developmental Equipment

The switch box connects to an Adaptive Firmware Card. Up to eight different switches can be attached to Apple II series computers. Each switch can be defined as a different computer key.

Device/Manufacturer(s)	Description

Muppet Learning Keys

Sunburst Communications

This is a touch-sensitive keyboard for Apple II series, Commodore, and IBM PC computers. The colorful keyboard can be used with software written specifically for the system.

Octima Chord Keyboard

TASH

The Octima Chord is a one-handed keyboard for Apple II series or IBM computers. The keyboard only has five keys, which are pressed alone or in combination to produce computer screen characters.

Opening Doors

Madenta Communications
Prentke Romich

Opening Doors is a keyboard emulator for Macintosh computers. It allows single- or dual-switch input via an on-screen keyboard and alternative keyboard input. Synthesized speech output is available. The accompanying software has word-prediction capabilities.

Paint Box Snap

Don Johnston
  Developmental Equipment

This colorful keyboard is designed for use with Apple *IIGS* computers and an Adaptive Firmware Card (model G32 or G32e). It has six large, colored keys and snaps on top of the standard keyboard. It includes a setup disk with applications written for many popular preschool programs.

PC A.I.D.

DADA
Don Johnston
  Developmental Equipment

The PC A.I.D. is a keyboard emulator for IBM PC computers. It attaches to the parallel printer port. Switches or assisted keyboards can be attached to the computer through the PC A.I.D. Talking scanning and customized scan lines can be developed.

PC King Keyboard

TASH

This IBM keyboard has large recessed microswitch keys. The keys provide auditory feedback when pressed. It plugs directly into the keyboard port of an IBM computer and requires no additional hardware or software.

Device/Manufacturer(s)	Description

PC Mini Keyboard

TASH

The PC Mini is a miniature IBM keyboard with a touch membrane surface. It plugs directly into the keyboard port of an IBM computer. No additional hardware or software is necessary.

PC Serial Aid

DADA
Don Johnston
  Developmental Equipment

The PC Serial Aid is a keyboard emulator for IBM PC computers which connects through a serial port. In addition to the features of the PC A.I.D., it allows the use of customizable matrix keyboards.

Porter

Don Johnston
  Developmental Equipment

The Porter is a multiple-input, game port extender that attaches to the Game I/O port of any Apple II series computer. Up to four different peripheral devices can be plugged into the Porter (9-pin and 16-pin ports). A dial selector is used to select the peripheral equipment being used at that time.

Power ^{N}

Dunamis

This keyboard emulator for IBM computers uses the Power Pad as a touch-sensitive computer input device.

Power Pad

Dunamis

The Powerpad is a 12×12-inch touch-sensitive computer input device which can be used with Apple II series, Atari, Commodore, VIC 20, and IBM computers. A wide variety of software is available for use with the Power Pad. The Power Pad Tool Kit software allows the design of custom programs including simple talking communication boards.

Power Port

Dunamis

The Power Port is used to connect the Power Pad to Apple II series computers. It connects to the 16-pin game I/O port.

SAR-100 Voice Plus Board

NEC America

This voice recognition system has a 250-word vocabulary and operates transparently with

Device/Manufacturer(s)	Description

SAR-100 Voice Plus Board
(continued)

most popular software programs. The user can customize the vocabulary. It operates on IBM series computers. Synthesized speech output is included in the system package.

Scanning WSKE II

Words+

Scanning WSKE II is a combination of hardware and software that runs on IBM series computers or compatibles. It provides a scanning method of keyboard emulation for single-switch users. In addition, it can be used as an augmentative communication aid with synthesized speech output. The software has word-prediction and alphabet-abbreviation expansion capabilities which run transparent to most software.

TetraScan II

Zygo

This device is a scanning keyboard emulator for Apple II series, Commodore, and IBM computers. The keyboard features alphanumeric characters arrayed according to frequency of use. Frequently used text can be stored for recall.

Touch Window

Edmark

The Touch Window is a transparent screen that mounts over the monitor display of Apple II series, IBM, and Tandy computers. Software written for the Touch Window allows the user to touch the screen to control the cursor.

T-TAM series

Prentke Romich
Words+

This keyboard emulator is designed for Apple II series, IBM series, and Macintosh computers. Any peripheral device that generates ASCII serial data in an RS-232 format can be used as the alternative keyboard. Prentke Romich augmentative communication aids can be used for keyboard emulation using this system.

Device/Manufacturer(s)	Description

Unicorn Expanded Keyboard Model II

Unicorn Engineering

The Unicorn Board is a popular expanded keyboard for Apple II series, Macintosh, and IBM computers. An Adaptive Firmware Card, Ke:nx system, or PC Serial Aid is needed to connect the keyboard to the computer. It consists of 128 large membrane-surface squares that can be arranged into various keyboard configurations. Programs and keyboard overlays are available for a wide variety of popular children's software.

Unicorn Expanded Keyboard Model 510

Unicorn Engineering

The Model 510 is a miniature version of the Unicorn Expanded Keyboard Model II. This touch membrane keyboard is only 5×10 inches.

Un Mouse

MicroTouch

The Un Mouse is a touch tablet surface that provides mouse emulation for Macintosh or IBM series computers.

Voice Key

TASH

Voice Key is a speech recognition system designed for IBM series computers. It has a 512-word or -phrase capacity.

Voice Master Key

Covox, Inc.

This voice-recognition system can be used to record and play back digitized speech on IBM computers. Up to 64 different words or phrases can be recognized by the system.

Voice Navigator

Articulate Systems

The Voice Navigator provides spoken voice control for Macintosh computers. It operates transparently and provides any keyboard function including mouse emulation. New voice commands can be added for special software applications.

Device/Manufacturer(s)	Description

Words+/Trace
Long Range Optical Pointer

Words+ Incorporated	This device provides keyboard emulation for IBM computers using an optical sensor. The sensor is pointed at a computer monitor which displays a keyboard. The software operates on a second monitor.

COMPUTER OUTPUT DEVICES

All computers provide output through a computer monitor or printer. The technology listed in this section includes devices that customize computer output options without the use of braille or synthesized speech. Devices that use braille and synthesized speech technology are listed separately in this chapter.

Device/Manufacturer(s)	Description

20/20+

Optalec	This high-resolution computer monitor for IBM series computers provides enlarged text output.

Compu-Lenz

Able Tech Connection	This device is a fresnel lens that more than doubles the size of computer screen characters with clear images even with color. The device has an adjustable holder which allows it to be attached to most computer visual display screens.

Diconix 150 Plus

Adhoc Reading Systems	The Diconix is a small ink jet portable printer which weighs less than 4 pounds. It can be attached to IBM computers and some communication aids.

DP-10, DP11, and DP11 Plus Large Print Display Processors

Telesensory/VTEK	These display processors enlarge dot-matrix video display text into solid proportional

Device/Manufacturer(s)	Description

DP Large Print Processors
(continued)

characters ranging from 2 to 16 times the original size. The DP-10 is for Apple II series computers. The DP11 and DP11 Plus are for IBM computers.

Universal Paper Loader

Extensions for Independence

The Universal Paper Loader gives a user the ability to independently load paper into a printer. The user must have some hand control or a direct-selection device such as a mouth stick or head stick.

Vista

Telesensory

Vista enlarges computer screen text and graphics 3 to 16 times. It is designed for use with IBM series computers. A three-button mouse is used to control the screen image and a screen cursor.

ENVIRONMENTAL CONTROLS

Environmental controls range from simple systems designed to operate one or two electronic appliances to sophisticated "smart homes" with computerized functions for controlling appliances, heating and cooling, door locking, and the phone system. This section lists environmental control systems and their components.

Device/Manufacturer(s)	Description

2 IR

TASH

This infrared environmental control receiver has two channels that work with TASH's Relax environmental control unit or any other trainable infrared transmitter system.

Control 1

Prentke Romich

The Control 1 environmental control system uses X-10 technology to operate up to 256 AC power devices. When a Control 1 Input Display (CID) is added, users can operate the

Device/Manufacturer(s)	Description

Control 1 (continued)

system using single-switch, dual-switch, or Morse code input. Adding a Wireless Data Transmission System (WTRS-1) to the unit gives a user the ability to send signals to the Control 1 Unit via radio signals. Without the WTRS-1, the user has to access the system through RS-232 cables.

Control Unit

AbleNet

Electric appliances can be plugged into the control unit and operated via adaptive switches. Two appliances with up to 1,700 watts of power can be operated.

Deuce

DU-IT Control Systems

This environmental control unit provides control of a standard phone or speaker phone, appliances, and door openers via a dual-control switch, direct selection, or infrared remote controls. It also can provide input to communication aids or computers through two-switch scanning or Morse code.

FRED

Don Johnston
  Developmental Equipment

FRED is an infrared transmitter and receiver system that can be operated with dual-switch access. It can operate up to two separate devices. The receiver can be attached to an Adaptive Firmware Card and Apple *IIGS* computer to provide infrared Morse code control of any software program.

GEWA Page Turner

Zygo

The GEWA Page Turner gives an individual independence in turning pages while reading. Single- or multiple-switch controls can be used. The device will turn pages forward and backward.

HAL-ES

Voice Connection

This environmental control system operates using voice recognition of up to 500 words. The system uses an IBM computer as an environmental control base. This lets the user switch between computer access through

Device/Manufacturer(s)	Description

HAL-ES *(continued)*

voice and environmental control options. Up to 36 different software applications and 16 different infrared-controlled electronic devices can be accessed.

MECCA

DU-IT Control Systems

MECCA is a portable environmental control system that can be integrated with a power mobility system. Its radio signals control up to 16 X-10 system receivers, the telephone, and up to ten other devices. Dual-switch input is required to operate the system.

MasterVoice

MasterVoice

This environmental control unit operates using voice-activation up to 20 feet from the control box. It can operate appliances, the telephone and can interface with computers.

Mini Environmental Control Unit

Arroyo & Associates

This low-cost environmental control system is operated via a single switch. It can operate only on a single electrical outlet and is usually used to reboot computers.

Power Minder

TASH

This is a switch-activated power cord with a built-in timer.

Relax

TASH

Relax is an infrared environmental control system that can be operated with single switches or an attached alternative keyboard. It can transmit signals to over six devices with over 50 control codes for those devices. The 2 IR infrared receiver can be used to adapt noninfrared appliances for control with the Relax system.

Scanning X-10 Powerhouse

Prentke Romich

The Scanning X-10 Powerhouse gives a user control over 16 appliances or lights using single or dual switches. The system uses X-10 technology with wireless radio control signals.

Device/Manufacturer(s)	Description

Kincontrol

TASH

Kincontrol is a single- or dual-switch environmental control system that can access any Ultra 4 transmitter or the Relax infrared system. Up to ten different appliances or functions can be accessed.

Ultra Power Bar

TASH

The Ultra Power Bar is a power strip that is activated by a single switch.

Ultra Series
4S, 4L, 4J, 2P, and 2T

TASH

The Ultra series of environmental control systems use X-10 technology with sound waves to operate appliances. The Ultra 4S has small keys for direct access. The Ultra 4L uses a wafer board. The Ultra 4J allows joystick control, and the Ultra 2P is accessed with sip-and-puff switches. Finally the Ultra 2T uses two single switches for access.

Unicontrol TV Converter

TASH

This single-switch system uses infrared signals to control television functions.

Wireless Data
Transmission System

Prentke Romich

This system transmits ASCII data from a portable computer or augmentative communication system to a stationary computer or environmental control unit via radio waves.

X-10 Control Systems

Heath
KY Enterprises
Radio Shack
Sears
Stanley Tools
X-10 (USA) Incorporated

This series of environmental controls operates by plugging appliances into receivers connected to the AC power system of a home. Infrared or radio signals are used to activate the receiver.

X-10 Home Control
Computer Interface

X-10 (USA) Incorporated

This device is a computer interface that can be used in Apple II series, Macintosh, Com-

Device/Manufacturer(s)	Description

X-10 Home Control
(continued)

modore, and IBM computers. It consists of eight rocking-lever switches, which can be used to operate up to eight different appliances, lights, or other devices. The device can be programmed to perform a series of events.

POWER MOBILITY SYSTEMS

Currently there are only four basic power mobility systems. Different manufacturers have developed their own variations for each system, but the basic technology remains the same across manufacturers.

Device/Manufacturer(s)	Description

Add-On Power Mobility Systems
ABEC

Add-On Power Mobility is available for converting standard manual wheelchairs into power systems. The Add-On system can accommodate a wide variety of control access and seating systems.

Modular Base Power Mobility Systems
Everest & Jennings
Fortress
Invacare

Modular Base systems are heavy and sit low to the ground. This makes them useful in rough terrain but limits their portability. Modular Bases can accommodate a wide variety of control access and seating systems.

Scooters and Three Wheelers
Everest & Jennings
Fortress
Invacare
Orthokinetics

Scooters are mobility bases with handlebars mounted on a central tiller. They are lightweight and easily transported. Scooters can be fitted with front- or rear-wheel drive systems. Control access methods and seating system options are limited.

Standard Power Mobility Systems
Everest & Jennings
Invacare

The large rear wheels of Standard Power Mobility Systems make them suitable for in-

Device/Manufacturer(s)	Description

**Standard Power
Mobility Systems** *(continued)*

door and outdoor terrain. These wheelchairs have limited portability. A wide variety of control access and seating systems can be accommodated.

SYNTHESIZED SPEECH

Synthesized speech provides individuals who cannot speak with a method of communicating with others. It gives persons with visual impairments a way to auditorily track work on the computer. Finally, it gives young children who are developing computer skills auditory feedback to enhance computer learning. The following list includes synthesized-speech systems that can be added as peripherals to micro-computer systems.

Device/Manufacturer(s)	Description

Artic D'Light
and Artic D'Light/Sonix

Artic Technologies

Both Artic D'Light systems are SynPhonix speech synthesizer systems designed to operate on Toshiba T-1000 laptop computers. The systems provide spoken computer output using off-the-shelf MS-DOS software.

Clarity

Innocomp

A speech synthesizer with human quality voice output that can be added to Innocomp communication aids.

DECtalk

Digital Equipment Inc.

DECtalk is a digitized speech synthesizer which can be altered for male or female, young or old speech qualities. Nine voices are predefined for ease of use. DECtalk can be purchased for use with Apple II series, Macintosh, IBM, Commodore, Texas Instruments, and Tandy computers. DECtalk is also available in many augmentative communication aids.

Device/Manufacturer(s)	Description

Echo Speech Synthesizers

Street Electronics

The Echo series of text-to-speech synthesizers provides low-cost speech output for a variety of computers. Versions are available for Apple II series, Tandy, Acorn, Atari, Commodore, IBM PC, and Texas Instruments computers.

Personal Speech System

Votrax

This synthesized-speech computer output system is available for a wide variety of computers, including Apple II series, Acorn, Macintosh, Atari, Commodore, IBM, Tandy, and Texas Instruments. It translates computer text into speech.

RealVoice PC

Adaptive Communication
Systems

The RealVoice is a diphone-based speech synthesizer with human voice qualities. It is available in male and female versions. The RealVoice PC connects to IBM computers through the serial port. It provides speech output for software applications.

SynPhonix
210, 220, and 240

Artic Technologies

This phonetic speech synthesizer is a plug-in card for IBM, Toshiba, and NEC computers. The system uses SONIX2 text-to-speech software.

Type N Talk

Votrax

Type N Talk is a text-to-speech synthesizer that can be connected to any computer with an RS232 serial port. The Votrax SC-01 speech synthesis chip is used in the system.

Vert Plus

Telesensory/VTEK

This speech synthesizer is a screen-reading program for IBM computers. It gives on-line information as well as tracking for menus, screen location, and formatting.

SOFTWARE

Many software programs have been written for users of assistive technology. These programs teach cognitive and academic skills through adaptive computer peripherals, train users of assistive technologies, offer assisted keyboard emulation through RAM-resident software, and serve as assistive technology evaluation tools. Because it is difficult to organize computer software into neat categories, the software programs included in this directory are listed alphabetically. Application programs that were not written specifically for disabled populations are not included in this listing unless the program is mentioned in the text of this book.

Software/Manufacturer(s)	Description
Abbreviation Expansion	
Zygo	This software lets a user store frequently used sentences or words under alphabet abbreviation expansion codes on Apple II series computers.
Access 190	
Adaptive Communication Systems	Access 190 is a RAM-resident software program written for IBM series computers. It offers one-key computer functions, variable keystroke timing delays, word and letter prediction, and voice output when an external synthesized-speech system is connected. It can be accessed by the standard keyboard, single-switch scanning, or joystick controls.
Action/Music Play	
PEAL Software	This software provides language intervention activities using action play and music. The Muppet Learning Keys are used to access Apple computers. An Echo II synthesizer provides voice output.
Adult Switch and Touch Window Progressions	
R. J. Cooper and Associates	This program has activities designed to teach adults with severe handicaps how to use switches, attend to the computer, and respond to visual cues given by an Apple II series computer.

Software/Manufacturer(s)	Description

AFC Access: TouchWindow

Don Johnston
  Developmental Equipment

AFC Access operates on Apple *IIe* or *IIGS* computers with an Adaptive Firmware Card and TouchWindow. It provides TouchWindow access for any Apple II software program.

APH/SEI Talking Software

American Printing House for the Blind

This software series for Apple II series computers includes talking programs for assessing knowledge of high school academic subjects.

Artic Crystal/Artic Vision

Artic Technologies

This software is designed for IBM series computers. It translates all keyboard activity and screen output into synthesized speech through the Artic Crystal speech synthesizer. It works transparently with most application software programs.

Artic Crystal Business Vision

Artic Technologies

This program is similar to the Artic Vision program, except it offers speech translation of business applications such as spreadsheets, menu entries, and special text such as row-column headings.

Artic Encore

Artic Technologies

Artic Encore offers spoken output through the Artic Crystal speech synthesizer on IBM series computers. This program includes a talking telephone book, calendar, checkbook, and other desk accessories.

Arctic Focus

Artic Technologies

This software program enlarges the text and graphics on IBM series computers. A graphics adaptor card is required.

Assistive Device Locator System (ADLS)

Academic Software

ADLS is a menu-driven program that lists thousands of assistive technology products in over 660 categories. It is currently available

Software/Manufacturer(s)	Description
ADLS *(continued)*	on floppy disks for Apple II series and IBM series computers. The program is updated annually for a minimal fee.
Audio Scan	
Don Johnston Developmental Equipment	Audio Scan provides a method of auditorily scanning simple communication overlays using a single switch and an Apple II series computer.
Bank Street Writer III	
Broderbund Software	Bank Street Writer is a simple word processing program designed for children. The newest version offers a spelling checker. The program is available for Apple II series, IBM series, and Tandy computers.
BEX	
Raised Dot Computing	BEX is a word processing program that provides grade II braille translation through a variety of computer-output devices such as braille printers, written text printers, and synthesized speech. The program is written for Apple II series computers.
Big Letters	
Lehigh Valley Easter Seal Society	This is a beginning word processing program for children. It prints large letters on the screen and speaks each selection through a speech synthesizer. Text-to-speech translation of printed words and sentences is available. The program is written for Apple II series computers.
Boardmaker	
Mayer-Johnson	Boardmaker, written for Macintosh computers, allows the user access to Picture Communication Symbols from Mayer Johnson, clip art, or other graphics applications. It can be used to easily make communication boards or picture-based educational activities.
Braille-Talk	
GW Micro	This program for Apple II series and IBM computers translates any text file into Grade I or II braille for printer output.

Software/Manufacturer(s)	Description

Brikeys Utility

Enabling Technologies
  Company

This RAM-resident utility gives a user a "pop up" braille keyboard that overides the regular keyboard. It operates on IBM series or Tandy computers.

Buddy's Body

UCLA Intervention Program for Handicapped Children

Buddy's Body is one of a series of software programs designed for children using Apple II series computers and the Power Pad. This program teaches the names of body parts.

Build-a-Scene

R. J. Cooper and Associates

This Apple II series software operates with a single-switch input box. Each activation of a switch adds another component to a real-life scene.

Catch the Cow

Computerade Products

This program teaches single-switch accessing skills through a progression of increasingly larger scanning arrays. It is designed for Apple II series computers with a single-switch input box.

Children's Switch and Touch Progression

R. J. Cooper and Associates

This program is similar to Adult Switch and Touch Progressions except that the content is designed for younger users. An Apple II series computer, Echo II speech synthesizer, and single-switch input or Touch Window are needed to operate the software.

CHPI Motor Training Games

Computers to Help People

Games are used to teach single-switch activation skills on Apple II series computers. Over 14 different games are available.

Close View

Apple Computer

Close View is a resident utility program included in every Macintosh System Folder. It provides the option of screen magnification.

Cognitive Rehabilitation Series

Hartley

Cognitive Rehabilitation consists of a series of programs used to train cognitive skills such

Software/Manufacturer(s)	Description

Cognitive Rehabilitation Series
(continued)

as attention, visual tracking, memory, and categorization. It was written for Apple II series computers.

COGREHAB

Life Science Associates

This software series has programs for evaluating and treating cognitive skills such as attention, memory, and perceptual disorders. The entire series consists of seven volumes of software and operates on Apple II series, IBM, and Tandy computers.

Communication Board Builder

Mayer-Johnson

This Macintosh HyperCard stack gives a user the ability to quickly make picture or text communication boards. The Picture Communication Symbols are included for use on the communication boards. Files with premade grids for common augmentative communication aids are available.

Communication Board SkillBuilder

Edmark Corporation

This Apple II series computer program works in conjunction with a Touch Window to teach early communication board use skills. The student touches the Touch Window screen or accesses the program through a single switch.

Cotton Tales

MindPlay

This is a word-processing program for children who are in the process of learning sight-word reading skills. The child combines picture graphics with whole words to "write" a story.

Creature Chorus

Laureate Learning Systems

This simple cause–effect software can be operated through a Touch Window or single switch on Apple II series computers. Six different programs offer bright graphics with varying sound effects.

Software/Manufacturer(s)	Description

DOS Helper

Aristo Computers, Inc.

This program is a help system for DOS commands. It is RAM-resident and can be called up within programming applications.

DU-IT Proportional Simulations Disk

DU-IT Control Systems Group

This series of programs for Apple II series computers simulates driving a power wheelchair, operating environmental control systems, and other activities which test use of proportional joystick input methods.

Early and Advanced Switch Games

R. J. Cooper and Associates

These single-switch games start at a cause–effect level and work up to programs that teach hitting a switch on time and matching tasks.

Easy Access

Apple Computer Inc.

This program is included in the system disk of Macintosh computers. It allows one-fingered typists a "Sticky Key" option that bypasses having to press multiple keys at once and a keyboard mouse emulation function.

Edmark Lesson Maker

Edmark Corporation

Lesson Maker software is an easy-to-use program for creating unique computer lessons using the TouchWindow and Apple II series computer. Graphics and words are contained in files which are used to create lessons.

Eency Weency Spider Games

UCLA Intervention Program for Handicapped Children

This Apple II series computer program operates with single-switch input. Up to four players can play a simple board game which moves the "spider" up a drain spout.

Electric Crayon

Merit Software

Electronic Crayon is a simple preschool drawing program for Apple II series, Macintosh, Commodore, IBM series, and Tandy computers. The child chooses pictures, then clicks on colors to fill in the pictures.

Software/Manufacturer(s)	Description

Equalizer

Words+

This augmentative communication software is designed to operate on IBM computers with single- or dual-switch Morse code input. Alphanumeric codes can be used as macros for preprogrammed words or text. The system has synthesized speech output when a separate synthesizer system is attached.

Exploratory Play

PEAL Software

This program uses the Muppet Learning Keys as an alternative computer input device with Apple II series computers. Special picture overlays are included with the software. There are two different early learning play activities with three levels of play complexity.

Explore-a-Story

Willam K. Bradford
  Publishing

This software series is written for Apple II series computers with high-resolution color graphic capabilities. Children can move animated characters through colorful background scenes. A simple word processor lets children write their own words to the story. In addition, story characters, objects, and backgrounds can be changed to create new story pictures.

EZ Keys/Key Wiz

Words+

This software program provides keyboard assistance for IBM series computers. This RAM-resident program offers word prediction and abbreviation expansion for slow typists. EZ Keys has synthesized speech output available for augmentative communication needs. Key Wiz does not have speech output capabilities but is otherwise identical to EZ Keys.

ezMorse

Regenesis Development Co.

This is a Morse code input program for IBM series or Tandy computers. It needs a dual switch or single switch for operation. The program is RAM-resident and has a mnemonic training system to teach Morse code skills.

Software/Manufacturer(s)	Description

EZ Talker

Words+

This computer access system is designed to run on IBM-compatible computers. It provides an augmentative communication system with synthesized speech output. Alphanumeric macros can be used as codes to retrieve preprogrammed words or text.

FaceMaker

Spinnaker

This software program is similar to Mr. Potato Head for computers. Users can select from an array of different heads, eyes, noses, and other body parts. When the face is completed users can command it to blink, stick out its tongue, or make other animated movements.

Filch 3.0 with Evaluate

Kinetic Designs

This program provides keyboard redefinition for IBM series computers. It has a key-repeat defeater, sticky key functions, and has auditory feedback for users.

Fire Organ

Colorado Easter Seal Society

This public domain program is written for Apple II series computers and single-switch use. It teaches cause–effect skills by giving the user colorful screen graphics each time the switch is pressed.

First Categories

Laureate Learning Systems

This program teaches children how to match objects into category groupings. Speech output is available through an Echo synthesizer. It can be used with the Touch Window on Apple II series and IBM computers.

First Words

Laureate Learning Systems

First Words is a vocabulary training program for young children with six levels of difficulty. It can run on any Apple II series computer or IBM, and has spoken output through a speech synthesizer. The Touch Window can be used with this program.

Software/Manufacturer(s)	Description

FreeBoard

Pointer Systems

This software provides keyboard emulation for IBM or Tandy computers. It requires 82K of RAM for operation. An image of the keyboard appears on the computer screen. The user moves a cursor around the screen using a joystick, mouse, or single switch.

FreeComm

Pointer Systems

FreeComm is a nondedicated augmentative communication system for IBM and Tandy computers. It provides spoken output through a speech synthesizer. Abbreviation-expansion features are included.

Fun with Drawing

Dunamis

This Power Pad software program lets the user create colorful computer pictures by selecting object shapes, colors, and sizes. It operates on IBM computers.

Gateway Stories

Don Johnston
   Developmental Equipment

Gateway Stories are written for single-switch use on Macintosh computers. The stories have talking text and let the user turn pages independently. A mouse button click or a single switch connected through a modified joystick will operate the program.

HandiCHAT

Microsystems Software Inc.

This RAM-resident IBM or Tandy software program has two synthesized speech capabilities. The first is a small pop-up screen that provides instant text-to-speech synthesized speech output without interrupting the main running program. The second option gives text-to-speech capabilities within the main running program.

HandiCHAT Deluxe

Microsystems Software Inc.

This software is a dedicated augmentative communication system for IBM, Tandy, and Texas Instruments computers. It has abbreviation-expansion features and a library of 1,296 phrases that can be combined to create messages.

Software/Manufacturer(s)	Description

HandiCODE

Microsystems Software

HandiCODE provides Morse code input for IBM and Tandy computers through a peripheral HandiWARE connector. Single or dual switches are connected to the connector. The program provides some user-definable options such as speed, auditory feedback, and automatic dash features. HandiCODE includes HandiWORD software.

HandiKEY and HandiKEY Deluxe

Microsystems Software

HandiKEY is a RAM-resident program that provides scanning matrices for computer access on IBM and Tandy computers. The HandiWARE connector is used to connect single or dual switches. In addition, joystick, mouse, trackball, and digitized tablet access is available. The scanning matrices are user-definable and have word-prediction capabilities. HandiKEY Deluxe adds the option of synthesized speech output and can be adapted for auditory scanning.

HandiSHIFT

Microsystems Software

This program is a RAM-resident utility that gives one-fingered users sticky key functions. It also has a "See Beep" option for users who are hearing impaired. Whenever the computer beeps an error code, the screen provides visual feedback. This program is written for IBM and Tandy computers.

HandiVIEW

Microsystems Software

HandiVIEW is a RAM-resident text enlarger for IBM and Tandy computers. It magnifies the screen up to eight times with true-color capability.

HandiWORD and HandiWORD Deluxe

Microsystems Software

This software has word-prediction features in a RAM-resident application that can be used with other programs. Application specific dictionaries can be defined by the user.

Software/Manufacturer(s)	Description

HandiWORD *(continued)*

Abbreviation expansion is available, but only through number codes. It can be used with IBM and Tandy computers. The Deluxe version also has foreign language dictionaries for French, Spanish, German, and Italian.

Help U Key

Bold World Computing

Help U Key displays an alternative keyboard on a computer monitor. A mouse, trackball, or other mouse emulation system is used to select keys on the monitor keyboard. Single-switch scanning options are also available. The software has word-prediction capabilities. It operates on any IBM series or Tandy computer.

Help U Keyboard

Bold World Computing

Help U Keyboard is similar to Help U Key except that single-switch scanning options are not available.

Help U Type

Bold World Computing

This is a RAM-resident program for one-fingered typists. It includes sticky key options, key accept delays, repeat-defeat functions, and other options. It was written for IBM and Tandy computers.

Help U Type and Speak

Bold World Computing

Help U Type and Speak is designed for one-fingered typists. It provides the features of Help U Type and also includes synthesized speech output, word prediction, and abbreviation-expansion capabilities.

Hyper ABLEDATA

Trace Research and
  Development Center

Hyper-ABLEDATA is an assistive technology database with over 15,000 products listed in hardware and software categories. The software is available in CD-ROM or in disk form for use on a hard drive system. Because Hyper ABLEDATA uses HyperCard stacks, it currently operates only on Macintosh computers.

Software/Manufacturer(s)	Description

inFocus

AI Squared

This RAM-resident program provides screen magnification for IBM and Tandy computers. It can enlarge the entire screen or portions of the screen.

inLARGE

Berkeley Systems

inLARGE is a RAM-resident program that magnifies Macintosh computer screens. Graphics and text can be enlarged from 2 to 16 times their normal size. It also tracks mouse and text cursor movements. When used in conjunction with outSPOKEN, it provides auditory speech output to track text and cursor information.

Interaction Games and Interaction Games II

Don Johnston
  Developmental Equipment

Both Interaction Games programs are written for single-switch users on Apple II series computers. The games, written for two users, range from simple cause–effect switch activation games to games that require scanning skills.

inTOUCH

Berkeley Systems

inTOUCH gives persons who are visually impaired tactile output of a Macintosh screen through the Optacon II's vibrating pin display surface. When combined with outSPOKEN software, synthesized speech output can be added to the system.

Join the Circus

Don Johnston
  Developmental Equipment

This Apple II series software works with a single switch to teach cause–effect skills. Colorful circus graphics and speech output make the software visually and auditorily motivating for children.

Joystick Games

Technology for Language
  and Learning

Joystick Games consists of various public domain programs designed to teach joystick use at varying complexity levels. It is designed for Apple II series computers with joystick input.

Software/Manufacturer(s)	Description

Joystick Mastery

ComputAbility Corporation

Joystick Mastery was developed to teach joystick control for power mobility systems. It includes six programs at varying complexity levels and an environmental simulation. It is designed to operate on Apple II series computers.

Joystick Trainer

R. J. Cooper and Associates

This program consists of nine programs designed to teach joystick control for power mobility systems. The programs offer increasingly more difficult joystick tasks for assessment and training. It was designed for Apple II series computers.

Katie's Farm

MCE

This software program was designed for preschool exploratory play on the computer. It is a continuation of the popular McGee software programs. Katie's Farm can be used with Apple *IIGS,* Macintosh, IBM series, and Tandy computers.

Keytalk

PEAL Software

Keytalk is an Apple II series program designed to teach beginning writing skills. It can work in conjunction with the Muppet Learning Keys keyboard. Children can write simple stories and receive synthesized speech feedback through an Echo II synthesizer.

KeyUp

Ability Systems Corporation

This IBM series and Tandy program is designed for one-fingered typists. It has options for eliminating repeating keystrokes and sticky key functions.

Large Print DOS

Optelec USA

This IBM program is a RAM-resident program that enlarges print up to 3 inches in height. It works in conjunction with most software programs. Zoom control and automatic cursor tracking are features of the program.

Software/Manufacturer(s)	Description

Learn to Scan

Don Johnston
  Developmental Equipment

Learn to Scan teaches simple single-switch scanning skills, then progresses to horizontal and vertical scanning formats. The program gives auditory commands and feedback to the user. To use higher levels of this program, the user must be able to recognize objects by name and match shapes and colors. It was developed for Apple II series computers with Echo II synthesizers.

Lotus 1-2-3

Lotus

This spreadsheet program is designed for business applications on IBM series, Tandy, and Macintosh computers.

LVE

Donald W. Ady

This Tandy TRS-80 program gives individuals who are visually impaired screen magnification. There are four screen magnification levels.

Magic and Magic Deluxe

Microsystems Software

Magic provides 2×2 screen magnification functions for IBM series computers. It enlarges both text and graphics. An EGA or VGA graphics card is needed. The programs have automatic cursor following and scrolling. Magic Deluxe is similar but offers different screen magnification sizes and the ability to change screen and text colors and fonts.

Magic Symbols

Enable

Magic Symbols is an augmentative communication program written for Apple II series computers. By adding an Echo II synthesizer and single-switch input method a user can scan semantically organized picture symbols to communicate a message.

Magic Slate and Magic Slate II

Sunburst Communications

Magic Slate and Magic Slate II are simple word-processing programs for Apple II series computers. They can be run in 20-, 40-, and

Software/Manufacturer(s)	Description

Magic Slate *(continued)*

80-column formats to provide large text for children who are visually impaired. Magic Slate requires only 64K of memory; Magic Slate II requires 128K.

Make It Happen

Don Johnston
   Developmental Equipment

This program is a cause–effect program designed to work with Apple II series computers and single-switch input. Eight activities teach switch use with colorful graphics and speech output through an Echo II synthesizer.

Make It in Time

Don Johnston
   Developmental Equipment

This program is a sequel to Make It Happen. It requires that the child activate a switch at a specific moment in time. It is designed for Apple II series computers with single-switch input and an Echo II synthesizer.

Math Scratchpad I and II

Zygo

These programs are designed as screen editing programs for math problems. The cursor automatically tracks to the next point in any given problem. The program does not do the calculations for the user. Program I is written for elementary-level math problems. Program II is written for advanced mathematics. The programs run on Apple II series computers.

McGee

MCE

This preschool program encourages exploratory play as children help McGee go exploring in the house while his mother is asleep. The program is written without words to promote independent exploration. It is designed for Apple *IIGS,* Macintosh, IBM series, and Tandy computers.

Morse Code and Scanning Practice Programs

ACS

This program has Morse code teaching activities in game formats. A scanning option can be adapted for several different scanning techniques. The program was written for Apple II series computers with switch input.

Software/Manufacturer(s)	Description

Motor Training Games

Don Johnston
Developmental Equipment

Motor Training Games teaches switch skills using 14 different games. It was written for Apple II series computers with single-switch input.

Mouse in the Toy Box

Don Johnston
Developmental Equipment

Nine colorful game activities are used to teach control of mouse accessing devices. The programs teach the concepts of clicking the mouse and dragging objects. It is written for Apple *IIGS* computers with mouse input.

Mousing Around

Unicorn Engineering

Mousing Around requires an Apple *IIe* or *IIGS* series computer, the Adaptive Firmware Card, Model G32 or G32e, and a Unicorn Board alternate keyboard. It consists of custom setups and keyboard overlays for operating mouse-controlled software through direct selection on the Unicorn Board. Programs such as Explore-a-Story, McGee, and Playroom can be used.

MultiScan

Words+

This IBM series program trains scanning skills for single-switch input. Linear and row-column scanning options can be trained. The computer screen illuminates sections within a scanning matrix. Handmade transparent symbol overlays are placed over the computer screen to give targets for scanning. Voice output is available if the computer has synthesized speech capabilities.

Muppets On Stage

Sunburst

Muppets On Stage is a preschool program designed to teach early letter, number, and color concepts using fun exploratory play activities. It operates on Apple II series computers through the Muppet Learning Keys keyboard.

Muppetville

Sunburst Communications

Muppetville teaches early shape, color, and number concepts. Activities take place in a

Software/Manufacturer(s)	Description

Muppetville *(continued)*

"town" and require learning simple direction skills. The program works on Apple II series with a Touch Window, or Muppet Learning Keys keyboard.

My House: Language Activities of Daily Living

Laureate Learning Systems

This Apple II series program was written to teach individuals with severe cognitive and communicative disabilities receptive and expressive language vocabulary centered around daily routines. Each activity program centers around a "room" which is displayed on the computer screen. A Touch Window or single switch can be used for computer access with this program.

NFBTRANS

Roudley Associates

NFBTRANS is a text-to-Braille program written for IBM computers. It requires a braille printer or other braille output device.

Old MacDonald I

UCLA Intervention Program for Handicapped Children

Old MacDonald uses a PowerPad with an Apple II series computer and Echo II synthesizer. Children can choose between six farm animals on the PowerPad and watch the computer animate the song with the animal.

One Finger

Trace Research and Development Center

This RAM-resident IBM series program is written for one-fingered typists. It has sticky key, key lock, and key repeat features. The program can be activated and deactivated easily using the keyboard.

outSPOKEN

Berkeley Systems

outSPOKEN provides speech output for Macintosh computer software. Rather than reading all text, the user selects letters, words, lines, menus, and icons to be read using key commands. When combined with inLARGE, large computer print display text can be added.

Software/Manufacturer(s)	Description

Overlay Express

Unicorn Engineering

Overlay Express lets a user easily make keyboard overlays or communication boards for the Unicorn Expanded Keyboard. It was written for Apple *IIe* or *IIGS* computers. Key-Pics, Core Picture Vocabulary, and Mayer Johnson Picture Communication Symbols are available graphic-symbol options.

PC Assisted Keyboard

DADA

The PC Assisted Keyboard is a software program that has functions for one-fingered typists. It has key redefinition, sticky key, and macro customization features. It operates on IBM series computers.

PC Lens

Arts Computer Products

This program is a screen enlarger for IBM series and Tandy computers. Text is enlarged, spaced farther apart, and colored for easier reading. The program has automatic cursor tracking.

Peripheral Tester

Don Johnston
  Developmental Equipment

Peripheral Tester was written to troubleshoot problems with assistive technology computer peripherals used with Apple II series computers. This software assists in determining whether problems with equipment are related to software or hardware.

Playroom

Broderbund

Playroom was written for preschool children. It has several different activities that teach time concepts, letter identification, sight word reading, and other skills. It can run on Apple *IIGS,* IBM series, Tandy, and Macintosh computers.

Point to Pictures Series

Don Johnston
  Developmental Equipment

The Point to Pictures software series consists of six different programs. At the earliest level, users learn to point to a choice of one to four different pictures. Additional programs add a variety of picture and word pointing choices. The programs are written for Apple *IIe* or

Software/Manufacturer(s)	Description

Point to Picture Series
(continued)

IIGS computers with access through a Power-Pad used with a Porter, Unicorn Expanded Keyboard with an Adaptive Firmware Card, or Touch Window.

PowerKey

Dunamis

This program combines the Adaptive Firmware Card with a Power Pad alternative keyboard. A cable is included to interface the two devices. PowerKey is written for the Adaptive Firmware Card, Models G12 and G32e.

PowerPad Tool Kit 3.0

Dunamis

The Power Pad Tool Kit version 3.0 lets a user design customized learning activities for the Power Pad alternative keyboard. The user can control speech output, computer graphics, and text. The Tool Kit can run on Apple *IIe* and *IIGS* computers.

Predict It

Don Johnston
　　Developmental Equipment

Predict It is a word processing program with word-prediction features written for Apple *IIe* and *IIGS* computers. It can be used with alternate-input devices through the Adaptive Firmware Card.

Rabbit Scanner

Exceptional Children's
　　Software

This Apple II series program teaches young children single-switch horizontal scanning skills. At the first level, a child presses a switch when a jumping rabbit reaches a carrot. At higher levels, the child matches shapes and colors.

Run Rabbit Run

Exceptional Children's
　　Software

This program is a companion to Rabbit Scanner. It teaches single-switch horizontal and vertical scanning skills by having the rabbit "jump" over obstacles when a switch, keyboard key, or joystick is activated.

Software/Manufacturer(s)	Description

Screen Doors

Madenta Communications
Prentke Romich

Screen Doors is a keyboard emulation program for Macintosh computers. It provides an on-screen keyboard that can be accessed using a mouse, joystick, or HeadMaster pointing system. Word-prediction features are included in the software.

ScreenKeys

Berkeley Systems

ScreenKeys is an alternate computer input program for Macintosh computers. A graphic image of the keyboard is pictured on the computer monitor. Any pointing access device, such as a mouse, joystick, or optical head pointer, can be used to access the screen keyboard.

Senior's Switch Progressions

R. J. Cooper and Associates

This program provides computer activities for senior citizens who have severe cognitive difficulties. Various activities train attention, following directions, responding to visual cues, and life skills simulations. The programs are written for Apple *IIe* and *IIGS* computers with single switch input.

Silly Sandwich

UCLA Intervention Program for Handicapped Children

Silly Sandwich is a preschool program that lets children build "sandwiches" by choosing between 6 to 12 different items. It was written for Apple II series computers with PowerPad input and Echo speech synthesis.

SimpleCom I: Yes/No Communication

Dunamis

This program teaches simple picture discrimination skills. The computer presents a symbol representing yes/no concepts that the user matches on a PowerPad keyboard overlay. The computer then reinforces the user with a teacher-selected reinforcer. The program is written for Apple II series computers.

Software/Manufacturer(s)	Description

SimpleCom II: Needs/Wants Communication

Dunamis

SimpleCom II follows SimpleCom I. The computer gives the user a teacher-selected yes/no activity choice that is presented verbally and graphically. The user then presses a yes/no symbol on the PowerPad to indicate a choice. Recognition of the yes/no symbols is trained using SimpleCom I.

Single Input Control Assessment

Hugh MacMillan Medical Centre
Easter Seal Communication Institute

This software was written to assist clinicians in the process of selecting single-switch control accessing methods. Factors of movement, body site, input device, and position of the input device are objectively compared using computer tasks that measure response time, autoscan control, and hold-release skills. The program runs on Apple II series computers.

Single Switch Assessment

Arthur Schwartz

In this program, an Apple II series computer is used with single switches to assess single-switch skills. The program stores data in mean response times for switch activation in a series of tasks.

Single Switch Game Library

Arthur Schwartz

Single Switch Game Library is a selection of early childhood games written for the Apple II series computer and single-switch access.

Single Switch Learning

Technology for Language and Learning

This software series consists of 14 volumes of software written for single-switch use on Apple II series computers. Various programs have scan assessment tools, cause–effect training, scanning training, and programs to teach concepts such as letter identification, counting, and clock skills.

SmoothTalker

First Byte

SmoothTalker is a software-driven speech synthesizer that does not require any additional computer hardware. Versions are available

Software/Manufacturer(s)	Description

SmoothTalker *(continued)*

for Apple *IIGS*, IBM series, Atari, Macintosh, Amiga, Tandy, and Commodore computers.

Soft Vert

Telesensory

Soft Vert works with IBM-series computers and an external speech synthesizer to provide spoken output for any software application program.

Switch Arcade

UCLA Intervention Program for Handicapped Children

Switch Arcade has a variety of interactive games written for up to two users using two single switches and an Apple *IIGS* computer.

Switch Assessment Program

Assistive Device Center, School of Engineering and Computer Science

This program is used by clinicians to objectively assess various switch-input, joystick, or switch-array accessing options. It is written for Apple II series and Macintosh computers.

Switch It-Change It

UCLA Intervention Program for Handicapped Children

This Apple II series program uses a single switch and Echo speech synthesizer to teach cause–effect switch-activation skills with colorful animated graphics.

Switch It-See It

UCLA Intervention Program for Handicapped Children

Switch It-See It teaches visual tracking in a variety of directions on the computer screen. It requires an Apple II series computer, Echo speech synthesizer, and single-switch input.

SynPhonix 215, 225, 235, 245, 255, MC 315 Artic Vision and Business Vision

Artic Technologies

This software program runs transparently to any application program and provides instant cursor-tracked, synthesized-speech output. A SynPhonix synthesizer is included with the program. The Business Vision version adds features to provide speech output with spreadsheets. The program is written for

Software/Manufacturer(s)	Description

Synphonix *(continued)*

IBM series, Toshiba laptops, and NEC Multi-speed computers.

Talking Screen

Words+ Incorporated

Talking Screen is designed to operate in IBM portable computers. It provides a dynamically changing graphic symbol display of up to 32 pictures per screen. Screens can be customized for the user. Direct selection with a mouse, trackball, or optical light pointer and a variety of single-switch scanning methods are supported. A variety of speech synthesizers can be used with the system, including Dec Talk.

Talking Touch Window

Edmark Corporation

This program is an authoring system for Apple II series computers, an Echo speech synthesizer, and Touch Window. Users can create picture screens with customized speech output for learning activities.

Talking Utilities for DOS 3.3 and ProDOS

American Printing House for the Blind

The Talking Utilities programs were written for users who are visually impaired and need to access DOS commands on Apple II series computers. The programs provide spoken output of all DOS operating system commands through an Echo speech synthesizer.

Tandy Combo Pak

Animated Voice Corporation

The Tandy Combo Pak is a program that takes advantage of the built-in digitized speech capabilities of the Tandy 1000SL and 1000TL computers. The program includes applications for augmentative communication.

Tea Party

UCLA Intervention Program for Handicapped Children

Tea Party is a preschool program that teaches classification skills through a pretend shopping trip. It was written for Apple II series computers using the Power Pad and Echo speech synthesizer.

Software/Manufacturer(s)	Description

Teenage Switch and TouchWindow Progressions

R. J. Cooper and Associates

This Apple II series program consists of five activities designed for adolescents with severe cognitive disabilities. The programs are written for single-switch scanning or TouchWindow applications.

TouchCom

Don Johnston
  Developmental Equipment

TouchCom gives the user the ability to create novel augmentative communication boards using the PowerPad connected to an Apple II series computer and an Echo speech synthesizer.

Up and Running

Unicorn Engineering

Up and Running consists of preprogrammed Unicorn Expanded Keyboard applications for popular software programs. The program comes with printed overlays ready to use with the Unicorn Board. It was written for Apple II series computers that have Adaptive Firmware Card and Unicorn Expanded Keyboard peripherals.

Verbal Operating System

Computer Conversations

This IBM-series program provides synthesized speech output of all keyboard and computer screen actions. The system tracks the program cursor throughout all application programs. It includes a word processor.

Verbal Star

Computer Conversations

Verbal Star is a word-processing program written for IBM computers. It includes spoken output when combined with a speech synthesizer. All program commands are executed with a single keystroke.

Verbal View

Computer Conversations

Verbal View is a computer screen magnification program. It can enlarge the print to fill six, three, or two lines and has options for changing character and background colors. It was written for IBM series computers equipped with color graphics boards.

Software/Manufacturer(s)	Description

Wheelchair Control Evaluation Program

Technical Resource Centre

This program assists in teaching joystick control to wheelchair users. The user can create custom room layouts in two or three dimensions. The program operates on Amiga and IBM series computers.

Wheels on the Bus I

UCLA Intervention Program for Handicapped Children

Wheels on the Bus is a software program that lets preschool children sing five different verses of the nursery song by touching a picture on a PowerPad or TouchWindow. The program runs on Apple II series computers with Echo speech synthesizers.

Where in the World is Carmen Sandiego?

Broderbund

This popular software program introduces children and adolescents to world geography in a mystery game that includes graphic adventures, arcade skill games, and trivia questions. It operates on Apple II series, Macintosh, Commodore, IBM series, and Tandy computers.

Word Perfect

Word Perfect Corporation

Word Perfect is a popular word-processing program written for IBM series and Macintosh computers.

Words+ Equalizer

Words+

The Equalizer is a nondedicated augmentative communication software program for individuals with written language skills. It has word-prediction features along with a drawing program, games, music, and a calculator. It can be operated with single-switch access.

Zoom Text

AI Squared

This RAM-resident program was written for IBM series and Tandy computers. It enlarges text and graphics characters up to eight times normal size. Split screen modes are available and the program has automatic cursor tracking. A graphics adaptor card is needed to run this program.

9

Assistive Technology Resources

■ Gregory Church, MS, MAS ■

This chapter is a U.S. and Canadian guide for the selection of product vendors, professional and nonprofit organizations, databases, professional journals, magazines, newspapers, and newsletters involved in the application of assistive technology. This resource directory also includes information on databases and telecommunication networks that disseminate information on assistive technology hardware, software, and service organizations.

HOW TO USE THIS CHAPTER

The search for specific hardware and software products listed in this text is available in the alphabetical product listings in Chapter 8. Each listing in the chapter indicates the product's name, provides a brief description, and identifies the manufacturer(s). To locate a specific hardware or software product in Chapter 8, the reader should identify the product and manufacturer or vendor. After identifying the product and vendor name in Chapter 8, the reader should then refer to the section entitled "Assistive Technology Vendors" in this Chapter for specific address and telephone information.

The lists of assistive technology information resources in this chapter are arranged in the following sections:

1. *Vendors:* This section provides an alphabetical listing of all vendors listed in the text, including addresses and telephone numbers.
2. *Organizations:* This listing is organized alphabetically by organization and includes addresses, telephone numbers, and the types of services offered by each organization.
3. *Publications:* This section lists technology resources available as printed material in newspapers, newsletters, magazines, professional journals, or textbooks.
4. *Databases:* This resource listing includes database information on assistive technology products, organizations, research, and related service delivery support. The information is available via on-line electronic networks, floppy disks, CD-ROM, audio cassette, or as printed hardcopy from an electronic source.

ASSISTIVE TECHNOLOGY VENDORS

The following is a list of assistive technology manufacturers and distributors that offer commercial hardware or software products to consumers. This detailed alphabetical listing provides a quick reference of assistive technology providers listed throughout this text.

A-BEC
20460 Gramercy Place
Torrance, CA 90501
(800) 421-2249

ABILITY SYSTEMS
1422 Arnold Ave.
Roslyn, PA 19001
(215) 657-4338

ABLENET
1081 10th Ave. S.E.
Minneapolis, MN 55414
(800) 322-0956

ABLETECH CONNECTION
P.O. Box 898
Westerville, OH 43081
(614) 899-9989

ACADEMIC SOFTWARE
331 W. 2nd St.

Lexington, KY 40507
(606) 233-2332

ACCESS UNLIMITED
535 Briarpark Dr., Ste. 102
Houston, TX 77042-5235
(713) 781-7441

ACS SOFTWARE
University of Washington
Dept. of Speech and Hearing
  Sciences JG-15
Seattle, WA 98195
(206) 543-7974

ADAMLAB
33500 Van Born Rd.
Wayne, MI 48184
(313) 467-1415

ADAPTIVE COMMUNICATION SYSTEMS, INC.
Box 12440

Pittsburgh, PA 15231
(412) 264-2288

ADHOC READING SYSTEMS, INC.
28 Brunswick Woods Dr.
E. Brunswick, NJ 08816
(908) 254-7300

AI SQUARED
1463 Hearst Dr., N.E.
Atlanta, GA 30319
(404) 233-7065

**AMERICAN PRINTING HOUSE
FOR THE BLIND**
P.O. Box 6085
Louisville, KY 40206-0085
(502) 895-2405

AMERICAN THERMOFORM CORPORATION
2311 Travers Ave.
City of Commerce, CA 90040
(213) 723-9021

AMIGO SALES INC.
6693 Dixie Highway
Bridgeport, MI 48722
(517) 777-0910

ANIMATED VOICE CORPORATION
P.O. Box 819
San Marcos, CA 92079-0819
(800) 942-3699

APPLE COMPUTER, INC.
Worldwide Disability Solutions Group
20525 Mariani Ave.
Cupertino, CA 95014
(408) 974-7910

ARISTO COMPUTERS, INC.
6700 S.W. 105th Ave., Ste 307
Beaverton, OR 97005
(503) 626-6333

ARROYO & ASSOCIATES, INC.
2549 Rockville Centre Pkwy.
Oceanside, NY 11572
(516) 763-1407

ARTHUR SCHWARTZ
Cleveland State University
Department of Speech and Hearing
Cleveland, OH 44115
(216) 371-3820

ARTIC TECHNOLOGIES
55 Park St., Ste. 2
Troy, MI 48083
(313) 588-7370

ARTICULATE SYSTEMS, INC.
600 West Cummings Park,
   Ste. 4500
Woburn, MA 01801
(617) 935-5656

ARTS COMPUTER PRODUCTS, INC.
121 Beach St., Ste. 400
Boston, MA 02111-2501
(800) 343-0095

ASAHEL ENGINEERING, INC.
S.E. 525 Water St.
Pullman, WA 99163
(509) 334-2226

BERKELEY SYSTEMS
1700 Shattuck Ave.
Berkeley, CA 94709
(415) 540-5537

BLAZIE ENGINEERING
3660 Mill Green Rd.
Street, MD 21154
(301) 879-4944

BOLD WORD COMPUTING
165 Old Meadow Rd.
Dracut, MA 01826
(508) 957-6148

BRODERBUND SOFTWARE, INC.
P.O. Box 6125
Novato, CA 94948-6125
(800) 521-6263

BURKHART TOYS
8503 Rhode Island Ave.
College Park, MD 20740
(301) 345-9152

CANON, INC.
One Canon Plaza
Lake Success. NY 11042
(516) 488-6700

COMPUTABILITY CORPORATION
4000 Grand River, Ste. 109
Novi, MI 48375
(800) 433-8872

COMPUTERADE PRODUCTS
2346 Wales Dr.
Cardiff, CA 92007
(619) 942-3343

COMPUTER CONVERSATIONS
6297 Worthington Rd. S.W.
Alexandria, OH 43001
(614) 924-2885

COMPUTERS TO HELP PEOPLE, INC.
1221 W. Johnson St.
Madison, WI 53715-1046
(608) 257-5917

COVOX, INC.
675 Conger St.
Eugene, OR 97402
(503) 342-1271

CRESTWOOD COMPANY
6625 N. Sidney Pl.
Milwaukee, WI 53209
(414) 352-5678

DADA
249 Concord Ave., Unit 2
Toronto, ON M6H 2P4
Canada
(416) 530-0038

DIGITAL EQUIPMENT CORPORATION
146 Main St.
Maynard, MA 01754-2571
(800) 832-6277

**DON JOHNSTON DEVELOPMENTAL
EQUIPMENT, INC.**
1000 North Rand Rd.
Building 115

Wauconda, IL 60084
(800) 999-4660

DONALD W. ADY
56 Oak Ridge Ave.
Summit, NJ 07901
(908) 277-3365

DRAGON SYSTEMS, INC.
320 Nevada St.
Newton, MA 02160
(617) 965-5200

DUFCO ELECTRONICS, INC.
2535-C Village Ln.
Cambria, CA 93428
(805) 927-5112

DU-IT CONTROL SYSTEMS GROUP, INC.
8765 Township Rd. 513
Shreeve, OH 44676
(216) 567-2906

DUNAMIS, INC.
620 Hwy. 317
Suwanee, GA 30174
(800) 828-2443

EASTER SEAL COMMUNICATION INSTITUTE
250 Ferrand Dr., Ste. 200
Don Mills, ON M3C 3P2
Canada
(416) 421-8377

EDMARK CORPORATION
P.O. Box 3903
Bellevue, WA 98009-3903
(800) 426-0856

EKEG ELECTRONICS CO. LTD.
P.O. Box 46199
Vancouver, BC V6R 4G5
Canada
(604) 273-4358

ENABLING TECHNOLOGIES CO.
3102 S.E. Jay St.
Stuart, FL 34997
(407) 283-4817

EVEREST & JENNINGS, INC.
3233 E. Mission Oak Blvd.
Camarillo, CA 93012
(805) 987-6911

EXCEPTIONAL CHILDREN'S SOFTWARE
P.O. Box 487
Hays, KS 67601
(913) 625-9281

EXCEPTIONAL COMPUTING, INC.
450 N.W. 58th St.
Gainesville, FL 32607
(904) 331-8847

EXTENSIONS FOR INDEPENDENCE
555 Veteran Blvd., #B-368
San Diego, CA 92154
(619) 423-7709

FIRST BYTE
3100 S. Harbor Blvd., Ste. 150
Santa Ana, CA 92704
(800) 523-8070

FIFTH GENERATIONS SYSTEMS, INC.
10049 N. Reiger Rd.
Baton Rouge, LA 70809
(800) 873-4384

FORTRESS SCIENTIFIC
61 Miami St.
Buffalo, NY 14204
(800) 869-4335

GW MICRO
310 Racquet Dr.
Fort Wayne, IN 46825
(219) 483-3625

HARTLEY COURSEWARE
133 Bridge St.
Dimondale, MI 48821
(800) 247-1380

HEATH COMPANY
P.O. Box 8589
Benton Harbor, MI 49022-8589
(616) 982-5950

HENTER-JOYCE, INC.
10901C Roosevelt Blvd., Ste. 1200
St. Petersburg, FL 33716
(813) 576-5658

HOOLEAN CORPORATION
P.O. Box 230
Cornville, AZ 86325
(602) 634-7515

HUGH MACMILLAN MEDICAL CENTRE
(Ontario Crippled Children's Centre)
350 Rumsey Rd.
Toronto, Ontario, M4G 1R8
Canada
(416) 425-6220

HUMANWARE, INC.
6245 King Rd., Ste. P
Loomis, CA 95650
(916) 652-7253

IBM NATIONAL SUPPORT CENTER FOR PERSONS WITH DISABILITIES
P.O. Box 2150
Atlanta, GA 30055
(800) 426-2133
(800) 284-9482

INNOCOMP
33195 Wagon Wheel Dr.
Sonon, OH 44139
(216) 248-6206

IN TOUCH SYSTEMS
11 Westview Rd.
Spring Valley, NY 10977
(914) 354-7431

INVACARE CORPORATION
P.O. Box 4028
Elyria, OH 44036
(216) 329-6000

JOSTENS LEARNING SYSTEMS, INC.
2860 Old Rochester Rd.
Springfield, IL 62703
(800) 323-7577

KINETIC DESIGNS
14231 Anatevka Ln. S.E.
Olalla, WA 98466
(206) 857-7943
(800) 453-0330

KOALA TECHNOLOGIES
70 N. Second St.
San Jose, CA 95113
(408) 287-6311

KURZWEIL IMAGING SYSTEMS, INC.
185 Albany St.
Cambridge, MA 02139
(800) 343-0311

KY ENTERPRISES
3039 E. 2nd St.
Long Beach, CA 90803
(213) 433-5244

LAUREATE LEARNING SYSTEMS, INC.
110 E. Spring St.
Winooski, VT 05404
(802) 655-4755

LAWRENCE PRODUCTIONS
1800 S. 35th St.
Galesburg, MI 49078
(800) 421-4157

LC TECHNOLOGIES
4415 Glenn Rose St.
Fairfax, VA 22032
(703) 425-7509

LEHIGH VALLEY EASTER SEAL SOCIETY
P.O. Box 33
1161 Forty Foot Rd.
Kulpsville, PA 19443
(215) 368-7000

LIFE SCIENCE ASSOCIATES
1 Fenimore Rd.
Bayport, NY 11705
(516) 472-2111

LOTUS DEVELOPMENT CORPORATION
5600 Glenridge Dr.

Atlanta, GA 30342
(800) 831-9679

LOVEJOY ELECTRONICS
35 Garrison St.
Portland, ME 04102
(207) 774-9421

LUMINAUD, INC.
8688 Tyler Blvd.
Mentor, OH 44060
(216) 255-9082

MASTERVOICE
10523 Humbolt St.
Los Alamitos, CA 90720
(213) 594-6581

MAYER-JOHNSON CO.
P.O. Box 1579
Solana Beach, CA 92075
(619) 481-2489

MCE
A Division of Lawrence Productions
1800 S. 35th St.
Galesburg, MI 49053
(800) 421-4157

MCINTYRE COMPUTER SYSTEMS
22809 Shagbark
Birmingham, MI 48010
(313) 645-5090

MED, INC.
3223 South Loop 289, #150
Lubbock, TX 79423
(806) 793-3421

MERIT SOFTWARE
13635 Gamma Rd.
Dallas, TX 75244
(214) 385-2353

MERRITT COMPUTER PRODUCTS, INC.
5565 Red Bird Ctr. Dr., Ste. 150
Dallas, TX 75237
(214) 339-0753

MICROTOUCH
55 Jonspin Rd.
Wilmington, MA 01887
(800) 866-6873

MICROSYSTEMS SOFTWARE, INC.
600 Worcester Rd., Ste. B2
Farmingham, MA 01701
(508) 626-8511

MINDPLAY
3130 N. Dodge Blvd.
Tuscon, AZ 85716
(800) 221-7911

MOBILITY PLUS
P.O. Box 391
291 N. 12th St.
Santa Paula, CA 93060
(800) 525-7165

NEC AMERICA
8 Old Sod Farm Rd.
Melville, NY 11747
(703) 753-7000

OPTELEC USA, INC.
P.O. Box 796
4 Lyberty Wy.
Westford, MA 01886
(800) 828-1056

ORTHO-KINETICS, INC.
W220 N507 Springdale Rd.
P.O. Box 1647
Waukesha, WI 53187
(800) 446-4522

PARALLEL SYSTEMS, CO.
P.O. Box 58435
Vancouver, BC V6P 6K2
Canada
(604) 943-6769

PEAL SOFTWARE
P.O. Box 8188
Calabasas, CA 91372
(818) 883-7849

PHONIC EAR, INC.
250 Camino Alto
Mill Valley, CA 94941
(800) 227-0735 in U.S.
(415) 383-4000

POINTER SYSTEMS, INC.
One Mill St.
Burlington, VT 05401
(800) 537-1562

POLYTEL COMPUTER PRODUCTS CORPORATION
1287 Hammerwood Ave.
Sunnyvale, CA 94089
(800) 245-6655
(408) 745-1540

PROGESSIVE COMPUTER SYSTEMS, INC.
P.O. BOX 8721
New Orleans, LA 70182
(800) 628-1131

PRENTKE ROMICH COMPANY
1022 Heyl Rd.
Wooster, OH 44691
(216) 262-1984
(800) 642-8255

RAISED DOT COMPUTING, INC.
408 S. Baldwin St.
Madison, WI 53703
(608) 257-9595

REACH
890 Hearthstone Dr.
Stone Mountain, GA 30083
(404) 292-8933

REGENESIS DEVELOPMENT CORP.
1046 Deep Cove Rd.
North Vancouver, BC V7G 1S3
Canada
(604) 929-6663

R. J. COOPER AND ASSOCIATES
24843 Del Prado, Ste. 283
Dana Point, CA 92629
(714) 240-1912

ROBOTRON ACCESS PRODUCTS, INC.
2101 Chestnut St. #518
Philadelphia, PA 19103
(800) 735-1031

ROUDLEY ASSOCIATES, INC.
Box 608
Owings Mills, MD 21117
(800) 333-7049

SCHOLASTIC INC.
2931 East McCarty St.
P.O. Box 7502
Jefferson City, MO 65102
(800) 541-5513

SEEING TECHNOLOGIES
7074 Brooklyn Blvd.
Minneapolis, MN 55429
(612) 560-8080
(800) 462-3738

SENTIENT SYSTEMS TECHNOLOGY, INC.
5001 Baum Blvd.
Pittsburgh, PA 15213
(412) 682-0144

SHEA PRODUCTS, INC
1721 W. Hamilton Rd.
Rochester Hills, MI 48309
(313) 852-4940

SPINNAKER SOFTWARE
201 Broadway
Cambridge, MA 02139
(617) 494-1200

STREET ELECTRONICS CORP.
6420 Via Real
Carpinteria, CA 93013
(805) 684-4593

SUNBURST COMMUNICATIONS
101 Castleton St.
Pleasantville, NY 10570
(800) 628-8897

SYNTHA-VOICE COMPUTERS, INC.
125 Gailmont Drive

Hamilton, Ontario, L8K 4B8
Canada
(416) 578-0565

TASH, INC.
70 Gibson Dr., Unit 12
Markham, Ontario, L3R 4C2
Canada
(416) 475-2212

TECHNICAL RESOURCE CENTER
200, 1201 5th St. S.W.
Calgary, AB T2R 0Y6 Canada
(403) 262-9445

TECHNOLOGY FOR LANGUAGE AND LEARNING
P.O. Box 327
East Rockway, NY 11518-0327
(516) 625-4550

TELESENSORY SYSTEMS, INC.
455 North Bernardo
P.O. Box 7455
Mountain View, CA 94039-7455
(415) 960-0920

TIGER COMMUNICATIONS SYSTEMS
155 E. Broad St. #325
Rochester, NY 14604
(716) 454-5134

TOYS FOR SPECIAL CHILDREN
385 Warburton Ave.
Hastings-On-Hudson, NY 10706
(914) 478-0960

TRACE RESEARCH AND DEVELOPMENT CENTER
Rm. S-151 Waisman Ctr.
1500 Highland Ave.
University of Wisconsin
Madison, WI 53705-2280
(608) 262-6966

UCLA INTERVENTION PROGRAM FOR HANDICAPPED CHILDREN
1000 Veteran Ave.
Rm. 23-10
Los Angeles, CA 90024
(213) 825-4821

UNICORN ENGINEERING, INC.
5221 Central Ave., Ste. 205-B
Richmond, CA 94704
(800) 899-6687

VTEC
1625 Olympic Blvd.
Santa Monica, CA 90404
(800) 345-2256

VOTRAX, INC.
24027 Research Dr.
Farmington Hills, MI 48335
(800) 521-1350

VOICE CONNECTION
17835 Skypark Circle, Ste. C
Irvine, CA 92714
(714) 261-2366

WM. K. BRADFORD PUBLISHING CO.
310 School St.
Acton, MA 01720
(508) 263-6996

WORDPERFECT CORPORATION
1555 North Technology Wy.

Orem, Utah 84057
(801) 225-5000

WORDS+, INC.
P.O. Box 1229
44421 10th St. West, Ste. L
Lancaster, CA 93535
(805) 949-8331

WORLD COMMUNICATIONS
245 Tonopah Dr.
Fremont, CA 94539
(415) 656-0911

X-10 (USA), INC.
185A LeGrand Ave.
Northvale, NJ 07647
(201) 784-9700
(800) 526-0027

XEROX IMAGING SYSTEMS, INC.
185 Albany St.
Cambridge, MA 02139
(617) 864-4700

ZYGO INDUSTRIES, INC.
P.O Box 1008
Portland, OR 97207-1008
(800) 234-6006

ORGANIZATIONS

The following directory of organizations has been included to provide professionals, consumers, and advocates with assistance in locating service delivery providers. Listings are organized alphabetically by organization name. Each listing includes address, telephone information, and the types of services offered by each organization.

4-SIGHTS NETWORK
c/o Greater Detroit Society for the Blind
16625 Grand River
Detroit, MI 48227
(313) 272-3900

This national, private agency serves the blind and is actively involved in information dissemination, referral, and advocacy services involving sensory aids. The organization is also involved in evaluations and equipment recommendations and training in the use of sensory aids for individuals with vision impairments.

ABLENET
1081 10th Ave. S.E.
Minneapolis, MN 55414
(612) 379-0956
(800) 322-0956

This private, nonprofit organization provides information on augmentative communication, environmental control, and automated learning devices. The organization also provides referral and technology training services for children and adults with severe and profound disabilities.

ACCESS TO OPPORTUNITY PROGRAM
c/o Community College of Rhode Island
400 E. Ave.
Warwick, RI 02886
(401) 825-2305

This college-based organization provides assistive technology information dissemination and training services. The program also maintains a resources center for computer hardware and software.

ACCESS UNLIMITED
3535 Briarpark Dr., Ste. 102
Huston, TX 77042-5235
(713) 781-7441

A nonprofit computer technology organization serving children and young adults with disabilities. Information, referral, training, and equipment recommendation services are provided.

ACCESSABILITY RESOURCE CENTER
1056 E. 19th Ave. B-410
Denver, CO 80218-1088
(303) 861-6250

This center supports a technology resource center that offers information dissemination and training services in computer applications and related technology areas.

ACTIVATING CHILDREN THROUGH TECHNOLOGY (ACTT)
c/o Western Illinois University
27 Horrabin Hall
Macomb, IL 61455
(309) 298-1634

This university-based center supports a technology resource center that offers information dissemination, training, and evaluation services to individuals who are disabled in microcomputer applications and related technology areas.

ALASKA CENTER FOR ADAPTIVE TECHNOLOGY

P.O. Box 6069
Sitka, AK 99835
(907) 747-6960

This center supports a technology resource center that offers information dissemination, training, equipment evaluation, and prescription services to disabled individuals who have microcomputer and related assistive technology needs.

ALLIANCE FOR TECHNOLOGY ACCESS

(formally the NATIONAL SPECIAL EDUCATION ALLIANCE)
Apple Computer, Inc.
20525 Nariani Ave., MS 43S
Cupertino, CA 95014
(415) 528-0747

The alliance was developed in association with the Disabled Children's Computer Group by Apple Computer's Office of Special Education Programs. The organization conducts research and provides information dissemination, database resources, referral services, and training related to the implementation of microcomputer technology with children and adults who are disabled. The alliance currently is developing model assistive technology sites across the United States.

ALOHA SPECIAL TECHNOLOGY ACCESS CENTER

1750 Kalakaua Ave.
P.O. Box 27741
Honolulu, HI 96827-0741
(808) 955-4464

This center supports a technology resource center that offers information dissemination, educational training, device evaluation and prescription services to individuals who are disabled and require assistive technology.

ALTERNATIVE COMMUNICATION TECHNOLOGY

c/o Central Michigan University
441 Moore Hall
Mt. Pleasant, MI 48859
(517) 774-3472

This university-based program provides augmentative communication information dissemination, referral, device evaluation, and prescription services. The program also maintains a resources center that provides education and training services.

AMERICAN FOUNDATION FOR TECHNOLOGY ASSISTANCE

Rt. 14, P.O. Box 230
Morgantown, NC 28655
(704) 433-9697

A comprehensive technology assistance organization offering assistive technology information, referral, advocacy, assessment, prescription, education, and training services.

AMERICAN FOUNDATION FOR THE BLIND
15 W. 16th St.
New York, NY 10011
(212) 620-2000

A network of local organizations for individuals who are blind or visually impaired. Services include rehabilitation, education, and employment.

AMERICAN OCCUPATIONAL THERAPY ASSOCIATION (AOTA)
1383 Piccard Dr.
P.O. Box 1725
Rockville, MD 20850
(301) 948-9626

AOTA is a national professional organization involved in all aspects of the occupational therapy field.

AMERICAN PHYSICAL THERAPY ASSOCIATION (APTA)
1111 North Fairfax St.
Alexandria, VA 22314
(703) 684-2782

APTA is a national professional organization involved in all aspects of the physical therapy field.

AMERICAN PRINTING HOUSE FOR THE BLIND
P.O. Box 6085
Louisville, KY 40206-0085
(502) 895-2405

A national organization dedicated to serving the needs of individuals who are visually impaired. The organization is actively involved in maintaining a database and resource center of technology for the blind. The organization also supports technology research efforts related to vision.

AMERICAN SPEECH-LANGUAGE-HEARING ASSOCIATION (ASHA)
10801 Rockville Pike
Rockville, MD 20852
(301) 897-5700

ASHA is a national professional organization involved in the application of assistive technology in the areas of speech and language, including administration, therapy, and research.

APPLE COMPUTER, OFFICE OF SPECIAL EDUCATION
20525 Mariani Ave., MS 43S
Cupertino, CA 95014
(408) 974-8601

Through this office, Apple Computer works with rehabilitation, education, and advocacy organizations nationwide to identify computer-related needs of individuals who are disabled and to assist in the development of responsive programs. Apple maintains a database of hardware, software, publications, and organizations involved in the use of assistive technology.

ARKANSAS DIVISION OF REHABILITATION SERVICES RESOURCE SYSTEMS
P.O. Box 3781
Little Rock, AR 72203
(501) 682-6689

This state agency supports rehabilitation services involving accessibility, environmental controls, driving aids, prosthetics, augmentative communication, computer applications, and seating and power mobility.

ASSISTIVE DEVICE ASSESSMENT PROGRAM (ADAP)
c/o San Diego State University
Interdisciplinary Center for Health and Human Services
San Diego, CA 92182
(619) 594-6121

This university-based program provides assistive technology information dissemination, referral, device evaluation, and prescription services. The program also maintains a technology resource center which provides education and training services.

ASSISTIVE DEVICE CENTER
c/o Assistive Device Center,
School of Engineering and Computer Science
California State University
Sacramento, CA 95819
(916) 278-6422

This university-based program provides assistive technology information dissemination, training, device evaluation, and prescription services. The program also maintains a technology resource center and supports research efforts in the area of assistive technology.

AUTISM SOCIETY OF AMERICA
8601 Georgia Ave. Ste. 503
Silver Spring, MD 20910
(301) 565-0433

This organization provides information dissemination and advocacy for children and adults who are autistic. The organization offers information relating to computers and children with autism.

BARKELEY MEMORIAL CENTER
University of Nebraska Lincoln
Lincoln, NE 68583
(402) 472-3956

This university service program emphasizes the application of augmentative communication, special education, and microcomputer use. The center provides information dissemination, evaluation, and prescription services in the areas listed above.

BLISSYMBOLICS COMMUNICATION INTERNATIONAL
250 Ferrand Dr., Ste. 200
Don Mills, ON M3C 3P2
Canada
(416) 421-8377

Organization dedicated to the development and dissemination of Blissymbolics as a communication system for people who do not speak.

BLOORVIEW CHILDREN'S HOSPITAL
c/o Communication & Assistive Technology Department
25 Buchan Ct.
Willowdale, ON M2J 4S9
Canada
(416) 494-2222

This nonprofit hospital serves children and young adults with multiple handicaps. The hospital provides assessment, prescription, and training services in the areas of augmentative communication, adaptive computer access, and environmental control.

BRAILLE INSTITUTE
741 N. Vermont Ave.
Los Angeles, CA 90029
(213) 663-1111

This institute acts as a technological resource center for individuals who are both visually and physically handicapped.

CARROLL CENTER FOR THE BLIND
770 Centre St.
Newton, MA 02158
(617) 969-6200

This nonprofit organization supports computer applications for individuals who are blind or visually impaired. Referral services, technology training, equipment evaluation, and prescription services are offered.

CENTER FOR APPLIED REHABILITATION TECHNOLOGY
c/o Rancho Los Amigos Medical Center
7601 East Imperial Hwy.
Downey, CA 90242
(213) 940-6800

This center is an evaluation and treatment program offering assistive technology services in augmentative communication, computer access, environmental control, seating and power mobility.

CENTER FOR COMPUTER ASSISTANCE TO THE DISABLED
617 Seventh Ave.
Fort Worth, TX 76104
(817) 870-9082

This center is a clearinghouse for user information on computer aids for disabled persons. The center also provides referral and advocacy services, training, diagnostic evaluations, and related support services in the area of computer-based assistive technology.

CENTER FOR INFORMATION RESOURCES
c/o University of Pennsylvania
4212 Chestnut St.
Philadelphia, PA 19104-3054
(215) 898-8108

This university-based center supports a technology resource center that offers information dissemination, training, equipment evaluation, and prescription services to individuals who are disabled.

CENTER FOR REHABILITATION TECHNOLOGY RESOURCES
c/o South Carolina Vocational Rehabilitation Dept.
1410-C Boston Ave.
P.O. Box 15
West Columbia, SC 29171
(803) 822-5362

This state agency supports rehabilitation services involving accessibility, environmental controls, driving aids, prosthetics, augmentative communication, computer applications, and seating and power mobility.

CENTER FOR SPECIAL EDUCATION TECHNOLOGY
1920 Association Dr.
Reston, VA 22091-1589
(703) 620-3660

A government-funded project of the Council for Exceptional Children, the program monitors new and existing assistive technology appropriate for use in special education. The center has a database and offers free searches.

CENTER FOR THERAPEUTIC APPLICATIONS OF TECHNOLOGY
c/o University of Buffalo
517 Kimball Tower
Buffalo, NY 14214
(716) 831-3141

This university-based program emphasizes the application of assistive technology with individuals who are disabled. The center provides information dissemination, evaluation, and prescription services, and supports a technology resource center for education and training.

CENTER FOR TECHNOLOGY AND HUMAN DISABILITIES
2301 Argonne Dr.
Baltimore, MD 21218
(301) 554-3046

The center's assistive technology services focus on research, training, direct service, and information dissemination. The center also offers a hands-on equipment demonstration center.

CLEARINGHOUSE ON COMPUTER ACCOMMODATION (COCA)
KGDO, 18th and F St. N.W., Rm. 2022
Washington, DC 20405
(202) 523-1906

COCA is a demonstration and technical resource center of the General Services Administration of the U.S. government. The center demonstrates hardware and software, provides technical assistance, and conducts workshops on computer accommodation for individuals with disabilities.

CLOSING THE GAP, INC.
P.O. Box 68
Henderson, MN 56044
(612) 248-3294

This organization offers regional and national conferences, workshops, and training. CTG also publishes a newspaper dedicated to the application of assistive technology with individuals who are disabled.

COLORADO EASTER SEAL SOCIETY, INC.
c/o Center for Adapted Technology
5755 W. Alameda
Lakewood, CO 80226
(303) 233-1666

This regional Easter Seal assistive technology center supports assistive device training, client evaluations, information dissemination, and support services.

COMMITTEE ON PERSONAL COMPUTERS AND THE HANDICAPPED (COPH-2)
P.O. Box 7701
Chicago, IL 60680-7701
(708) 866-8195

This consumer organization disseminates information, provides technical consultations, and sells adaptive computer devices. The organization also publishes information resources and supports an electronic bulletin board.

COMMUNICATION ASSISTANCE RESOURCE SERVICE
2140 Arbor Blvd.
Dayton, OH 45439
(515) 294-8086

This advocacy organization focuses on the needs of individuals who are unable to communicate, speak, or write. The organization supports computer applications that have the potential to address the needs of its constituency. Information dissemination, referral, and networking services are provided.

COMPUTE ABLE NETWORK
P.O. Box 1706
Portland, OR 97207
(503) 645-0009

The organization provides information dissemination, training, research, and evaluation and supports services to individuals with disabilities.

COMPUTER ACCESS CENTER
2425 16th St. Rm. 23
Santa Monica, CA 90405
(213) 450-8827

The center disseminates assistive technology information and offers individualized and group workshops on the use of hardware and software. The center also maintains an assistive technology library of related materials.

CONNECTICUT SPECIAL EDUCATION NETWORK FOR SOFTWARE EVALUATION
University of Connecticut
Special Education Lab
249 Glenbrook Rd. U-64
Storrs, CT 06269
(203) 486-0165

The center provides information on hardware and software for use with special education populations. The center also supports a software lab for training and demonstration activities.

CONNECTICUT REHABILITATION ENGINEERING CENTER
78 Eastern Boulevard
Glastonbury, CT 06033
(203) 657-9954

The center provides assistive technology information and referral, education, and technical assistance to individuals with disabilities. The center also coordinates workshops on assistive technology for consumers, their families, employers, and professionals.

COUNCIL FOR EXCEPTIONAL CHILDREN (CEC)
1920 Association Dr.
Reston, VA 22091
(703) 620-3660

CEC is a national association of special education teachers, administrators, and advocacy groups. The organization provides information dissemination, conferences, and publications related to the use of technology with children.

CSUN OFFICE OF DISABLED STUDENT SERVICES
California State University Northridge
1811 Nordhoff St.-DVSS

Northridge, CA 91330
(818) 885-2795

The center provides assistive technology referral, advocacy, training, evaluation, and prescription services. In addition, the organization is involved in technology research and database networking activities.

DELAWARE LEARNING RESOURCE SYSTEM CENTER FOR TECHNOLOGY
University of Delaware
012 Willard Hall
Newark, DE 19716
(302) 451-2084

The center is a state resource center that provides diagnostic and prescriptive services to individuals who are disabled and require assistive technology. Equipment can be used on-site or requested by an outlying area for staff development or short-term loan.

DIRECT LINK FOR THE DISABLED
P.O. Box 1036
Solvang, CA 93463
(805) 688-1603

An information referral service that links the disabled with direct service agencies. Direct Link also provides resources for computer technology and training programs.

DISABLED CHILDREN'S COMPUTER GROUP
2095 Rose St. 1st Fl.
Berkeley, CA 94709
(415) 841-3224

This nonprofit resource center provides information, referral, and training services. The organization serves children with physical, sensory, mental, and learning disabilities.

DIVISION OF REHABILITATION SERVICES
878 Peachtree St., Rm. 706
Atlanta, GA 30309
(404) 894-6744

A state program offering vocational technology information, referral, advocacy, assessment, prescription, education, and training services.

DU PAGE EASTER SEAL TREATMENT CENTER, INC.
830 S. Addison
Villa Park, IL 60181
(312) 620-4433

The center provides assistive technology information dissemination, training, evaluations, and prescriptions to individuals who are disabled.

EAST TENNESSEE SPECIAL TECHNOLOGY ACCESS CENTER, INC.
5719 Kingston Pike
Knoxville, TN 37919
(615) 584-4465

This center supports a technology resource center that offers information dissemination, educational training, and referral services to individuals who are disabled and require assistive technology.

EASTERN REGIONAL ASSISTIVE DEVICE CLINIC
2413 W. Vernon Ave.
Kinston, NC 28501
(919) 559-5371

This organization provides assistive technology information dissemination, equipment modification, training, and diagnostic and prescriptive services to individuals who are disabled.

EASTER SEAL REHABILITATION CENTER
2203 Babcock Rd.
San Antonio, TX 78229
(519) 699-3911

This Easter Seal regional assistive technology center supports assistive device training, maintains a technology resource center, and provides referral services.

EASTER SEAL SOCIETY OF DADE COUNTY
1475 N.W. 14th Ave.
Miami, FL 33125
(305) 325-0470

This Easter Seal regional assistive technology center provides information dissemination, referral, and assistive device training services to individuals with disabilities.

EASTER SEAL SOCIETY OF METROPOLITAN CHICAGO
c/o Gilchrist-Marchman Center
2345 W. North Ave.
Chicago, IL 60647
(312) 276-4000

This Easter Seal regional assistive technology center disseminates technology information, provides client referrals, furnishes assistive device training services, and maintains a technology resource center for individuals with disabilities.

EASTER SEAL SOCIETY OF RHODE ISLAND
c/o Assistive Device Resource Center
667 Waterman Ave.
East Providence, RI 02914
(401) 438-9500

This Easter Seal regional assistive technology center disseminates technology information, supplies client referrals, furnishes assistive device training services, provides client evaluations and device prescriptions, and maintains a technology resource center for individuals with disabilities.

EASTER SEAL SOCIETY OF THE MONTEREY REGION
c/o Easter Seal Society of Santa Cruz and Monterey Counties
621-A Water St.
Santa Cruz, CA 95060
(408) 427-3360

This Easter Seal regional assistive technology center disseminates technology information, provides client referrals, and maintains a technology resource center for individuals with disabilities.

EASTER SEAL SYSTEMS' COMPUTER ASSISTED TECHNOLOGY SERVICES (CATS)
c/o Technology Related Loan Fund Officer
5120 South Hyde Park Blvd.
Chicago, IL 60615
(312) 667-8400

This national technology loan program assists persons with disabilities in purchasing computers and other technological aids. CATS focuses on loans to adults, children, or elderly individuals with disabilities. Applicants are required to pay the loan within a 1- to 3-year period.

EASTERN REGIONAL ASSISTIVE DEVICE CLINIC
2415 W. Vernon Ave.
Kinston, NC 28501
(919) 559-5371

This technology resource center offers services in environmental control, seating and power mobility, augmentative communication, and computer access. The clinic maintains a technology resource center that provides information dissemination, equipment evaluation and prescription services, and training.

EDUCATIONAL TECHNOLOGY CENTER
1313 N.E. 134th St.
Vancouver, WA 98685
(206) 574-3215

This center supports a technology resource center that provides education and training services to individuals with sensory, learning, physical, speech, or mental disabilities.

ELECTRONIC INDUSTRIES FOUNDATION
Rehabilitation Engineering Center
1901 Pennsylvania Ave. N.W., Ste. 700
Washington, DC 20006
(202) 955-5826

A government think-tank for rehabilitation technology policy, the organization has helped agencies set up revolving low-interest loan funds for technology needs of patients.

FEDERATION FOR CHILDREN WITH SPECIAL NEEDS
312 Stuart St., 2nd Fl.
Boston, MA 02116
(617) 482-2915

Network of parent organizations offering technical assistance, referral services, and a resource center for children with disabilities.

FLORIDA DIAGNOSTIC LEARNING RESOURCES SERVICES (FDLRS)
9220 S.W. 52 Terrace
Miami, FL 3316
(305) 274-3501

This state agency provides information, referral, advocacy, assessment, and prescription services. The agency also provides education and training in the use of technology.

GEORGIA TECH CENTER FOR REHABILITATION TECHNOLOGY
Georgia Institute of Technology
Atlanta, GA 30332-0156
(404) 894-4960

This university-based research facility specializes in adaptive equipment design, development, and evaluation for the individuals who are disabled and elderly. The center also supports a data and information clearinghouse with networking capabilities. The network offers information about laws, products, services, resources, and related technology for the disabled.

HEATH RESOURCE CENTER
1 Dupont Circle, Ste. 800
Washington, DC 20036-1193
(202) 727-3866

A federally funded resource center that operates the National Clearinghouse on Postsecondary Education for Handicapped Individuals, the center provides information dissemination, database, and referral services.

HEAR OUR VOICES
105 W. Pine St.
Wooster, OH 44691
(212) 262-4681

A national patient advocacy group run by Prentke Romich Company. Any augmentative communication aid user or family member can join this organization.

HIGH TECHNOLOGY CENTER FOR THE DISABLED
c/o Foothill-DeAnza Community College
2105 McClellan Rd.
Cupertino, CA 95014
(408) 996-4636

This community college program maintains a technology resource center that provides technology information, referral, and training services to individuals with physical, learning, and sensory disabilities.

HUGH MACMILLAN MEDICAL CENTRE
c/o Microcomputer Applications Programme
350 Rumsey Rd.
Toronto, Ontario M4G 1R8
Canada
(416) 425-6220

This nonprofit hospital provides assessment, prescription, education, and training services in personal vehicle and driving aids, seating and power mobility, prosthetics, augmentative communication, and computer applications.

IBM NATIONAL SUPPORT CENTER FOR PERSONS WITH DISABILITIES (IBM–NSCPD)
P.O. Box 2150
Atlanta, GA 30055
(800) 426-2133

This IBM support center provides information, referral, advocacy, and demonstration center services. The center provides specific IBM computer applications and resources for individuals who are disabled.

INFORMATION CENTER FOR INDIVIDUALS WITH DISABILITIES
2743 Wormwood St.
Boston, MA 02210
(617) 727-5540

The center provides assistive technology information dissemination and referral services.

INTERDISCIPLINARY TECHNOLOGY CENTER
c/o University of Kansas Medical Center
39th and Rainbow
Kansas City, KS 66103
(913) 588-7195

The center offers assistive technology information, advocacy, assessment, prescription, education, and training services. The center also provides a database for assistive technology applications.

INTERNATIONAL SOCIETY FOR AUGMENTATIVE AND ALTERNATIVE COMMUNICATION (ISAAC)
P.O. Box 1762, Sta. R.
Toronto, Ontario M4G 4A3
Canada
(416) 737-9308

An information and referral organization whose focus is the international advancement of augmentative and alternative communication techniques and aids.

JOB ACCOMMODATION NETWORK (JAN)
West Virginia University
809 Allen Hall, P.O. Box 6122
Morgantown, WV 26506
(800) 526-7234

This organization is an international information network and consulting resource to enable qualified workers with disabilities to be hired or retrained. JAN offers information on methods and available equipment needed for employment of an individual with disabilities.

KENNEDY INSTITUTE
Assistive Technology Center
707 North Broadway
Baltimore, MD 21205
(301) 550-9519

A nonprofit hospital that provides interdisciplinary technology information, referral, advocacy, assessment, and prescription services. Equipment modification and fabrication services are also offered. The institute also provides education and training in the use of assistive technology.

LIVING AND LEARNING RESOURCE CENTRE
601 West Maple St.
Lansing, MI 48906
(517) 371-5897

A private, nonprofit organization that provides assistive technology information, referral, advocacy services, and training in the use of technology.

MARYLAND REHABILITATION CENTER
Technology Resource Center
2301 Argonne Dr.
Baltimore, MD 21218
(301) 554-3116

A state program offering vocational technology information, referral, advocacy, assessment, prescription, education, and training services.

MASSACHUSETTS SPECIAL TECHNOLOGY ACCESS CENTER (MASTAC)
P.O. Box J
Bedford, MA 01730
(617) 275-2446

MASTAC seeks to promote increased access to microcomputer technology and other assistive technology. The organization provides information regarding new and existing products, professional services, and potential funding sources.

MINNESOTA STAR PROGRAM
300 Centennial Bldg., 3rd Fl.
658 Cedar St.
St. Paul, MN 55101
(612) 297-1554

This program provides assistive technology referral, advocacy, training, evaluation, and prescription services. In addition, the program provides information dissemination on uses of technology with disabled individuals.

NATIONAL ASSOCIATION OF HEARING AND SPEECH ACTION (NAHSA)
10801 Rockville Pike
Rockville, MD 20852
(301) 897-8682

A consumer advocacy group for persons with speech and hearing impairments. The group provides information dissemination and referral services.

NATIONAL BRAILLE PRESS, INC.
88 Saint Stephens St.
Boston, MA 02115
(617) 266-6160

This organization provides information dissemination on assistive technology applications for individuals who are blind or visually impaired. It publishes books and magazines in braille, and provides transcription services for books, magazines, and pamphlets.

NATIONAL CENTER FOR YOUTH WITH DISABILITIES
c/o University of Minnesota
Box 721
Minneapolis, MN 55455
(612) 626-2825

This center maintains a technology resource center that supports information dissemination on the application of technology with individuals who are disabled.

NATIONAL DOWN SYNDROME CONGRESS
1800 Dempster
Park Ridge, IL 60068-1146
(312) 823-7550

An organization of parents and professionals providing information dissemination, referral services, and resources for persons with Down syndrome.

NATIONAL EASTER SEAL SOCIETY
5120 S. Hyde Park Blvd.
Chicago, IL 60615-1146
(312) 667-8400

This national organization provides information dissemination, education, and training. The organization is also developing regional assistive technology centers that support assistive device training, client evaluations, and support services.

NATIONAL FEDERATION FOR THE BLIND
1800 Johnson St.
Baltimore, MD 21230
(301) 659-9314

A national organization with more than 500 state and local chapters. The organization provides information dissemination, advocacy, referral services, database, and resource support services to persons who are visually impaired.

NATIONAL INFORMATION CENTER FOR CHILDREN AND YOUTH WITH HANDICAPS
P.O. Box 1492
Washington, DC 20013
(703) 893-6061

This center supports a resource center that offers technology information dissemination and referral services to individuals who are disabled.

NATIONAL INSTITUTE FOR REHABILITATION ENGINEERING (NIRE)
P.O. Box 841
Butler, NJ 07405
(201) 838-2500

This organization is an information and referral center for persons with disabilities seeking computer-based rehabilitation. This interdisciplinary organization also provides research, and training, as well as a service organization that provides assessment, prescription, training, and device modification and fabrication services.

NATIONAL LEKOTEK CENTER
CompuPlay
711 E. Colfax
South Bend, IN 46617
(219) 233-4366

CompuPlay provides computer play sessions for parents and children with special needs ages 2 to 14. Adaptive equipment and software are employed to allow children to play and learn. The organization provides a software lending library and computer demonstration center.

NATIONAL ORGANIZATION ON DISABILITY (NOD)
910 16th St., N.W., #600
Washington, DC 20006
(202) 293-5968

NOD provides information and referral services to all individuals with handicaps. The organization's local groups support a national network of people who are disabled for information dissemination and advocacy.

NATIONAL SPINAL CORD INJURY ASSOCIATION
600 W. Commings Park, Ste. 2000
Woburn, MA 01801
(617) 935-2722

This organization provides information and referrals for the direct care of persons with para- or quadriplegia. The organization also disseminates publications for rehabilitation professionals and persons with spinal cord injuries.

NATIONAL TECHNOLOGY CENTER
c/o American Foundation for the Blind
15 West 16th St.
New York, NY 10011
(212) 620-2000

A nonprofit organization that provides technology-related information, referral, and advocacy services to persons with vision impairments. The organization also supports research efforts related to vision impairments.

NEIL SQUIRE FOUNDATION
4381 Gallant Ave.
North Vancouver, BC V7G 1L1
Canada
(604) 929-3316

A nonprofit foundation that provides technology training, assessment, and prescription services to disabled adults. The foundation is also involved in technology research.

NEVADA TECHNOLOGY CENTER
2880 E. Flamingo Rd., Ste. A
Las Vegas, NV 89121
(702) 735-2922

The center provides a training environment for employment of children and adults who are disabled. The center offers technology information dissemination, referral, assessment, and prescription services.

NEW HAMPSHIRE ADAPTED TECHNOLOGY AND EQUIPMENT CENTER
P.O. Box 370
Laconia, NH 03246
(603) 524-5373

This assistive technology resource center provides training, equipment evaluation, and prescription services to individuals with physical, mental, and speech disabilities.

NEW JERSEY DIVISION OF VOCATIONAL REHABILITATION SERVICES
CN 398, Rm. 1005 Labor Bldg.
Trenton, NJ 08625-0398
(609) 292-5987

This state agency provides vocational technology referral services, assistive technology device evaluation and prescription services, and training support to individuals with disabilities.

NORTHERN ILLINOIS CENTER FOR ADAPTIVE TECHNOLOGY
3615 Louisiana Rd.
Rockford, IL 61108
(815) 229-2163

This regional technology center offers technology information dissemination, referral, training, equipment evaluation, and prescription services to individuals with disabilities.

OHIO RESOURCE CENTER FOR LOW INCIDENCE AND SEVERELY HANDICAPPED
470 Glenmont Ave.
Columbus, OH 43214
(614) 262-6131

This organization provides technology training, information dissemination, and networking services to disabled individuals. The center also maintains a technology resources center.

PACER COMPUTER RESOURCE CENTER
4826 Chicago Ave.
Minneapolis, MN 55417-1055
(612) 827-2966

Parent-based center provides access to assistive technology hardware and software, offering children and adults who are disabled the opportunity to try these devices and evaluate their effectiveness. The center also provides technology information dissemination and training.

PARENT ADVOCACY COALITION FOR EDUCATIONAL RIGHTS
4826 Chicago Ave. South
Minneapolis, MN 55417

This advocacy organization offers publications and newsletters about special education, technology, and supported employment.

PENNSYLVANIA ASSISTIVE DEVICE CENTER
150 South Progress Ave.
Harrisburg, PA 17109
(717) 657-5840

A state agency that provides information, referral, and advocacy services to disabled school-age children. The center provides technology training and supports a technology equipment library.

PROJECT TECH
c/o Massachusetts Easter Seal Society
484 Main St., 6th Fl.
Worcester, MA 01608
(508) 757-2756

This Easter Seal regional assistive technology center provides information dissemination, referral, and assistive device training services to individuals with disabilities.

RECORDING FOR THE BLIND
20 Roszel Rd.
Princeton, NJ 08540
(609) 452-0606
(800) 221-4792

This nonprofit service organization provides recorded educational books and related library services to people with blindness, low vision, learning disabilities, or other physical impairments that affect reading. The organization records educational books on all subjects and at all academic levels.

REHABILITATION TECHNOLOGY CENTER
6535 E. 82nd St.
Indianapolis, IN 46250
(317) 845-3408

This center provides technology training, device assessment and prescription, and training services to individuals with disabilities. The center also supports a technology database on technology for the handicapped.

REHABILITATION TECHNOLOGY RESOURCE CENTER
354 S. Broad St.
Trenton, NJ 08608
(609) 392-4004

This center provides technology training, device assessment and prescription, and referral services to individuals with disabilities. The center also supports a technology database and provides information dissemination activities.

REHABILITATION TECHNOLOGY SERVICES
1 S. Prospect St.
Burlington, VT 05401
(802) 656-2953

This center disseminates technology information related to augmentative communication, computer access, and related technology to aid disabled individuals. The center also offers client evaluations and technology training services.

RESNA
1101 Connecticut Ave. N.W., Suite 700
Washington, DC 20036
(202) 857-1199

This interdisciplinary association is devoted to the advancement of rehabilitation and assistive technology. The organization offers conferences, publications, and networking services to professionals, advocates, and consumers on practical applications of technology in vocational, educational, and independent living settings.

ST. LOUIS EASTER SEAL SOCIETY
c/o Computer Resource Center
5025 Northrup
St. Louis, MO 63110
(314) 776-1996

This Easter Seal regional assistive technology center supports assistive device training, maintains a technology resource center, and provides referral services.

TECHNOLOGY ACCESS CENTER OF MIDDLE TENNESSEE
Fountain Sq. 2222 Metro Ctr., Ste. 110
Nashville, TN 37228
(615) 248-6733

This program maintains a technology resource center and supports referral, advocacy, and networking efforts supporting the application of assistive technology with individuals who have disabilities.

TECHNOLOGY AND MEDIA DIVISION (TAM)
Council for Exceptional Children
1920 Association Dr.
Reston, VA 22091-1589
(816) 276-1041

This division of the Council for Exceptional Children keeps abreast of advances in special education technology. The organization provides information dissemination, referral services, and offers several publications on the use of technology.

TECHNOLOGY RESOURCE CENTER
c/o Arkansas Easter Seal Society
2801 Lee Ave.
Little Rock, AR 72225
(501) 663-8331

This Easter Seal regional assistive technology center supports assistive device training, maintains a technology resource center, and provides referral services.

TECHNICAL AIDS AND SYSTEMS FOR THE HANDICAPPED (TASH)
70 Gibson Dr., Unit 12
Markham, Ontario L3R 4C2
Canada
(416) 475-2212

This organization offers books and publications on the use of technology with individuals who are severely handicapped. The organization also manufactures assistive technology devices.

TECHNICAL AIDS AND ASSISTANCE FOR THE DISABLED CENTER
1950 W. Roosevelt
Chicago, IL 60608
(312) 421-3373

The center provides information to individuals who are disabled about personal computer technology. The center maintains a database, part of a nationwide network that gives users the ability to exchange information on new and existing technology. The center has an equipment loan program and a technology information library.

TRACE RESEARCH AND DEVELOPMENT CENTER
1500 Highland Ave., Rm. S-151 Waisman Ctr.
Madison, WI 53705
(608) 262-6966

The Trace Center develops and disseminates information related to nonvocal communication, computer access, and technology to aid individuals who are disabled. The center also conducts research and training in technology.

UCLA INTERVENTION PROGRAM FOR HANDICAPPED CHILDREN
1000 Veteran Ave. Rm. 23-10
Los Angeles, CA 90024
(213) 825-4821

This university-based technology program has developed software for use with individuals who are disabled. The program also supports a resource center and is actively involved in technology training activities.

UNIVERSITY OF CONNECTICUT SPECIAL EDUCATION CENTER TECHNOLOGY LAB
c/o University of Connecticut
U-Box 64249 Glenbrook
Storrs, CT 06269-2064
(203) 486-0172

This university-based center supports a resource center that provides assistive technology information dissemination, referral, networking, research, education, and training services.

UNIVERSITY OF NORTH CAROLINA, DIVISION OF SPEECH & HEARING SCIENCES
c/o University of North Carolina
CB #7190
Chapel Hill, NC 27599-7190
(919) 966-1006

This university-based center furnishes research, training, and diagnostic services in the area of augmentative communication for individuals with speech, hearing, and learning disabilities.

VARIETY CLUB
c/o Temple University
National Computer Institute

Ritter Hall 301, 13th & Montgomery Ave.
Philadelphia, PA 19122
(215) 787-5632

This university-based technology program is involved in field-based technology training, research, and the maintenance of a rehabilitation database. The program also provides device evaluation and prescription services to individuals with disabilties.

VOLUNTEERS FOR MEDICAL ENGINEERING
c/o UMBC TEC
5202 Westland Blvd.
Baltimore, MD 21227
(301) 455-6395

A volunteer organization made of professional engineers dedicated to improving the lives of individuals who are disabled. The organization actively provides technical expertise to solving hardware and software problems for children and adults with disabilities.

DATABASES

Database resources are large clearinghouses for information on a wide variety of assistive technology including new and existing hardware, software, and related resources. These databases provide information via on-line electronic networks, floppy disks, CD-ROM, audio cassette, or printed material.

ABLEDATA
181 E. Cedar St.
Newington, CT 06111
(203) 667-5405

The database is maintained by Newington Children's Hospital in Newington, Connecticut, and is funded by the National Institute on Disability and Rehabilitation Research (NIDRR). The computerized listings cover more than 16,000 commercially available assistive technology products from over 2,000 companies. Access to the database is available through subscription to BRS Information Technologies or through libraries and rehabilitation programs that offer search services. The database is updated monthly.

ACCENT ON INFORMATION
P.O. Box 700
Bloomington, IL 61702
(309) 378-2961

A computerized database of product, publication, and related resource information on how to adapt assistive technology equipment. The database contains over 6,000 product entries.

ACCESS/ABILITIES
P.O. Box 458
Mill Valley, CA 94942
(415) 388-3250

A database of technology resources for individuals who are physically handicapped. The database contains information on services, hardware, and software aids.

ASSISTIVE DEVICE DATABASE SYSTEM
Assistive Device Center
California State University
Sacramento, CA 95819
(916) 278-6422

This database contains information on assistive devices and related resource listings. This database focuses on the educational implications of using assistive technology with disabled populations.

ADAPTIVE DEVICE LOCATOR SYSTEM
Academic Software, Inc.
331 West Second St.
Lexington, KY 40507
(606) 233-2332

This floppy-disk-based system provides descriptions and pictures of assistive devices and lists of sources for products and product information. The system can generate mailing labels and form letters to vendors. The database includes over 600 generic device descriptions, categorized by over 350 functional goal descriptions, and cross-indexed with over 300 vendors.

COMPUSERVE
5000 Arlington Centre Blvd., P.O. Box 20212
Columbus, OH 43220
(614) 457-8600

The system contains a users' database that contains information on all aspects of technology used by individuals who are disabled.

DEAFNET
508 Bremer Bldg., 7th & Roberts Sts.
St. Paul, MN 55101
(612) 223-5130

DEAFNET is a nonprofit organization that serves technology users who are hearing impaired. It has a nationwide electronic mail service with international links.

ECER
Council for Exceptional Children
1920 Association Dr.
Reston, VA 22091-1589
(703) 620-3660

ECER is the ERIC database for technology users who are disabled. The database contains bibliographic information on books, articles, teaching materials, and reports on the education of individuals who are disabled.

HANDICAPPED EDUCATION EXCHANGE (HEX)
11523 Charlton Dr.
Silver Spring, MD 20902
(301) 681-7372

The HEX database offers resource information on the use of technology with individuals who are disabled. The database contains information on products, organizations, and related information on training and service.

HYPER-ABLEDATA-PLUS
Trace Center Reprint Service
1500 Highland Ave., S-151 Waisman Ctr.
Madison, WI 53706
(608) 263-6966

The CD-ROM version of the on-line version of ABLEDATA. This disk provides information on over 16,000 assistive technology products. The system also provides pictures and sound samples of many database items, and it has an access system for users who are blind or visually impaired.

NATIONAL TECHNOLOGY CENTER
American Foundation for the Blind, Inc.
15 W. 16th St.
New York, NY 10011
(212) 620-2000

The center maintains three database systems: National Technology Database, Evaluations Database, and Research and Development Database. Each database focuses on resources for individuals who are blind or visually impaired and professionals who work with them.

SOLUTIONS
Apple Computer, Inc.
20525 Mariani Ave., MS 43S
Cupertino, CA 95014
(408) 973-2732

The database contains information on hardware, software, organizations, and publications maintained by Apple Office of Special Education Programs. The database can be accessed via SpecialNet or AppleLink.

SPECIALNET
2021 K. St. N.W., Ste. 215
Washington, DC 20006
(202) 835-7300

The largest computer network in the United States devoted exclusively to the information needs of professionals in special education. The database includes information on service providers, new and existing products, bulletin boards, and national forums for information exchange.

PUBLICATIONS

The following technology resources are additional publications in the form of newsletters, magazines, professional journals, or textbooks covering a wide variety of assistive technology issues, such as service planning and delivery, funding, equipment and service agency directories, research, and professional literature.

APPLE COMPUTER RESOURCES IN SPECIAL EDUCATION AND REHABILITATION
DLM Teaching Resources
One DLM Park
Allen, TX 75002
(800) 527-5030

A comprehensive resource guide of assistive technology hardware and software for disabled individuals. The guide also provides resource directories on organizations and related technology resources.

ASSISTIVE DEVICE NEWS
Central Pennsylvania Special Education Regional Resource Center
150 S. Progress Ave.
Harrisburg, PA 17109
(717) 657-5840

A newsletter that focuses on information regarding new and existing technology products.

ASSISTIVE TECHNOLOGY
Demos Publications
156 5th Ave., Suite 1018
New York, NY 10010
(202) 857-1199

A quarterly interdisciplinary journal dedicated to the advancement of rehabilitation and assistive technologies. This professional journal provides information on applied research, technology reviews, practical implementations of technology, and reports on small studies with informal protocols.

ASSISTIVE TECHNOLOGY: A FUNDING WORKBOOK
RESNA Press
1101 Connecticut Ave. N.W., Ste. 700
Washington, DC 20036
(202) 857-1199

A textbook that provides information on ways to facilitate a better understanding of funding sources and creative ways to eliminate funding barriers for the payment of assistive technology devices and services.

AUGMENTATIVE COMMUNICATION NEWS
One Surf Way, Ste. 215
Monterey, CA 93940
(408) 649-3050

A bimonthly newsletter on augmentative communication issues. Each newsletter examines a special topic. Updates on funding, local resources, and related information are also included.

AUGMENTATIVE AND ALTERNATIVE COMMUNICATION JOURNAL
Williams & Wilkins
428 E. Preston St.
Baltimore, MD 21202
(800) 638-6423

A professional journal that focuses on nonverbal communication, integration theory, technology, assessment, treatment, and education of users who rely on augmentative communication systems.

BEGINNER'S GUIDE TO PERSONAL COMPUTERS FOR THE BLIND AND VISUALLY IMPAIRED
National Braille Press
88 Stephen St.
Boston, MA 02115
(617) 266-6160

This text is available in print or on audiotape. It provides information on the application of microcomputers for users who are blind or visually impaired. It also includes hardware and software resources.

CHILDHOOD POWERED MOBILITY: DEVELOPMENTAL, TECHNICAL, AND CLINICAL PERSPECTIVES
RESNA Press
Department 4813
Washington, DC 20061-4813
(202) 857-1199

This textbook consists of proceedings of the RESNA First Northwest Regional Conference. Topics include clinical conditions for prescribing powered mobility, spatial understanding with respect to power mobility, perceived self-motion and sensory organization, and interdisciplinary technology team programming issues related to the client and the family.

CLOSING THE GAP
P.O. Box 58
Henderson, MN 56044
(612) 248-3294

A bimonthly newsletter devoted exclusively to assistive technology and its application in special education and rehabilitation. Technology reviews, a resource directory, and device application information are included in the publication.

COMMUNICATION OUTLOOK
Artificial Language Laboratory
Michigan State University
East Lansing, MI 48824
(517) 353-0870

This quarterly international magazine covers new products and developments in the area of augmentative and alternative communication.

COMPUTER ACCESS IN HIGHER EDUCATION FOR STUDENTS WITH DISABILTIES
The High-Tech Center for the Disabled of the California Community Colleges
Chancellor's Office
1109 Ninth St.
Sacramento, CA 95814
(916) 322-4636

This textbook discusses computer applications for use with individuals who are disabled. It covers hardware and software systems that can be used to augment microcomputer systems.

COMPUTER-DISABILITY NEWS
National Easter Seal Society
5120 S. Hyde Park Blvd.
Chicago, IL 60615
(312) 667-8400

This periodical focuses on the use of microcomputers for all individuals who are disabled. It also includes general interest articles on the application of microcomputers.

COMPUTING TEACHER (THE)
International Society for Technology in Education
1787 Agate St.
Eugene, OR 97403-1923
(503) 346-4414

This periodical offers feature articles on the use and integration of technology in education. It also includes hardware and software reviews.

DISABILITY BOOKSHOP CATALOG
P.O. Box 129
Vancouver, WA 98666
(206) 694-2462

This shop-by-mail bookstore stocks 375 hard-to-find titles covering a wide range of topics related to individuals who are disabled. The books available cover visual, hearing, physical, and mental impairments.

DIRECTORY OF COMPUTER AND HIGH TECHNOLOGY GRANTS
Research Grant Guides
Dept. 3A P.O. Box 1214
Loxahatchee, FL 33470
(407) 795-6129

This resource lists over 600 funding sources for computers, software, and technology-related grants. The publication also provides profiles on foundations, corporations, and federal programs. Guidelines for grant writing are also included.

DIRECT LINK
Independent Living Center
617 Seventh Ave.
Fort Worth, TX 76104
(817) 870-9082

A quarterly publication available in print, braille, and audio-cassette versions from the Center for Computer Assistance to the Disabled. It provides information about existing products and techniques and modifications for computer-based assistive technology applications.

EDUCATIONAL TECHNOLOGY
720 Palisade Ave.
Englewood Cliffs, NJ 07632
(201) 871-4007

A monthly publication covering the application of computers in education, literature and product reviews, and abstracts from ERIC Clearinghouse of Information Resources.

FINANCIAL AID FOR THE DISABLED AND THEIR FAMILES
References Services Press
1100 Industrial Rd., Ste. 9
San Carlos, CA 94070
(415) 594-0743

This textbook provides funding information on scholarships, loans, grants, and awards that are available for individuals who are disabled.

FINANCING ADAPTIVE TECHNOLOGY: A GUIDE TO SOURCES AND STRATEGIES
FOR BLIND AND VISUALLY IMPAIRED USERS
Smiling Interfaces
P.O. Box 2792, Church Street Station
New York, NY 10008-2792

This resource guide focuses on service systems and sensory aids for individuals who are visually impaired. The book covers assistive technology legislation, delineates resources, and describes procedures for paying for sensory aids. It also covers sources of technology funding on the federal, state, and local levels.

FUNDING BOOK: THE MANY FACES OF FUNDING
Phonic Ear, Inc.
250 Camino Alto
Mill Valley, CA 94941
(415) 383-4000

This textbook focuses on funding strategies for communication devices. The information it gives is also applicable to funding for other types of assistive technology aids. It highlights sources of funding on the federal, state, local, educational, and private levels.

MOBILITY LTD.
401 Linden Center Dr.
Fort Collins, CO 80524
(303) 484-7969

This bimonthly magazine provides articles and news for people with mobility impairments. Features include reviews of new products and services, an events calendar, equipment classifieds, and specialty articles.

PRINTER CONNECTIONS BIBLE
Howard W. Sims & Co., Inc.
4300 West 62nd St.
Indianapolis, IN 46268

This textbook provides technical data on how to make printer cable and similar connections to different microcomputer systems. It includes detailed diagrams for making the proper wiring connections.

REHABILITATION TECHNOLOGY SERVICE DELIVERY: A PRACTICAL GUIDE
RESNA
Association for the Advancement of Rehabilitation Technology, Publishers
1101 Connecticut Ave. N.W., Ste 700
Washington, DC 20036
(202) 857-1199

This textbook addresses the development of rehabilitation technology service delivery systems. It covers planning, developing, and implementing a technology service program.

REHABILITATION TECHNOLOGY SERVICE DELIVERY DIRECTORY
RESNA Press
Department 4813
Washington, DC 20061-4813
(202) 857-1199

This book is a comprehensive directory of rehabilitation resources available throughout the United States and Canada. The directory includes a detailed information on service delivery providers through geographic and alphabetical listings.

RESOURCE GUIDE FOR PERSONS WITH SPEECH OR LANGUAGE IMPAIRMENTS
IBM National Support Center for Persons with Disabilities
P.O. BOX 2150
Atlanta, GA 30055
(800) 426-2133

This guide presents information about technology products and services that are available to aid persons with disabilities. The major focus of the guide is on IBM and compatible devices that allow a disabled individual to function more independently.

TEACHING WITH COMPUTERS: A CURRICULUM FOR SPECIAL EDUCATORS
Pro-Ed 8700 Shoal Creek Blvd.
Austin, TX 78758-6897
(512) 451-3246

A comprehensive textbook that gives professionals basic information on computer hardware, functions, adaptability, and peripheral equipment. Software listings, publishers, productivity tools, and glossaries are also included.

TRACE RESOURCE BOOK ON ASSISTIVE TECHNOLOGY FOR COMMUNICATION, CONTROL AND COMPUTER ACCESS
Trace Center Reprint Service
1500 Highland Ave., S-151 Waisman Ctr.
Madison, WI 53706
(608) 263-6966

This book includes information on over 1,400 selected products, including written descriptions and pictures. It also includes other resources, such as publications and programs doing research or service delivery in assistive technology.

Glossary of Assistive Technology

■ Gregory Church, MS, MAS ■

Assistive technology has great potential for improving the quality of life for individuals with disabilities. The application of assistive technology can be found in seating and positioning equipment, mobility devices, communication devices, and computer access. The tremendous growth of technology has made it difficult, if not impossible, to keep abreast of new products and effective strategies for their use. As an added help to individuals, professionals, and advocates working with assistive technology who may require a brief review of some of the basic terminology of hardware and software systems, an assistive technology glossary has been added to this book. It is not meant to be an all-inclusive list, but it can serve as a way of familiarizing oneself with terms that are often used to promote the value of one product over another.

AAC. An acronym for augmentative and alternative communication.

Abbreviation expansion. Memory resident utility software that provides keyboard assistance. A short acronym is used to represent a larger, expanded set of keystrokes. When the acronym is activated, the expanded stream of keystrokes replace the acronym. The expansion can be of any type of data, such as words, phrases, salutations, or computer commands.

Abduction. The movement of an extremity (an arm or a leg) away from the midline of the body. The muscles that perform such a function generally are called abductors.

Acceleration techniques. Communication aid and computer techniques used to speed up system use. Prestored messages, word prediction, and abbreviation expansion are methods of input acceleration.

Access software. Software that supports input to the computer by devices other than the standard keyboard or supports output from the computer in formats other than those normally provided by the standard monitor.

Adaptive computer access. Hardware and/or software created or modified to allow persons to use a computer with or without its standard input or output devices. For example, adaptive access may be accomplished via alternative keyboards, touch boards, braille, screen enlargement, speech synthesis, voice recognition, switch access through the game port, or switches with scanning.

Address bus. A communication channel internal to a computer by which the central processing unit can access particular input and output devices or locations in memory.

Adduction. A movement that draws a displaced body part, usually an arm or a leg, toward the center or midline of the body. The muscles that perform such a function generally are referred to as adductors.

Aided communication. Communication modes that require equipment in addition to the communicator's body. Examples are pencil and paper, typewriters, computers, headsticks, and augmentative communication aids.

Alternative communication. Communication modes, such as sign language, gestures, and communication aids that are used to replace oral language skills.

Alternative keyboard. A hardware device that replaces or works in conjunction to the standard keyboard and is positioned to meet the specific needs of the user.

Analog signal. A signal that varies continuously over time. Examples of analog signals include sound, light, and heat.

Anterior. Situated before or toward the front of a structure.

Aphasia. A general language deficit affecting the ability to read, write, listen, and talk, usually secondary to a cerebrovascular accident (stroke) or traumatic injury to the left cerebral hemisphere of the brain.

Application software. Computer programs designed for a particular purpose, such as education, word processing, database management, finance/accounting, or drawing and graphics.

Apraxia. The inability to voluntarily perform a learned motor movement in the absence of paralysis or paresis.

Array. A selection of letters, numbers, punctuation marks, or computer commands commonly used with scanning input.

ASCII. American Standard Code for Information Exchange. A standardized system that assigns a unique decimal value from 0 to 127 to each of 128 letters, numbers, punctuation marks, and various other computer control characters. For example, the letter "A" is represented by the ASCII code 65, while ASCII code 49 is the number "1." ASCII file formats provide a standardized method for transferring information from one computer to another (or peripheral).

Associative play. The fourth stage of play development in which children make brief contact with one another while playing.

Asymmetrical. Different on each side of the body. Opposite of symmetrical.

Ataxia. Total or partial inability to coordinate voluntary bodily movements, especially muscular movements.

Athetosis. Constantly recurring series of purposeless motions of the hands and feet, usually the result of a brain lesion.

Augmentative communication. Communication modes such as sign language, gestures, and communication aids that are used to supplement oral language skills.

Automatic linear scanning. A common scanning method in which the user presses the switch to bring up the array. A cursor then starts moving across the array of selections using either one-item-at-a-time or group-item scanning. The user waits until the cursor is on the desired item and then presses the switch.

Bandwidth. The difference between the lowest and highest frequencies that can be transmitted by an analog or digital communication channel. Analog signals are expressed in hertz (Hz) or cycles per second. Digital pulses are expressed in bits per second (baud rate).

Barrier game. A communication game in which a speaker knows something that is not known by the listener. The speaker has to successfully communicate a message to the listener to accomplish a task.

Baud. The rate of transmission used in exchanging information between a computer and peripheral devices or between two computers. The rate refers to the number of bits per second that can be transmitted between devices. For example, "300 baud" is a transmission speed of 300 bits per second.

Binary system. A numbering system in which a place holder can assume the value 0 or the value 1. The binary system is used by the computer's microelectronics because a binary signal can easily be characterized by the presence or absence of an electrical voltage. On is usually represented as 1, off as 0.

Bit. The smallest unit of useful information a computer can handle, usually represented as a single binary digit, 1 or 0. Eight bits equal one byte.

Blissymbols. A pictographic symbol system developed by Charles Bliss.

Braille. A system of writing for individuals who are visually impaired that uses letters, numbers, and punctuation marks made up of raised dot patterns. Braille software translates from English to braille, braille to English, or functions as a braille training program.

Braille input. A hardware device that allows input to the computer via a braille-style keyboard or specific keys on a standard keyboard that function in braille patterns.

Braille output. A hardware device that produces hard copy braille, or paperless refresh braille as output from the computer.

Buffer. Hardware or software that temporarily holds information in memory until the computer or peripheral device is ready to use it. For example, a print buffer accepts information from a computer at high speed, then passes the information to a lower speed printer.

Bus. Electrical circuits inside a computer that transmit information from one part of the computer to another or between a computer and its peripheral devices.

Byte. A sequence of eight bits that represent a fundamental unit of storage, such as a letter, a number, a punctuation mark, or computer instruction. Also indicates the relative capacity of computer memory and storage.

Cathode-ray tube (CRT). A display device in which an electronically aimed stream of electrons strikes a light sensitive material, such as phosphorus, to create a visible image. Television and computer monitors commonly use CRTs.

Central nervous system. Comprised of the brain and the spinal cord, as well as the nerve trunks and fibers connected with them; also known as the cerebrospinal system.

Central processing unit (CPU). The CPU is the "central control center" of the computer. CPUs process logical and mathematical functions, store the intermediate results of data manipulations, and direct the flow of data and instructions to and from peripheral devices. Also called a microprocessor. Microprocessors commonly use 8-, 16-, and 32-bit configurations.

Centronics interface. A parallel transmission system developed by Centronics, Inc., in support of the company's printers. The Centronics interface has become a standard for interfacing computers with parallel peripherals.

Cognitive ability. The ability to accumulate and retain new knowledge.

Communication acts. The pragmatic function of a message. For example, messages may function as requests, answers, statements, or descriptions.

Communication board. Allows expressive communication by pointing or gazing at printed word, symbol, or picture. These systems do not have spoken or written output.

Communication mode. The modality of communication. Gestures, facial expressions, vocalizations, communication boards, and speaking are all modes of communication.

Compatibility. The condition allowing hardware devices or software to work with each other.

Composite color monitor. A monitor that uses a video signal that includes both display information and the synchronization signals needed to display it.

Computer system. A collective term for a computer and all peripherals attached to it.

Configure. A general-purpose term used to refer to the way a user sets up a computer system. The configuration process involves changing hardware and software settings. The configuration process allows various hardware components of a computer system to communicate with each other.

Contractures. Shortening of the tissues surrounding a joint, preventing full range of motion of the joint.

Cooperative play. The fifth stage of play development in which children begin to take turns and play together cooperatively.

Coprocessor. An auxiliary processor designed to relieve demands on the central processing unit (CPU) by performing specialized tasks. For example, mathematical coprocessors handle math functions that could be performed by the CPU but much more slowly.

Cranial nerves. Nerves that originate in the brain, including the 12 cranial nerves proper, their branches, and their ganglia.

Cursor. A special display screen character which indicates the location at which the next keyboard character will appear. The cursor can take the form of a blinking square, a bar, or an underlined character.

Cursor keys. Special keys on the computer keyboard that permit the cursor to be moved up, down, right, or left on the display screen.

Data bus. A communication channel internal to a computer by which the central processing unit can exchange data with peripherals.

Dedicated augmentative communication aids. Communication systems specifically designed to operate as communication aids.

Default. A set of standard settings in hardware or software that remain in effect until explicitly changed by the user. Defaults are preset to common responses or settings that minimize time required for setup and operation.

Digital signal. A signal that is transmitted and received as a sequence of discrete values and can assume only limited values. Examples of digital signals include the presence or absence of an electric voltage or a magnetic field.

Digitized speech. This technique stores a real person's actual words and sentences in the form of "digitized" sounds. These sounds are recorded by a peripheral device that converts sound input from a stereo system, an instrument, or a microphone into a form that the computer can process, store, and play back. The sound quality is excellent, but this technique requires large amounts of RAM and storage space to sample and convert words and phrases into digitized speech.

Direct selection. An access method that allows the user to indicate choices directly by pointing with a body part or technology aid to make a selection. Direct selection is the most rapid method of entering information into the computer.

Disk drive. A hardware device that holds a disk, receives information from it, and saves information on it. Disk drives are controlled by means of a disk-operating system.

Disk operating system (DOS). A generic term for system software programs that manage communication between a central processing unit, disk drives, printers, and other peripheral devices. For example, MS-DOS is an operating system developed for IBM and IBM-compatible computers. ProDOS and DOS 3.3 are operating systems used with Apple II series computers.

Distal. Situated away from a point of origin or attachment, such as of a bone or a limb; opposite of proximal. For example, the shoulder is proximal and the hand is distal.

Dorsal. Pertaining to the back or a position toward or on the back side of a structure (posterior).

Dvorak keyboard. A keyboard layout designed to increase typing speed and efficiency by locating the keys used most often in the home row.

Dynamic display. Communication aid or computer displays of symbols that change constantly based on previous system selections.

Dysarthria. An incoordination of the muscles of respiration, phonation, articulation, and resonation leading to slurred and imprecise speech.

Environmental control unit (ECU). A hardware device that allows the user programmed or spontaneous control over remote, electrically operated appliances.

Expanded keyboard. An alternative keyboard designed for persons who can select keys on a larger keyboard. These keyboards provide users with enlarged touch-sensitive keys that can be grouped together to create larger keys. Expanded keyboards often use paper overlays to define the layout of particular keys. Expanded keyboards differ in such properties as the size, spacing, and sensitivity of the keys. In general, expanded keyboards require a "keyboard emulator" interface to communicate with a computer.

Expansion card. A removable circuit board that plugs into the expansion slots in some models of computers. These computers are termed "open bus" systems. Expansion cards expand the computer's capabilities.

Expansion slot. A long, thin socket used on the mother board of open bus computers into which the user can install an expansion card.

Exploratory play. The first stage of play development, consisting of sensory and causative exploration with toys.

Expressive language. An individual's ability to communicate to others using language.

Extension. Straightening or unbending of a joint. This movement is the opposite of flexion.

File. Any named, ordered collection of data stored on a disk. Application software and user documents are examples of files.

Firmware. Software stored permanently in read-only memory (ROM).

Fixed memory. Communication aid memory that cannot be altered or programmed by a user. This is ROM memory.

Flexion. Bending at a joint, such as the elbow or knee. Opposite of extension.

Floppy disk. A secondary storage system for computers. A disk is a flat, circular, magnetic surface on which information can be recorded in the form of small magnetized spots. The magnetic spots are organized on the disk's surface via concentric tracks and radial sectors. Floppy disks are housed in rigid, plastic jackets for support and protection. Two common sizes of floppy disks are the 3.5-inch or 5.25-inch disk format. The maximum amount of data a disk can hold is usually measured in kilobytes (K) or megabytes (MB).

Format. The physical division of space on a disk into concentric tracks and radial sectors where information can be stored. A disk's format is established as part of the initialization process.

Frequency-of-use scanning. A scanning method that uses statistics and frequency counts to determine which items in the array are used most often by the user. Special software then dynamically changes the order of items from the most frequently used to the least frequently used. The idea behind this approach is to reduce scanning time by grouping together commonly used items in the array.

Game I/O switch interface. A hardware device that connects to the computer's game port or socket. The interface can include one or more jacks that allow switches to be connected to it. To use the switch interface with a computer, the application software must be written to detect game port or socket input.

Game port. A connector, socket, or plug on the computer into which joysticks, game paddles, game I/O switch interfaces, and touch tablets or pads connect Software must be specifically written to work with these devices.

Graphics tablet. A hardware device used to draw pictures. A special pen or stylus is used to draw images. The tablet senses the position of the stylus, converts positional information into X–Y coordinate values, and sends those values to the computer.

Group–item scanning. Scanning procedures that move the cursor by highlighting groups of symbols, then single items in the selected groups.

Handshaking signal. A signal that regulates the flow of data between the computer and peripheral devices.

Hard copy. A paper copy of an electronic file or image.

Hard disk. A secondary storage device that can hold more information than a 3.5-inch disk or a 5.25-inch disk. A hard disk stores very large amounts of information (20 MB to 600 MB) and operates much faster than a floppy disk. The disk usually is permanently mounted inside a disk drive.

Hardware. The physical part of a computer or peripheral device that you can touch: the computer, peripheral devices, and cables used to connect them.

Head stick. Adaptive pointers that attach to helmets or other bracing systems on the head.

Hemiparesis. Muscular weakness of one side of the body.

Hertz (Hz). The unit of frequency of vibration or oscillation defined as the number of cycles per second. Hertz is often used to characterize CPUs and monitors.

High-technology augmentative communication aids. Computerized AAC systems that use specifically written software and have either printed or spoken output, or both.

Home row. The row of keys on the keyboard where the fingers rest when they are not reaching for other keys. In the standard (Qwerty) keyboard layout, the home row contains A, S, D, F, G, and so on. With the Dvorak keyboard layout, the home row contains the most frequently used keys (A, O, E, U, I, etc.).

Hyperextension. Movement of a joint to a position of more extension than natural alignment.

Icon. An image that represents an object, a concept or a message. For example, icons on a screen can represent a disk, a file, or something else the user can select.

Impact printer. A printer that uses an inked ribbon and a striker mechanism to place images on paper. Daisy wheel printers use a wheel system with discrete characters. Dot matrix printers create images using a matrix of dots.

Independent play. The second stage of play development in which children begin to use objects for appropriate functions.

Indirect selection. An input method that involves intermediate selection steps between indicating the choice and actually sending a keystroke or command to the computer. Indirect selection schemes replicate the computer's keyboard characters by using a variety of display formats. For example, indirect methods can appear as a graphical keyboard image, a textual scanning array of keyboard characters, or a menu of computer commands.

Individualized education program (IEP). P.L. 94-142 requires that an IEP be developed by the educational team for each exceptional child; the IEP must include a statement of present educational performance, instructional goals, educational services to be provided. and criteria and procedures for determining that the instructional objectives are being met.

Initialize. To prepare a blank disk to receive information by organizing its surface into tracks and sectors.

Innervate. Furnish with nerves; grow nerves into.

Input. Information transferred into a computer from some external source, such as the keyboard, the mouse, a disk drive, switch, or alternative keyboard.

Input/output (I/O). Refers to the means by which information is exchanged by the computer and its peripheral devices.

Intercostal. Between the ribs.

Interface. The physical point of communication between the computer and peripheral devices. For example, a printer interface allows a computer to direct information to a printer. Two common computer interfaces are the serial and parallel interfaces.

Interrupt. A signal that causes a computer to pass control to a special interrupt-handling routine. Interrupts are used to signal computers that peripheral devices need attention.

Inverse scanning. A scanning method in which the user is required to hold the switch closed to start the cursor moving across an array. The user continues to press and hold the switch until the cursor reaches the desired item. Only then does the user release the switch.

Item-by-item scanning. Scanning procedures that move the cursor one by one through every item in the scanning array.

Joystick. A peripheral device with a movable stick used to provide two-dimensional control to computers for applications ranging from games to graphics software.

Keyboard. A peripheral device that provides a common way to communicate with the computer. Computer keyboards are arranged in a variety of layouts with different numbers, sizes, and shapes of keys.

Keyboard emulator. A hardware device that interfaces with a computer and allows input from a source other than the standard keyboard. Examples of other input devices include switches and alternative keyboards. Keyboard emulators allow alternative input devices to run standard software without modification.

Keyguard. A hardware device that covers a standard or alternative keyboard. Keyguards allow users to slide a pointer over the surface without accidentally activating keys.

Kilobyte (K). A unit of measure for computer memory or storage. One kilobyte consists of 1,024 bytes.

Large print display. A hardware device that enlarges the image on the computer monitor.

Large print software. Software that provides large print on either the computer monitor or paper.

Laser printer. A printer that produces high-quality text and graphics. A directed laser beam burns the image onto the surface of a page.

Lateral. Relating to the side of a structure; situated on, directed toward, or coming from the side.

Least restrictive environment (LRE). A legal term referring to the fact that exceptional children must be educated in as "normal" an environment as possible.

Linear predictive coding (LPC). A method of speech output that utilizes a combination of speech digitizing and mathematical modeling to reconstruct and produce high-quality voice. Special hardware and software are used to reconstruct and simulate the original speech signal. This technology is often referred to as custom-encoded speech.

Liquid crystal display (LCD). An image technology used in calculators, computer displays, and digital watches. LCDs are lightweight and low-power displays made for portable and laptop computers.

Low-technology augmentative communication aids. Simple devices without written or spoken output and without programming capabilities. They may be nonelectronic or electronic.

Lower motor control. Pathway from the anterior horn cell to the muscle fiber.

Macro command. A group of computer commands treated as a unit. When activated, macros execute the set of commands as if entered by the keyboard.

Mainstreaming. The practice of placing students with handicaps in classes that are predominantly composed of nonhandicapped students.

Megabyte (MB). A unit of measure for computer memory or storage. One megabyte equals 1,048,576 bytes, or approximately one million bytes.

Megahertz (MHz). One million cycles per second. This term is commonly used to measure CPU clock speed.

Memory. Storage systems used by a computer to store and recall data and programs. Memory size is expressed in numbers of bytes. Primary memory is memory that can be directly addressed and controlled by the CPU. Examples of primary memory include RAM, ROM, and PROM. Secondary memory is memory that can be indirectly accessed by the CPU through the disk drive system.

Menu. A list of options from which the user can choose, typically shown on the screen. An option may be selected by keystrokes or mouse actions. Menus are used to make application software easier to use.

Minikeyboard. These keyboards provide a smaller key surface area for input, reducing the motor requirements for making keystrokes. Minikeyboards use a matrix of touch-sensitive membrane switches that can be grouped together to form larger keys. Minikeyboards often use paper overlays to define the layout of particular keys. Minikeyboards differ in properties such as the size, spacing, and sensitivity of the keys. In general, minikeyboards require a "keyboard emulator" interface to communicate with a computer.

Minspeak. A pictographic retrieval code system that relies on the concept of multimeaning symbols.

Modem. Short for modulator/demodulator. A hardware device that allows computers to communicate with each other over telephone lines. Modems can operate at different speeds — from 300 to 9600 baud.

Molded seat. A seat insert for a chair that is made from a mold of the individual.

Monitor. A display device that can receive video signals by direct connection. Monitors are available as monochrome (one color) and color systems. Some color monitors employ composite video signals. Others require separate signals for red, green, and blue information (RGB monitors).

Mother board. A large circuit board that holds RAM, ROM, the central processing unit, custom integrated circuits, and other computer components that make the computer work. Also called main circuit board or main logic board.

Motor neurons. Usually refers to the lower motor neurons that carry action potential impulses from the spinal cord to the muscles.

Mouse. A small hardware device used to position a cursor on the computer screen. The mouse is rolled around on a flat surface next to the computer. When the user moves the mouse, the cursor on the screen moves correspondingly.

Mouse button. The button on top of the mouse. Users press the mouse button to choose commands from menus or move items around on the screen.

Mouse emulator. An alternative access method that replaces the physical movement tasks associated with the mouse. The alternative input method can include alternative keyboards, touch tablets, or switches. Alternative keyboards usually require the use of paper overlays to indicate mouse functions. Switches usually require an indirect selection method.

Mouth stick. An adaptive pointer that attaches to a mouth guard that is held by clamping it between the teeth.

MS-DOS. An acronym for Microsoft Disk Operating System. This disk operating system is used with IBM and compatible computers.

Muscle tone. Continual flow of nerve impulses to muscle which keeps the muscle ready for activity.

Musculoskeletal deformity. Limitation in movement of a joint due to problems with muscle and bone.

Network. A group of computers linked together so that their users can share information and peripheral devices.

Nondedicated augmentative communication aids. Communication systems that consist of standard microcomputers that have been adapted for use as augmentative communication aids by adding special software, speech synthesizers, and other peripherals.

Open bus architecture. A computer that provides expansion slots which allow users to expand the capabilities of the computer.

Open memory. Computer or communication aid memory that can be altered or programmed by a user. This is RAM memory.

Output. Information transferred from the computer to an external device, such as the display screen, a disk drive, a printer, or a modem.

Parallel play. The third stage of play development in which children play independently yet near each other.

Parallel transmission. A method of sending data between a computer and a peripheral device. Parallel transmission exchanges information several bits (usually eight) at a time along separate wires. Parallel transmission is very fast. Parallel communication is often used with high-speed printers and external disk drives.

Peer tutoring. A method that can be used in integrating students with handicaps in regular classrooms, based on the notion that students can effectively tutor one another. The role of learner or teacher may be assigned to either the student with handicaps or a nonhandicapped peer.

Pelvic obliquity. Position of the pelvis in which one side of the pelvis is higher than the other.

Pelvic rotation. Position of the pelvis in which one side of the pelvis is more forward than the other side.

Pelvic tilt. Associated with incline of the pelvic girdle in a forward or backward alignment.

Peripheral device. A piece of hardware that is physically separate from a computer. Examples include video monitors, disk drives, printers, alternative keyboards, and touch tablets.

Pictographic symbols. Symbol sets that have picture representations of concrete concepts as well as abstract concepts.

P.L. 94-142. The Education for All Handicapped Children Act, which contains a mandatory provision stating that, beginning in September 1978, to receive funds under the Act, every school system in the nation must make provision for a free, appropriate education for every child between the ages of 3 and 18 years old (extended to ages 3 to 21 by 1980), regardless of how or how seriously the youngster may be handicapped.

P.L. 101-476. 1990 Education of the Handicapped Act Amendments, known as the Individuals with Disabilities Education Act (IDEA). Includes the same provisions as P.L. 94-457 with additions in: accepted handicapping conditions that qualify for services, transition services for children 16 years and older, provisions for the use of assistive technology, addressing the infant and toddler population, and other specific amendments to services and service provision.

Port. A socket on the back panel of the computer where users plug in a cable to connect a peripheral device, another computer, or a network.

Posterior. Pertaining to the back or a position toward or on the back side of a structure (Dorsal).

Prestored messages. Preprogramming frequently used words, phrases, and sentences into a computer or AAC system for quick retrieval with symbol codes.

Prognosis. A prediction of the probable course of an individual's disease and chances of recovery.

Program. A set of instructions describing actions required for a computer to perform a task, conforming to the rules and conventions of a particular programming language.

Pronation. A turning down or outward. For example, turning the palm of the hand downward. The muscles used to perform this function are called pronators.

Proximal. Situated nearest to the center of the body. Opposite of distal. Thus, the shoulder is proximal and the hand is distal.

Qwerty keyboard. The most commonly used keyboard layout in the United States, named for the first six letters in the top row of letter keys.

Radio frequency (RF) modulator. A hardware device that converts the video output of a computer into a signal detectable by the tuner of a standard television.

RAM cache. A portion of primary memory (RAM) that users set aside for special use. RAM cache often is used by the disk operating system to store frequently used data. Because this information is stored in memory, the operating system can access the information more quickly, improving computer performance.

RAM disk. A portion of primary memory (RAM) allocated as a storage area for data and program files. The computer treats this section of RAM as if it were a floppy disk drive. The advantage of RAM disk is that the computer can get information from RAM much faster than from a floppy disk in an actual disk drive.

Random-access memory (RAM). Primary memory where application software and data are stored temporarily for the CPU. Anything stored in RAM is erased when the computer's power is turned off.

Read-only memory (ROM). Primary memory whose contents can be read but not changed. Information is placed into read-only memory only once, during manufacturing. The contents of ROM are not erased when the computer's power is turned off.

Receptive language. An individual's ability to understand language.

Resolution. The detail and clarity of an image on the display screen. An RGB color monitor has better resolution than a composite color monitor.

Retrieval codes. Picture or letter symbol codes used to retrieve prestored communication aid or computer messages, text, or macros.

RGB monitor. A type of color monitor that receives separate signals for each color (red, green, and blue). These three primary colors are used to generate all screen colors.

Rotation. Movement that turns a body part on its own axis; for example, the turning of the head. The muscles that perform this function are called rotators.

Row-column scanning. This scanning method is commonly used with AAC systems. These scanning procedures quickly move the cursor by first highlighting an entire row of symbols, then single symbols in the selected row.

Scanning. An indirect method of computer access. The process entails stepping through choices that the user selects by switch activation. In general, scanning involves the use of an array, a keyboard emulator, and one or more switches. The four most common scanning methods are automatic linear scanning, step linear scanning, inverse scanning, and frequency-of-use scanning.

Screen. The part of the computer monitor that displays information.

Serial transmission. A method of sending data between a computer and a peripheral device. Serial transmission exchanges information one bit at a time along a single wire. Serial transmission is much slower than parallel transmission. Serial communication is often used with printers and modems.

Software. Instructions, usually stored on disks, that give the computer directions on what to do. Also called programs and application software.

Spasticity. A condition usually associated with stroke or spinal cord disease whereby stretch reflexes are exaggerated and may even occur spontaneously, producing involuntary muscle contractions.

Speech recognition. A process whereby the computer learns to understand discrete sounds or words. This is accomplished by training the recognition system with repetitions of individual words or phrases. A template for each word is stored and then saved to a vocabulary file which can contain up to several thousand words. Also called voice input.

Step linear scanning. This is a manual scanning method of moving the cursor through an array and selecting items. A user presses a switch to bring up the array. The user then presses and releases the switch to move the cursor across the array item by item. This process is repeated until the cursor reaches the desired item.

Static display. Communication aid or computer displays of symbols that never change or vary.

Sticky key. Memory-resident utility software that provides keyboard assistance. Sticky key features allow head-stick users and single-finger typists to simultaneously depress two or more keys. A single keystroke can then be used to capitalize letters or to enter multiple control key sequences.

Subcutaneous. Beneath the skin. Usually refers to the region between the skin and underlying fat layer.

Suboccipital ledge. Contour to the back of the head.

Supination. A turning upward; for example, turning the palm upward. The muscles that perform this function are called supinators.

Symbols. Language units that have shared meaning between the user and listener. Photographs, drawings, letters, and written text can serve as symbols.

Symbolic play. The final stage of play development in which children begin to participate in make-believe and pretend play.

Synthesized speech. Spoken computer or communication aid output that uses partial numerical waveform parameters representing the formant frequencies of speech.

Switch. A hardware device that either opens or closes an electronic circuit, controlling the flow of electricity to an electronic device — much like a light switch in the home turns the lights on (closed circuit) or off (open circuit). Switches are connected to a computer using either a game I/O switch interface or a keyboard emulator.

Switch toys. Battery- or radio-controlled toys that have been adapted for use with a single switch.

System unit. A box or case in which the major components of the computer are located. The system unit consists of three major elements: the microprocessor, primary memory, and input/output interfaces.

Symmetrical. The same on both sides of the body. Opposite of assymetrical.

Taped speech. Cassette tapes with prerecorded speech output for use in AAC systems.

Terminate-and-stay-resident (TSR). A software program that remains RAM-resident and active in the background while other application software runs in the foreground. TSR programs operate in conjunction with application software. Typical TSR programs include word-prediction and abbreviation-expansion software.

Text-to-speech synthesis. A synthesized speech technique that defines and stores the phonemes or sounds of the English language as a set of mathematical rules and procedures. Typically, text-to-speech systems include hundreds of such pronunciation rules to describe the English language. The voice quality of text-to-speech synthesizers is not as good as digitized or LPC methods.

Touch screen. An input device that senses the position of a finger on the computer monitor.

Touch tablet. An input device that senses the position of a finger or stylus on a flat, touch-sensitive surface. Touch tablets can be used to control cursor movements, act as an alternative keyboard, or replace a mouse or a joystick.

Traditional orthography. Written language text.

Transceiver. A hardware device that is capable of transmitting and receiving information. Commonly found in environmental control applications.

Unaided communication. Communication modes that use only the communicator's body. Vocalizations, gestures, facial expressions, and head nods are examples.

Upper motor neurons. All of the descending fibers in the brain and spinal cord that can influence and modify the activity of the lower motor neurons.

Utility software. Software programs designed to handle specialized tasks, for example, enhancements to the disk operating system, improvements to the general operation of the computer, or augmentations to standard computer input methods.

Visual-motor. Pertaining to the performance of a function in response to visual input.

Word. The smallest unit of information that can be addressed by a computer. Most microcomputers use 8-, 16-, or 32-bit words.

Word prediction. Memory-resident utility software that provides keyboard assistance. As the user inputs each keystroke, the software presents a list of possible words or phrases that it thinks the user is typing. The user then selects the appropriate word from the prediction list. Statistical weighting is often incorporated into the software to improve prediction tasks.

Yes/No verbal scanning. A scanning method in which the listener points to all possible choices while the speaker responds yes or no to each selection.

Index

750.364 LARCENY; FROM LIBRARIES

SEC. 364. LARCENY FROM LIBRARIES--
ANY PERSON WHO SHALL PROCURE, OR
TAKE IN ANY WAY FROM ANY PUBLIC
LIBRARY OR THE LIBRARY OF ANY
LITERARY, SCIENTIFIC, HISTORICAL
OR LIBRARY SOCIETY OR ASSOCIATION,
WHETHER INCORPORATED OR UNINCOR-
PORATED, ANY BOOK, PAMPHLET, MAP,
CHART, PAINTING, PICTURE, PHOTO-
GRAPH, PERIODICAL, NEWSPAPER,
MAGAZINE, MANUSCRIPT OR EXHIBIT
OR ANY PART THEREOF, WITH INTENT
TO CONVERT THE SAME TO HIS OWN
USE, OR WITH INTENT TO DEFRAUD
THE OWNER THEREOF, OR WHO HAVING
PROCURED OR TAKEN ANY SUCH BOOK,
PAMPHLET, MAP, CHART, PAINTING,
PICTURE, PHOTOGRAPH, PERIODICAL,
NEWSPAPER, MAGAZINE, MANUSCRIPT
OR EXHIBIT OR ANY PART THEREOF,
SHALL THEREAFTER CONVERT THE SAME
TO HIS OWN USE OR FRAUDULENTLY
DEPRIVE THE OWNER THEREOF, SHALL
BE GUILTY OF A MISDEMEANOR.

MICHIGAN COMPILED LAWS.